Health Economics for Nurses

PRENTICE HALL NURSING SERIES

A series of comprehensive textbooks and reference manuals for nurses and other health care professionals.

Other titles in the series include:

Teaching and Assessing in Clinical Nursing Practice
edited by Peter L. Bradshaw

Clinical Nursing Manual
edited by Jennifer E. Clark

Nursing Research: A Skills-Based Introduction
Collette Clifford and Stephen Gough

Legal Aspects of Nursing, second edition
Bridgit Dimond

Nursing Care of Women
Dinah Gould

Drugs and Nursing Implications
Laura E. Govoni and Janice E. Hayes (adapted by Jill A. David)

Research and Statistics: A Practical Introduction for Nurses
Carolyn M. Hicks

Becoming a Staff Nurse: A Guide to the Role of the Newly Registered Nurse
edited by Judith Lathlean and Jessica Corner

Nursing Concepts for Health Promotion
Ruth Beckman Murray and Judith Proctor Zentner (adapted by Cindy Howells)

Body Image: Nursing Concepts and Care
Bob Price

Clinical Nursing Practice: The Promotion and Management of Continence
Brenda Roe

The Art and Science of Midwifery
Louise Silverton

Nursing the Patient with Cancer, second edition
edited by Verena Tschudin

Health Economics for Nurses:
An Introductory Guide

Stephen Morris

PRENTICE HALL EUROPE

London   New York   Toronto   Sydney   Tokyo   Singapore
Madrid   Mexico City   Munich   Paris

First published 1998 by
Prentice Hall Europe
Campus 400, Maylands Avenue
Hemel Hempstead
Hertfordshire, HP2 7EZ
A division of
Simon & Schuster International Group

Typeset in 10/12 pt Times
by Photoprint, Torquay, Devon

Printed and bound in Great Britain by
TJ International Ltd

Library of Congress Cataloging-in-Publication Data

Morris, Stephen.
    Health economics for nurses : an introductory
guide / Stephen Morris.
       p.   cm. – (Prentice Hall nursing series)
    Includes bibliographical references and index.
    ISBN 0–13–255993–5 (pbk. : alk. paper)
    1. Medical economics–Great Britain.
    2. Nursing–Economic aspects–Great Britain.
    I. Morris, Stephen. II. Title. III. Series.
    [DNLM: 1. Economics, Medical–nurses'
instruction. W 74 M8767h 1998]
RA410.55.G7M67   1998
338.4'33621'0941–dc21
DNLM/DLC
for Library of Congress   97–41281
                             CIP

British Library Cataloguing in Publication Data

A catalogue record for this book is available from
the British Library

ISBN 0–13–255993–5

---

1 2 3 4 5 02 01 00 99 98

Contents

To Mum and Dad

Preface

In recent years there has been a growing interest in the application of economics to the health care sector. Increasingly, attention is being given to the role of health economics for nurses, as efficient and cost-effective use of resources is seen to be necessary for the provision of a high-quality nursing service. Moreover, as the number of nursing degrees and diplomas increases, the incorporation of formal tuition in health economics and related issues in the training of nurses is becoming more common.

This book is specifically designed for and aimed at nurses and will provide a foundation upon which teaching of the economic concepts relevant to the National Health Service in general and the nursing profession in particular can be based. This book has then two primary objectives: (1) to explain the economic theory underlying health care policy in the National Health Service, particularly with reference to nursing; and (2) to explore the use of a number of economic techniques which can be used to improve the understanding of issues of efficiency and cost-effectiveness in the health care sector for the nursing profession. Particular attention has been paid to providing a text that is comprehensive, comprehensible and directly relevant to nurses, and various issues are discussed, such as the NHS reforms, the nursing labour market, and the economic evaluation of health care programmes and nursing services. No prior knowledge of economics is assumed, and clear and concise explanation of the various economic concepts is provided. The intention is to make the text as user-friendly as possible and, where appropriate, detailed worked examples are provided to highlight relevant issues.

The scope of the text is primarily directed towards individuals training to be nurses, at both diploma and degree levels. However, the topics covered are equally relevant to those studying for postgraduate degrees in nursing, to nurses undergoing post-qualification training, and to any other parties interested in the application of economics to nursing. There are, of course, a great many nursing textbooks currently available, and there are also a fair number of health economics textbooks. There is, as yet, no health economics textbook specifically oriented towards nurses and nursing.

Finally, in writing this book I would like to express my gratitude to a number of friends from whom I have received valuable assistance and advice. I would especially like to thank Ali McGuire, Ed Godber and Debbie Rowntree for their thoughts, comments, suggestions and support.

1   Scarcity and health care

In this chapter we provide a foundation for the application of economics to the health care sector. We examine the existence of scarcity in the context of the UK National Health Service, and evidence is provided which forms the basis of the analysis and discussion of the following chapters.

Summary

1. The fundamental problem that economics attempts to address is that of scarce resources. This is the basic economic problem, and it provides the foundation and justification for economic theory and analysis.

2. The three basic problems that we are interested in as economists are: What goods and services shall we produce? How shall we produce these goods and services? Who will receive these goods and services?

3. It is often argued that the basic economic problem of scarcity is exceptionally acute in the UK National Health Service (NHS). This is because the need and demand for health care in the UK are thought by far to exceed the resources available to the NHS. It is difficult to quantify the exact size and nature of the problem of scarcity in the NHS though evidence is available which may be used to draw some general conclusions. Such evidence includes data on: expenditure on health care; quantity of resources to provide health care; size of the population; utilisation of the NHS; waiting lists; length of stay; and utilisation of private health insurance.

4. The United States spends nearly three and a half times more on health care per person than the UK (£2,816 versus £808), and the only countries in the developed world to spend less on health care per person than the UK are Ireland, New Zealand, Spain, Portugal and Greece.

5. In 1994 there were 61,331 fewer nurses and midwives working in the NHS than there were in 1989 (429,214 versus 490,545 nurses and midwives).

6. In 1994 there were just over half the number of beds available in NHS hospitals than there were in 1975 (497,000 versus 285,000 beds). The number of available

hospital beds in the NHS per 100,0000 individuals in the population has also fallen (8.8 beds per 100,000 individuals in the population in 1975 versus 4.9 beds per 100,000 individuals in the population in 1994).

7. In 1994 there were 58.4 million individuals of all ages living in the UK, and the population of the UK is rising continuously.

8. In 1975, 5.0 per cent of the population of the UK was aged 75 years or more (2.8 million individuals). In 1994, this figure had risen to 7.1 per cent of the population (4.1 million individuals).

9. In 1975, 24 per cent of the population of Great Britain reported chronic ill health and 15 per cent reported acute ill health. In 1993 these figures had risen to 32 per cent and 19 per cent, respectively.

10. Across all ages, the average number of NHS consultations per person per year is increasing. In 1975, the average number of NHS consultations was three. In 1993 this figure had risen to five.

11. Across all specialities in 1994 there were 608,000 individuals on a waiting list for treatment as an inpatient in England.

12. In 1975 the average length of stay in an NHS hospital was 23 days. This was nearly three times longer than the average length of stay in 1994, which was eight days.

13. In 1975 approximately 1.1 million individuals subscribed to private health insurance and 2.3 million individuals were insured. In 1996, 4.0 million individuals subscribed to private health insurance and 8.0 million individuals were insured.

14. Evidence suggests that the NHS is underfunded and that health care resources in the UK are scarce. Unfortunately, this evidence may also be interpreted quite differently to show that the NHS, rather than being underfunded, is in fact adequately meeting the demands placed upon it. Given the available evidence, it is therefore difficult to draw any firm conclusions as to whether there are scarce resources in the NHS because the extent of the problem depends upon the way in which the available evidence is interpreted.

15. If we assume that the problem of scarcity does exist in the NHS, the key issue then becomes what to do about it. Specifically, three issues need to be addressed: What treatments should be made available? How should these treatments be provided? Who should receive these treatments?

Scarcity

The fundamental problem that economics attempts to address is that of *scarce resources*. This is called the *basic economic problem*, and it provides the foundation and justification for economic theory and analysis.

By resources we refer to all the things which are used in the production of goods and services. This includes not only natural resources such as oil, trees, land and water, but also human resources, such as labour, and capital resources, such as machines and factories. These are the things which are used to produce the goods and services which we desire. Unfortunately, these resources are scarce.

With only limited resources, we are unable to provide all the goods and services which ideally we would like. Therefore, we must make a choice between competing uses of limited resources in terms of what to produce, how to produce it and who shall receive it.

Economics is concerned with evaluating the choices between different uses of scarce resources, and therefore the three basic questions that we are interested in as economists are:

1. What goods and services shall we produce?

In the presence of scarcity, the resources available are too few to satisfy the total 'wants' desired by society, and, inevitably, producing more of one good means producing less of another. Therefore, some form of choice or prioritisation is inevitable, and we are required to decide what goods and services we should produce, given that there are not enough resources to produce the total quantity of goods and services that we would ideally like.

2. How shall we produce these goods and services?

Even after it is decided what goods and services to produce, we still need to decide on how to produce them. This decision too is an important one because the production of goods and services also requires the use of limited resources.

3. Who will receive these goods and services?

Because of the problem of scarcity, individuals may not be able to obtain everything that they would ideally like. Therefore, it will be necessary to develop some mechanism for dividing among all individuals the goods and services which have been produced using the limited available resources. This will inevitably lead to some discussion of whether this division is a 'fair' one.

There is an economic element to the production of all goods and services because resources are generally thought to be scarce in all aspects of society, including in the production of: food; clothing; education; housing; employment; defence; transport; the environment; and health care.

Scarcity and the UK National Health Service

It is often argued that the basic economic problem of scarcity is exceptionally acute in the UK National Health Service (NHS). This is because the demand for health care in the UK is thought by far to exceed the resources available to the NHS. In the context of the NHS, by resources we refer to all the things which go into the production of health care, including nurses, midwives, doctors, hospitals, hospital beds, X-ray machines, medicines and all the other things which are used to provide health care.

It is difficult to quantify the exact size and nature of the problem of scarcity in the NHS. Evidence is available which may be used to draw some general conclusions, and this may take one of two forms:

1. evidence on the quantity of resources devoted to the NHS;
2. evidence that the burdens imposed on the NHS are likely to increase.

More specifically, data are available on the following:

1. expenditure on health care;
2. quantity of resources to provide health care;
3. size of the population;
4. utilisation of the NHS;
5. waiting lists;
6. length of stay;
7. utilisation of private health insurance.

Such evidence suggests that the NHS is underfunded and that health care resources in the UK are scarce. Unfortunately, this evidence may also be interpreted quite differently to show that the NHS, rather than being underfunded, is in fact performing efficiently and adequately meeting the demands placed upon it. In the following sections we examine the evidence in greater detail.

Expenditure on health care

UK health care expenditure

Total health care expenditure in the UK is presented in Table 1.1. This is comprised of NHS expenditure, private health care expenditure and expenditure by individuals on over-the-counter purchases of pharmaceuticals not available on NHS prescriptions. In 1995, total UK health care expenditure was £47,266 million. Eighty-eight per cent of this total (£41,517 million) consisted of NHS expenditure. Every year, both expenditure on the NHS and total health care expenditure in the UK have increased.

The average health care expenditure per person in the UK is also presented in Table 1.1. This is calculated by dividing total UK health care expenditure by the total population of the UK. In 1995, average health care expenditure per person in the UK was £808. This sum is an average, and the actual proportion of health care services received will differ widely across individuals. Some individuals will require and receive no health care, and health care expenditure on these individuals will be negligible. Other individuals will be seriously ill and accordingly will receive large

Table 1.1 Total UK health care expenditure.

Year	Health expenditure (£ million)				Average per person (£)
	NHS	Private	Other[1]	Total	
1974	3,970	120	235	4,325	77
1975	5,315	134	276	5,725	102
1976	6,303	166	313	6,782	121
1977	7,001	205	349	7,555	134
1978	8,032	231	403	8,666	154
1979	9,321	263	502	10,086	179
1980	11,954	355	615	12,924	229
1981	13,768	463	689	14,920	265
1982	14,543	593	787	15,923	283
1983	16,470	672	904	18,046	320
1984	17,417	623	1,080	19,120	339
1985	18,578	738	1,190	20,506	362
1986	19,901	846	1,364	22,111	390
1987	21,700	1,066	1,432	24,198	425
1988	23,829	1,246	1,596	26,671	467
1989	26,193	1,353	1,787	29,333	512
1990	28,900	1,623	1,920	32,443	565
1991	32,394	1,969	2,294	36,657	634
1992	36,261	2,015	2,728	41,004	707
1993	38,211	2,138	2,964	43,313	745
1994	39,968	2,377	3,102	45,447	779
1995	41,517	2,536	3,214	47,266	808

Note:
[1] Consumer expenditure on over-the-counter purchases of
pharmaceuticals without NHS prescriptions.
Source: OHE (1995).

quantities of health care. Health care expenditure on these individuals will be large.

The proportion of total NHS expenditure spent on each service is presented in Table 1.2. For example, in 1995, of the £41,517 million spent on the NHS (Table 1.1), 54.2 per cent was spent on hospital services, 8.6 per cent was spent on community health services, and 24.2 per cent was spent on family health services (comprising pharmaceuticals available on prescription [11.2 per cent], general medical services provided by general practitioners [8.4 per cent], general dental services provided by dentists [4.0 per cent], and general ophthalmic services provided by opticians [0.6 per cent]). Clearly, the bulk of NHS expenditure is therefore spent on hospital services.

A breakdown of expenditure on those hospital services combined with expenditure on community health services is presented in Table 1.3. This is revenue expenditure and does not include expenditure on capital such as large pieces of equipment and machinery, buildings and motor vehicles. Easily the largest component of expenditure on the NHS is salaries and wages. In 1994, 63.9 per cent of total expenditure on hospital and community health services was spent on the salaries and wages of

Table 1.2 Proportion of total UK NHS expenditure spent on each service.

Year	Hospital services	Community health services	Family health services				
			Pharmaceuticals	General medical services	General dental services	General ophthalmic services	Other services[1]
1975	62.0	6.1	8.5	6.5	4.1	1.4	11.2
1976	60.7	6.0	9.0	6.1	3.9	1.2	12.9
1977	60.8	6.0	9.9	6.1	3.7	1.2	12.0
1978	59.6	5.8	10.3	5.9	3.5	1.1	13.5
1979	60.6	6.0	9.9	6.1	3.9	1.1	12.1
1980	60.0	6.1	9.4	6.3	3.8	1.0	13.3
1981	60.2	6.1	9.3	6.5	3.9	1.0	13.0
1982	61.6	6.4	10.1	6.9	4.1	1.1	9.8
1983	57.6	6.0	9.9	6.7	3.9	1.6	14.3
1984	57.6	6.2	10.0	7.1	4.1	1.1	13.9
1985	57.1	6.4	10.1	7.2	4.2	0.9	14.1
1986	56.4	6.7	10.2	7.2	4.1	0.8	14.6
1987	55.1	7.5	10.5	7.5	4.2	0.8	14.3
1988	54.9	8.2	10.7	7.4	4.4	0.8	13.6
1989	54.1	8.4	10.4	7.6	4.2	0.6	14.5
1990	53.0	8.4	10.3	8.1	4.1	0.5	15.7
1991	53.3	8.4	10.3	8.0	4.5	0.5	15.0
1992	53.5	8.5	10.3	7.9	4.3	0.6	15.0
1993	54.4	8.6	10.7	8.1	4.0	0.6	13.7
1994	54.2	8.6	10.9	8.2	3.9	0.6	13.6
1995	54.2	8.6	11.2	8.4	4.0	0.6	13.0

Note:
[1] Including headquarters administration, central administration, ambulance services, mass radiography services, and centrally financed items such as laboratories and vaccination programmes and research and development.
Source: OHE (1995).

workers employed in the NHS (£15,267 million). This includes salary payments to nurses and midwives, hospital doctors and dentists, ambulance staff, administrative and clerical staff and managers.

Comparison with other countries

In Table 1.4, average health care expenditures per person for countries in the developed world are presented. The country that spends the most on health care per person is the United States, which in 1995 spent £2,816 per person on health care. Average health care expenditure per person in the UK was £808.

Quantity of resources to provide health care

Evidence on the quantity of resources devoted to the NHS may also be obtained from:

Table 1.3 Hospital and community health services revenue fund expenditure for England.

Component	1985	1987	1988	1989	£ million (%) 1990	1991	1992	1993	1994
Salaries and wages[1]	6,778	7,685	8,468	9,562	10,255	11,212	12,562	13,639	15,267
	(74.1)	(74.5)	(75.0)	(76.2)	(75.6)	(76.2)	(63.7)	(62.9)	(63.9)
Clinical supplies[2]	835	966	1,040	1,108	1,191	1,307	1,640	1,836	2,076
	(9.1)	(9.4)	(9.2)	(8.8)	(8.7)	(8.9)	(8.3)	(8.4)	(8.7)
General supplies[3]	293	320	334	343	372	386	451	439	496
	(3.2)	(3.1)	(3.0)	(2.7)	(2.7)	(2.6)	(2.2)	(2.0)	(2.0)
Establishment[4]	306	346	382	292	421	61	540	599	678
	(3.3)	(3.3)	(3.3)	(3.1)	(3.1)	(3.1)	(2.7)	(2.7)	(2.8)
Transport[5]	54	56	63	71	91	101	94	101	114
	(0.5)	(0.5)	(0.6)	(0.6)	(0.7)	(0.7)	(0.4)	(0.4)	(0.4)
Premises[6]	809	828	854	897	982	95	1,211	1,329	1,504
	(8.8)	(8.0)	(7.6)	(7.1)	(7.2)	(6.1)	(6.1)	(6.1)	(6.3)
Capital charges	0	0	0	0	0	0	1,859	1,748	1,977
	(0.0)	(0.0)	(0.0)	(0.0)	(0.0)	(0.0)	(9.4)	(8.0)	(8.2)
Non-NHS purchases	0	0	0	0	0	0	208	247	279
	(0.0)	(0.0)	(0.0)	(0.0)	(0.0)	(0.0)	(1.0)	(1.1)	(1.1)
External contracts[7]	0	0	0	0	0	0	80	122	138
	(0.0)	(0.0)	(0.0)	(0.0)	(0.0)	(0.0)	(0.4)	(0.5)	(0.5)
Agency services	54	59	70	83	108	140	0	0	0
	(0.5)	(0.5)	(7.6)	(0.7)	(0.8)	(0.9)	(0.0)	(0.0)	(0.0)
Miscellaneous	185	260	293	354	425	516	1,088	1,205	1,363
	(2.0)	(2.5)	(2.6)	(2.8)	(3.1)	(3.5)	(5.5)	(5.5)	(5.7)
Total[9]	9,135	10,317	11,277	12,555	13,573	14,710	19,733	21,693	23,893

Notes:
[1] Including nursing, medical, dental, professional, and technical staff, ambulance, administrative and clerical staff, and managers.
[2] Including medicines, dressings, medical, surgical and laboratory equipment, and patient appliances.
[3] Including purchases of provisions, staff uniforms, patient clothing, laundry, and bedding and linen.
[4] Including printing and stationery, postage, telephone, advertising, travelling and subsistence.
[5] Including fuel and oil, maintenance, and hire of transport.
[6] Including energy, furniture, office and computer equipment, rent and rates, and maintenance.
[7] Including consultancy services.
[8] Including student bursaries and auditors' remuneration.
[9] Inexact totals due to rounding error.
Source: OHE (1995).

1. the number of staff;
2. the number of available beds.

Number of staff

The numbers of nurses and midwives, hospital doctors and general practitioners working in the NHS in Great Britain are presented in Table 1.5. In 1994, there were 429,914 nurses and midwives working in the NHS, 53,787 hospital doctors and 34,421 general practitioners. Clearly, a large number of individuals are employed by the NHS to provide health care to the population of the UK and this is reflected in

Table 1.4 Average total health care expenditure per person by countries in the developed world in 1995.

Ranking	Country	Average per person (£)
1	United States	2,816
2	Switzerland	2,176
3	Germany	1,677
4	Japan	1,650
5	Austria	1,513
6	Canada	1,447
7	France	1,435
8	Norway	1,367
9	Sweden	1,317
10	Denmark	1,249
11	Belgium	1,214
12	Italy	1,122
13	Finland	1,001
14	Australia	949
15	UK	808
16	Ireland	659
17	New Zealand	659
18	Spain	643
19	Portugal	337
20	Greece	295

Source: OHE (1995).

Table 1.5 Nurses and midwives, hospital doctors and general practitioners working in the NHS in Great Britain.

Year	Nurses and midwives	Hospital doctors	General practitioners
1974	377,633	31,486	25,844
1975	405,817	33,017	26,128
1976	414,961	33,909	26,418
1977	415,694	34,821	26,810
1978	424,304	35,815	27,227
1979	433,490	37,102	27,696
1980	448,824	38,235	28,414
1981	474,497	39,012	29,252
1982	481,873	39,618	29,806
1983	483,061	40,382	30,422
1984	482,215	40,564	30,976
1985	486,607	43,499	31,465
1986	487,273	43,833	31,854
1987	489,044	43,784	32,422
1988	489,574	45,438	32,888
1989	490,545	46,906	33,310
1990	487,012	48,435	33,058
1991	483,507	49,620	33,463
1992	467,723	50,793	33,833
1993	446,056	52,476	34,135
1994	429,214	53,787	34,421

Source: ONS (1997).

Table 1.6 Number of NHS hospital beds available in the UK, and per 100,000 population.

Year	Available beds ('000s)	Available beds (per 100,000 population)
1975	497	8.8
1976	489	8.7
1977	480	8.5
1978	471	8.4
1979	463	8.2
1980	458	8.1
1981	455	8.1
1982	453	8.0
1983	446	7.9
1984	431	7.6
1985	421	7.4
1986	410	7.2
1987	388	6.8
1988	372	6.5
1989	356	6.2
1990	339	5.9
1991	323	5.6
1992	309	5.3
1993	294	5.1
1994	285	4.9

Source: ONS (1997).

the large proportion of NHS expenditure devoted to salaries and wages (see Table 1.3).

Number of available hospital beds

The number of NHS hospital beds available in the UK is presented in Table 1.6. In 1994 there were 285,000 hospitals beds available in the NHS. The number of available NHS hospital beds per 100,000 individuals in the UK population is also presented. This is calculated by dividing the number of available beds by the total population of the UK. In 1994, there were 4.9 available hospital beds in the NHS per 100,000 individuals in the UK.

Size of the population

Evidence that the burdens imposed on the NHS are likely to increase may be obtained from:

1. the size of the population;
2. the proportion of the population who are elderly.

Table 1.7 UK population in millions by age group.

Year	Age group							As % of all ages	
	0–14	15–29	30–44	45–64	65–74	75+	All ages	0–74	75+
1975	13.1	12.2	9.9	13.1	5.1	2.8	56.2	95.0	5.0
1976	12.9	12.4	10.0	13.0	5.1	2.9	56.2	94.9	5.1
1977	12.6	12.3	10.3	13.0	5.1	3.0	56.3	94.8	5.2
1978	12.3	12.4	10.5	12.9	5.2	3.0	56.3	94.6	5.4
1979	12.1	12.5	10.7	12.7	5.2	3.1	56.4	94.5	5.5
1980	11.8	12.7	10.9	12.6	5.2	3.2	56.4	94.3	5.7
1981	11.6	12.9	11.0	12.5	5.2	3.3	56.4	94.2	5.8
1982	11.4	13.0	11.0	12.5	5.1	3.4	56.3	94.0	6.0
1983	11.2	13.1	11.1	12.5	5.0	3.4	56.3	93.9	6.1
1984	11.0	13.3	11.2	12.6	4.8	3.5	56.4	93.7	6.3
1985	10.9	13.4	11.3	12.4	4.9	3.6	56.6	93.6	6.4
1986	10.8	13.5	11.5	12.3	5.0	3.7	56.8	93.5	6.5
1987	10.7	13.5	11.6	12.2	5.0	3.8	56.9	93.4	6.6
1988	10.8	13.5	11.7	12.2	5.0	3.9	57.1	93.2	6.8
1989	10.8	13.3	11.8	12.3	5.0	3.9	57.2	93.1	6.9
1990	10.9	13.2	12.0	12.3	5.0	4.0	57.4	93.1	6.9
1991	11.1	13.0	12.2	12.4	5.1	4.0	57.8	93.1	6.9
1992	11.2	12.8	12.2	12.7	5.1	4.0	58.0	93.0	7.0
1993	11.3	12.5	12.3	12.8	5.1	4.1	58.2	93.0	7.0
1994	11.4	12.3	12.5	13.0	5.1	4.1	58.4	92.9	7.1

Source: ONS (1997).

Size of the population

The size of the population of the UK in millions by age group is presented in Table 1.7. In 1994 there were 58.4 million individuals of all ages living in the UK, and the population of the UK is rising continuously.

Proportion of the population who are elderly

We can also see from Table 1.7 that whilst the total size of the population is increasing, so too is the proportion of individuals in the total population who are aged 75 years or more. In 1975, 5.0 per cent of the population of the UK was aged 75 years or more (2.8 million individuals). In 1994, this figure had risen to 7.1 per cent of the population (4.1 million individuals aged 75 years or more).

Utilisation of the NHS

Evidence on the quantity of resources used in the NHS may also be obtained from data on the utilisation of health care services, specifically:

1. level of morbidity;
2. NHS consultations.

Level of morbidity

Table 1.8 shows the proportion of the population of Great Britain reporting chronic ill health and acute ill health. In 1993, 32 per cent of the population of Great Britain reported suffering from chronic ill health; 19 per cent reported suffering from acute ill health. In more recent years, both the level of reported chronic ill health and the level of reported acute ill health in the population have stayed fairly constant. Compared with 1975, however, the level of morbidity in the population has increased (in 1975, 24 per cent of the population reported chronic ill health and 15 per cent reported acute ill health).

NHS consultations

The average number of NHS consultations per person per year in Great Britain is presented in Table 1.9. In 1993, every individual in Great Britain had an average of five NHS consultations. For the very young and the elderly the average number of consultations was higher: for individuals aged less than 5 years, the average number of NHS consultations was seven; for individuals aged 65 to 74 years, the average number of NHS consultations was six; and, for individuals aged 75 years or more, the average number of NHS consultations was seven.

Table 1.8 Percentage of population of Great Britain reporting illness.

Year	Proportion (%) of population	
	Reporting chronic ill health[1]	Reporting acute ill health
1975	24	15
1980	30	19
1982	30	18
1984	31	18
1985	30	17
1986	33	19
1987	33	21
1988	33	18
1989	32	18
1990	34	21
1991	31	18
1992	32	19
1993	32	19

Note:
[1] Defined as long-standing sickness, disability or infirmity.
Source: OPCS (1995).

Table 1.9 Average number of NHS consultations per person per year in Great Britain.

Year	0–4	5–15	16–44	45–64	65–74	75+	All ages
1975	4	2	3	4	4	6	3
1980	6	3	4	4	6	7	4
1982	7	3	4	5	5	6	4
1984	6	3	4	4	5	7	4
1985	7	3	4	4	5	6	4
1986	7	3	4	4	5	7	4
1987	8	4	4	5	6	7	5
1988	7	3	4	4	5	6	4
1989	8	3	4	5	6	7	5
1990	8	4	5	5	6	7	5
1991	7	3	4	4	6	6	5
1992	7	3	4	5	6	7	5
1993	7	3	4	5	6	7	5

Source: OPCS (1995).

Across all ages, the average number of consultations per person is slowly increasing. In 1975, the average number of NHS consultations was three. In 1993 this figure had risen to five.

Waiting lists

The size of the NHS hospital inpatient waiting list in England is presented in Figure 1.1. Across all specialities in 1994 there were 608,000 individuals on a waiting list for treatment as an inpatient in England.

Length of stay

In 1975 the average length of stay in an NHS hospital was 23 days. This was nearly three times longer than the average length of stay in 1994, which was eight days. The fall in the average length of stay in NHS hospitals over time is presented in Figure 1.2.

Utilisation of private health insurance

The utilisation of private health insurance may be demonstrated by the number of individuals who subscribe to private health insurance and the number of individuals who are insured privately. This information is presented in Figure 1.3. In 1975, approximately 1.1 million individuals subscribed to private health insurance and 2.3 million individuals were insured. In 1996, 4.0 million individuals subscribed to private health insurance and 8.0 million individuals were insured.

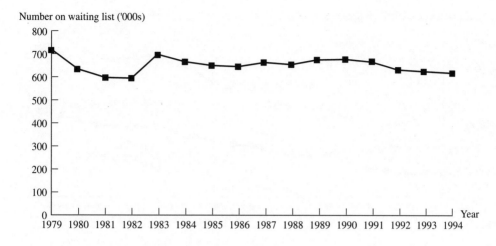

Figure 1.1 NHS hospital inpatient waiting list in England (*source*: OHE, 1995).

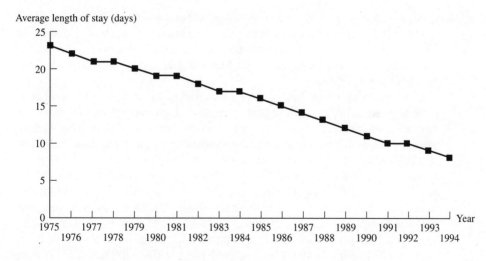

Figure 1.2 Average length of stay in NHS hospitals (*source*: OHE, 1997).

Interpreting the evidence

Interpretation 1: scarce resources and underfunding in the NHS

Evidence presented above may be used to support the existence of scarce resources and underfunding in the NHS:

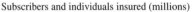

Subscribers and individuals insured (millions)

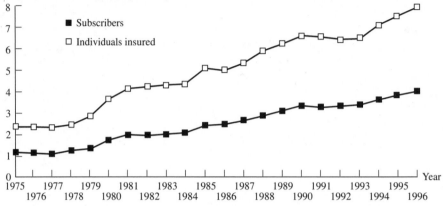

Figure 1.3 Subscribers to private health insurance and individuals insured in the UK (*source*: OHE, 1995).

1. Comparison of total UK expenditure with other countries. The United States spends nearly three and a half times more on health care per person than the UK (£2,816 versus £808), and the only countries in the developed world to spend less on health care per person than the UK are Ireland, New Zealand, Spain, Portugal and Greece.
2. Number of staff. Both the number of hospital doctors and the number of general practitioners has increased over time. However, in recent years, the number of nurses and midwives working in the NHS has fallen. In 1994 there were 61,331 fewer nurses and midwives working in the NHS than there were in 1989 (429,214 versus 490,545 nurses and midwives).
3. Number of available hospital beds. Both the total number of beds available and the number of beds available per 100,000 individuals in the population have fallen considerably in recent years. In the UK there are now just over half the number of beds available in NHS hospitals than there were twenty years ago (497,000 beds in 1975 compared with 285,000 beds in 1994). The number of available hospital beds in the NHS per 100,0000 individuals in the population has also fallen (8.8 beds per 100,000 individuals in the population in 1975 compared with 4.9 beds per 100,000 individuals in the population in 1994).
4. Size of the population. In 1994 there were 58.4 million individuals of all ages living in the UK, and the population of the UK is rising continuously. With this increase, burdens imposed on the NHS are likely to rise.
5. Proportion of population who are elderly. In 1975, 5.0 per cent of the population of the UK was aged 75 years or more (2.8 million individuals). In 1994, this figure had risen to 7.1 per cent of the population (4.1 million individuals). This increase in the proportion of individuals aged 75 years or

more is significant because it is generally the case that older individuals require more health care than younger individuals. Therefore, an increase in the number and proportion of older individuals in the UK is likely to impose a greater burden on the NHS.

6. Level of morbidity. In 1975, 24 per cent of the population of Great Britain reported chronic ill health and 15 per cent reported acute ill health. In 1993 these figures had risen to 32 per cent and 19 per cent, respectively. As the level of morbidity in the population increases, the demands placed on the NHS will also increase.

7. NHS consultations. Across all ages, the average number of consultations per person is slowly increasing. In 1975, the average number of NHS consultations was three. In 1993 this figure had risen to five. Therefore, the use of NHS resources is increasing over time.

8. Waiting lists. Across all specialities in 1994 there were 608,000 individuals on a waiting list for treatment as an inpatient in England. In recent years, the size of the waiting list has fluctuated. Currently, the waiting list is decreasing from its recent high in 1990 of 671,000 individuals. However, whilst the number of individuals waiting for treatment may be falling, the total number is still high.

9. Length of stay. In 1975 the average length of stay in an NHS hospital was 23 days. This was nearly three times longer than the average length of stay in 1994, which was eight days. Every year, the average length of stay has fallen.

10. Utilisation of private health insurance. Evidence of the quantity of resources used in the NHS may also be obtained from data on the utilisation of private health insurance as an alternative to receiving health care via the NHS. This may reflect the level of scarcity in the NHS as individuals turn to private health care rather than relying on the NHS for the provision of health care. Both the number of individuals who have subscribed to private health insurance and the number of individuals insured have increased substantially in recent years.

Interpretation 2: efficiency and adequate funding in the NHS

The evidence may also be used to support the claim that the NHS is not underfunded and is, in fact, performing well:

1. Comparison of total UK expenditure with other countries. Whilst the United States may spend nearly three and a half times more on health care per person than the UK (£2,816 versus £808), and whilst most countries in the developed world may spend more on health care per person than the UK, this may suggest that resources are being used more efficiently in the UK than in other

countries and that there is less wastage because health care is being provided at lower cost.

2. Number of staff. Whilst the number of nursing and midwifery staff is decreasing this may be because staff are better trained and used more efficiently so that fewer staff are needed to provide high quality health care.

3. Number of available hospital beds. The number of available hospital beds is falling, but this may indicate that patients are being treated more efficiently. For example, more patients are treated on a day case or an outpatient basis, thus reducing the need for hospital beds.

4. Size of the population. Whilst the population of the UK is rising continuously, in line with this increase there has also been a rise in health care expenditure. From Table 1.1 we can see that not only total health care expenditure but also average health care expenditure per person has increased. This implies that the increase in health care expenditure has more than matched the increase in the size of the population.

5. Proportion of population who are elderly. Whilst the proportion of the population who are elderly has increased, so too has the average health care expenditure per person to accommodate this.

6. Level of morbidity. The level of morbidity may be increasing, but so too is average expenditure on health care per person to meet this increase.

7. NHS consultations. The average number of consultations per person is increasing. However, rather than indicating scarce health care resources, what this in fact may be showing is that the NHS is coping well with increased demands placed on it by increasing the quantity of health care provided to each individual.

8. Waiting lists. Waiting lists for treatment do exist, but in recent years these have fallen significantly (approximately 10 per cent in four years). It could be argued that it is unlikely that waiting lists will ever be completely removed because the demand for health care will always increase with the increased productivity of the NHS.

9. Length of stay. Rather than being a sign of underfunding, reductions in the length of stay may in fact be a sign of efficiency because due to improvements in the quality of health care individuals are required to spend less time in hospital following treatment. Additionally, reductions in the length of hospital stay mean that throughput may increase so that the number of individuals who are treated will rise.

10. Utilisation of private health insurance. The number of individuals who subscribe to private health insurance and the number of individuals insured are increasing, but this may not necessarily be due to dissatisfaction with the NHS. Instead, this may simply be a result of increases in income and the standard of living which allow more individuals to obtain health care privately. Furthermore, increases in the number of individuals utilising private health insurance may be advantageous for those who continue to receive their health care via the NHS if it means that average NHS expenditure per patient will rise.

Addressing the problem of scarce health care resources

Evidence suggests that the NHS is underfunded and that health care resources in the UK are scarce. Unfortunately, this evidence may also be interpreted quite differently to show that the NHS, rather than being underfunded, is in fact adequately meeting the demands placed upon it. Given the available evidence, it is therefore difficult to draw any firm conclusions as to whether there are scarce resources in the NHS. Whilst many people do believe the NHS to be underfunded, the extent of the problem depends upon the way in which the available evidence is interpreted.

If we assume that the problem of scarcity does exist in the NHS, the key issue then becomes what to do about it. This is exactly the issue that health economics seeks to address, and it is the subject of this book. Specifically, some decision is needed regarding the appropriate allocation of resources. The questions which need to be addressed correspond roughly with those presented at the beginning of the chapter:

1. What treatments should be made available?

In the presence of scarcity, the health care resources available are too few to satisfy the total health care needs of the population. Therefore, some form of choice or prioritisation is inevitable so that we may decide what health care services we should provide. For example, should prenatal screening for Down's syndrome be made available to all pregnant women? Should condoms be provided free by the NHS? Which drug should be used to treat patients with hypercholesterolaemia?

2. How should these treatments be provided?

Even after it is decided what treatments to provide, we still need to decide how to provide them. This decision too is an important one because the provision of health care also requires the use of scarce resources. For example, should more inpatients be treated on a day case basis, and should more day case patients be treated on an outpatient basis? Should mentally ill patients be cared for through traditional institution-based methods or in the community? To what extent should nurses be able to prescribe medications?

3. Who should receive these treatments?

Because of the problem of scarcity, individuals may not be provided with all the health care that they would otherwise like. Therefore, it will be necessary to develop some mechanism for allocating health care among all individuals. For example, what priority should be given to treating the elderly compared to, say, the young, or the terminally ill? Should preference be given to non-smokers over smokers in the treatment of lung cancer?

Methods for answering these three questions and for deciding how health care resources should be allocated in the NHS are the subject of this book. In the next few chapters we examine a first possible solution to these problems, namely, the market solution.

References

Office of Health Economics (OHE) (1995) *Compendium of health statistics*. London: OHE.
Office for Population Censuses and Surveys (OPCS) (1995) *General household survey, 1993*.
    London: HMSO.
Office for National Statistics (ONS) (1997) *Annual abstract of statistics*. London: HMSO.

Suggested further reading

For a general discussion of the problem of scarcity and the basic economic problem see any of the following:

Lipsey R.G. and Chrystal K.A. (1995) *An introduction to positive economics*. Eighth edition.
    Oxford: Oxford University Press. Pages 4–9.
Parkin M. and King D. (1992) *Economics*. Wokingham: Addison-Wesley. Pages 5–11.
Begg D., Fischer S. and Dornbusch R. (1994) *Economics*. Fourth edition. London: McGraw-
    Hill. Pages 2–9.

For data on resource use in the NHS see:

Office of Health Economics (OHE) (1995) *Compendium of health statistics*. London: OHE.

2 Basic theory of economics: demand, supply and the market solution

In this chapter we examine the basic aspects of economic theory which lay the foundation for the analysis of the following chapters. The discussion concentrates on the development and explanation of the basic tools of economics: demand, supply and markets, and how they may be used in response to the problem of scarcity. The discussion is general in nature, and is not specifically related to health care or nursing at this stage. These issues will be examined in following chapters.

Summary

1. The basic problem which economics attempts to address is that of scarce resources. Because of scarcity, all economic decisions necessarily involve a choice in terms of what goods to produce, how to produce them and who shall receive them.

2. One way of addressing these issues is to use the notion of a market, in which resource allocation decisions are determined by the independent decisions of consumers and producers, and signals in the form of prices are used to allocate resources.

3. There are two components of a market: demand and supply.

4. The quantity of a good that consumers are willing and able to buy in a specific time period is called the demand for a good, and is influenced by many variables including the price of the good, income, the prices of other goods and tastes.

5. There is, in general, an inverse relationship between the price of a good and the quantity demanded of that good.

6. The demand curve may be derived using the Law of Diminishing Marginal Utility and the assumption that consumers wish to maximise their utility.

7. By supply we mean the quantity of a good that producers will wish to offer for sale at a particular price per time period.

8. The quantity supplied of a good is also influenced by a number of variables, such as the price of the good, the prices of other goods and the costs of production.

9. There is, in general, a positive relationship between the price of a good and the quantity supplied of that good.

10. The supply curve may be derived using the Law of Increasing Costs and the assumption that producers wish to maximise their profits.

11. The equilibrium price is the price at which the wishes of consumers and producers coincide.

12. If the market price is different from the equilibrium price, then either an upward or downward pressure on price, exerted by market forces and caused by excess demand or excess supply, will cause the market price to tend towards the equilibrium price.

13. Changes in the demand and supply curves, caused by changes in the determinants of demand and supply, will cause the equilibrium price to change.

14. There are four basic changes which can occur to the equilibrium price: a rise in demand; a fall in demand; a rise in supply; and a fall in supply.

15. The intuitive reason for using the market framework to address the issue of scarcity is that markets provide a means of allocating resources which is efficient.

16. Aiming to maximise their utility, consumers will spend the amount of money which will maximise their well-being, resulting in allocative efficiency. At the same time, producers, seeking to maximise their utility through maximising their profits, will compete for custom by producing goods most highly valued by consumers at least cost, thus behaving in a technically efficient manner.

17. Consumers in the market have the knowledge and ability to determine the level of price at which demand equals supply. The dominance of consumer preferences is known as consumer sovereignty, and is a necessary condition for the market to allocate resources efficiently.

Scarce resources

Because of the problem of resource scarcity, all economic decisions necessarily involve a choice in terms of what to produce, how to produce it and who shall receive it. Therefore the three basic problems that we are interested in as economists are:

1. What goods and services shall we produce?
2. How shall we produce these goods and services?
3. Who will receive these goods and services?

The method by which these three questions are addressed may be referred to as the allocation of resources, or how the resources in society are divided among the various outputs, among the various methods of producing these outputs, and among the members of society.

Although every society has to decide how to allocate the resources available to it, societies differ in how these decisions are made. One means of addressing the basic economic problem and allocating resources is using the notion of a market. In a market system, resource allocation decisions are determined by independent decisions of individual consumers and producers.

The market

A market may be defined as any institution where parties can communicate with each other in order to buy and sell goods and services. More obvious examples of what we might mean by markets include street markets, supermarkets and the stock exchange. Other, perhaps more obscure, examples include the nursing labour market and the NHS internal market.

The reason why markets are appealing as a means of addressing the problem of scarcity is that, under certain perfect conditions, markets will allocate resources in an efficient manner. Efficiency is a state where the costs of producing any given output are minimised and the benefits of that output are maximised. It is possible to distinguish between three different types of efficiency which may be achieved in markets:

1. technical efficiency;
2. productive efficiency;
3. allocative efficiency.

Technical efficiency

Technical efficiency is achieved when the inputs used in producing a given output are minimised or where output is maximised for a given set of inputs. A particular method of producing a good is technically inefficient if there exists some other way of producing the output that will use fewer resources in the process.

Productive efficiency

Productive efficiency is achieved when the costs of producing a given output are minimised or where output is maximised for a given cost. Productive efficiency is not achieved in the production of a good if there exists some other method of producing the good that is less costly.

Allocative efficiency

Allocative efficiency exists when it is not possible to change the allocation of resources in such a way as to make one individual better off without making another individual worse off. From an allocative point of view, resources are said to be allocated inefficiently when using them to produce a different bundle of goods makes it possible for one person to be made better off without another person being made worse off.

The existence of markets can be shown, under ideal conditions, to lead to the existence of technical, productive and allocative efficiency. Markets are therefore desirable in that they obtain the best outcomes from limited resources. Before discussing the processes by which this occurs, it is useful to first distinguish between the terms cost, price and value.

Costs relate to the costs incurred by producers in the production of a good. Prices relate to the price of a good that consumers are required to pay in order to obtain the good. Values relate to the value of a good to consumers, and this may be higher or lower than the price.

Markets work by the interaction of decisions made by individual buyers and sellers of goods and services acting in their own self-interest. This interaction of buyers and sellers ensures that the quantity of a good that people wish to buy is the same as the quantity that people wish to sell. A perfect market delivers maximum consumer satisfaction with the resources available to society. The role of prices is crucial to the market system, since prices perform the important function of providing signals to buyers and sellers that help to allocate resources. Therefore, in a market scenario, resources are allocated using the medium of prices.

The price system

The basis of any market is the price system. A market price is the result of the interaction between the consumers' demand for a good and the supply of that good by producers. Therefore, two basic concepts necessary for a market are:

1. demand;
2. supply.

We shall now examine each of these in turn.

Demand

In a market situation, those parties that demand goods or services are often known as buyers or consumers. In this discussion we will use the term consumers to refer to parties or individuals who demand goods.

The demand for a particular good is defined as the quantity of a good that consumers are willing and able to buy in a specific time period.

The amount of a good that consumers will be willing and able to buy in any one time period will be influenced by many variables. As has been already indicated, perhaps the most important variable that will have an effect on the quantity demanded of a good is its price.

In the case of almost all goods, as the price of a good increases, the quantity demanded will fall. Conversely, if the price falls, then the quantity demanded will rise. We therefore say that there is an inverse relationship between price and quantity demanded.

We can demonstrate this relationship between price and quantity demanded graphically, by constructing a demand curve (see Figure 2.1).

The demand curve D is downward sloping from left to right. We say that it has a negative slope, reflecting the negative relationship between price and quantity demanded. At a relatively high price such as P_1 a relatively low quantity will be demanded, Q_1. As the price falls to a lower value, such as P_2, then the quantity demanded will increase to Q_2.

The simple explanation for this is that when the price of a good falls, the good becomes cheaper. Therefore, all other things being equal, we will wish to buy more of this good. This occurs for two reasons: the substitution effect; and the income effect.

1. The substitution effect: if the price of a good falls we buy more of it because it is cheaper.

This is the effect of a price change on the quantity demanded due exclusively to the fact that its relative price has changed. For instance, suppose two goods, A and B. If the price of good A falls, it becomes relatively cheaper compared with good B and consumers are likely to substitute good A for the relatively more expensive alternative, B. Therefore the quantity demanded of the cheaper good A will increase.

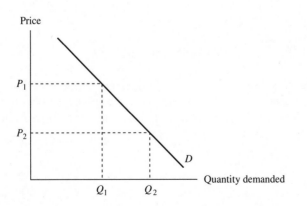

Figure 2.1 The demand curve, D.

2. The income effect: if the price of a good falls we buy more of it because it leaves more income to spend.

This is the effect of a price change on the quantity demanded due exclusively to the fact that the consumers' real disposable income has changed so that they have greater purchasing power. If the price of good A falls, consumers are likely to buy more of good A, but also more of good B, even though the price of good B does not change. This is because the fall in the price of good A means that more income is left to buy both goods.

These two effects provide intuitive reasons why there is a negative relationship between price and quantity demanded. A more involved explanation of why the demand curve has a negative slope is provided by what is known as Utility Theory.

Utility

The satisfaction that consumers derive from the goods they consume is called their utility. The term utility may also be used synonymously with welfare, satisfaction or happiness. The concept of utility enables us to construct a theory of consumer behaviour and explain the shape of the demand curve.

Consider the utility that one consumer derives from purchases of a good such as chocolate bars. Let us assume that if one chocolate bar is eaten each day then it will be enjoyed a great deal. If two chocolate bars are eaten in one day then the second may be enjoyed a little less than the first, and the third even less. Each subsequent chocolate bar eaten in a single day will give less pleasure. At a certain point, the consumer may have had enough of chocolate bars and may want no more, even if chocolate bars are free. Ultimately, eating more chocolate bars will cause displeasure, as too much consumption may even make the individual ill.

This demonstrates the relationship between utility and quantity consumed. The principle on which this is based is called the Law of Diminishing Marginal Utility.

The Law of Diminishing Marginal Utility

In order to explain the principle of diminishing marginal utility we can make a distinction between the total utility derived from the consumption of all units of a good consumed over a period of time, and the marginal utility of an additional unit of a good consumed over that period of time.

Total utility

In general, the more of a good that an individual consumes the greater the total utility that they enjoy. After a certain saturation point, further consumption may cause total utility to fall, though individuals will not usually consume units of a good beyond this point. This may be compared with marginal utility, where the marginal utility from each successive unit of consumption decreases.

Marginal utility

Marginal utility is defined as the difference in utility arising from the consumption of one more or one less unit of a good. It is the rate at which total utility changes as we change our consumption of a good by one unit. For instance, if consuming 20 chocolate bars yielded 100 units of utility, and 21 chocolate bars yielded 102 units of utility, then the marginal utility of consuming the twenty-first chocolate bar is 2 units of utility. Algebraically, if TU_n is the total utility from consuming n units of a good, and TU_{n+1} is the total utility from consuming $n + 1$ units of a good, then the marginal utility from consuming the $n + 1$th unit (MU_{n+1}) is the difference between T_n and T_{n+1}:

$$MU_{n+1} = T_{n+1} - T_n \tag{2.1}$$

The principle of diminishing marginal utility states that while total utility increases with consumption, marginal utility falls. In other words, the extra satisfaction obtained from eating more and more chocolate bars leads to smaller and smaller rises in satisfaction. As consumption increases, total utility increases at a diminishing rate. Ultimately, marginal utility may even become negative, though it is unlikely that an individual would consume so much of a good that it would cause disutility.

This relationship between quantity demanded, total utility and marginal utility may be seen more clearly using a numerical example.

Table 2.1 presents a hypothetical example illustrating the relationship between the quantity of chocolate bars consumed, total utility and marginal utility. It can be seen that, up to a certain point, as the quantity of chocolate bars eaten per day rises so total utility rises also. Note that after consuming the ninth chocolate bar, however, total utility falls. At this point the individual will only receive displeasure or disutility

Table 2.1 The relationship between quantity, total utility and marginal utility.

Bars of chocolate eaten per day, Q	Total utility, TU	Marginal utility, MU
0	0	
1	80	80
2	150	70
3	205	55
4	240	35
5	265	25
6	280	15
7	290	10
8	295	5
9	290	−5
10	275	−15

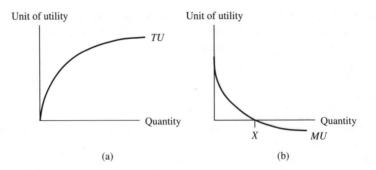

Figure 2.2 Total utility (*TU*) and marginal utility (*MU*).

from consuming more bars of chocolate. Marginal utility decreases as the quantity of chocolate bars eaten increases. For example, 35 units of utility is obtained from consuming the fourth bar of chocolate, but only 25 units of utility is gained from consuming the fifth bar of chocolate. This same data may be seen graphically in Figure 2.2.

Figure 2.2(a) shows the total utility schedule and demonstrates how total utility increases at a diminishing rate as the quantity consumed increases. Figure 2.2(b) shows a diminishing marginal utility curve. Should more than *X* units of the good be consumed then the marginal utility becomes negative. If individuals were forced to consume more of the good than quantity *X* then the additional units would actually reduce total utility.

Using the Law of Diminishing Marginal Utility we can now formally derive the demand curve for a particular good, and demonstrate why it slopes downwards from left to right. When an individual buys a good, they become better off by the amount of utility which the good yields. Also, however, they become worse off by paying a price for the good and therefore forgoing other goods that could have been obtained with the same money. In order to decide how much of a good to buy, therefore, it is necessary to examine the nature of these gains and losses and to define some decision-making criterion, which in this case is utility maximisation.

Utility maximisation

We assume that all consumers seek to maximise their total utility. This maximisation is, however, constrained by their limited resources, taken here to be measured by their income. Therefore, it is assumed that individuals maximise their utility subject to their income.

The method for achieving utility maximisation is to distribute expenditure between available goods and services until the last penny spent on each good and service yields the same marginal utility. This has commonsense appeal. If the last penny spent on chocolate bars yielded more utility than the last penny spent on, say, bread, then total utility could be increased by transferring a penny of expenditure from bread to chocolate bars. For instance, if the last penny spent on chocolate bars yielded ten units of utility and the last penny spent of bread yielded six units of utility, by spending a penny less on bread, six units of utility are lost. However, by spending that penny instead on chocolate, ten units are gained. Therefore, the net gain from the transfer is four units of utility.

However, in this situation we have already seen that as we buy more of a good (or as quantity increases), so the marginal utility falls. Conversely, as we buy less of a good (or as quantity falls), so marginal utility increases.

We reallocate our spending by buying less bread and therefore the marginal utility of bread rises. Conversely, we buy more chocolate bars, and as we do the marginal utility of chocolate bars falls. As this reallocation continues, so the marginal utilities of the two alternatives converge on each other. This transfer of expenditure between the two goods will continue until the marginal utility of a penny spent on chocolate bars is the same as the marginal utility of a penny spent on bread. At this point there is nothing to be gained from further reallocations. For instance, if enough chocolate bars have been consumed such that the marginal utility of the last penny spent on chocolate bars consumed is eight units, and the marginal utility of the last penny spent on bread is eight units, both marginal utilities are identical. There is now nothing that can be gained from further reallocations of expenditure between the two goods.

More formally, suppose two goods, A and B. We reallocate expenditure between bread and chocolate bars until

$$MU \text{ of 1p spent on bread} = MU \text{ of 1p spent on chocolate bars} \qquad (2.2)$$

This is therefore the condition for maximising utility.

More generally, the marginal utility of a penny spent on a good is calculated by dividing the marginal utility of the good by the price of the good. For example, if a chocolate bar costs 30p and yields a marginal utility of 60 units of utility, then the marginal utility per one penny spent is $60/30 = 2$ units of utility per penny spent. We can therefore rewrite Equation 2.2, so that it now becomes:

$$MU \text{ of A } / \text{ Price of A} = MU \text{ of B } / \text{ Price of B} \qquad (2.3)$$

This can be rearranged and also written as:

$$MU \text{ of A } / MU \text{ of B} = \text{Price of A } / \text{ Price of B} \qquad (2.4)$$

Equation 2.4 basically states that in order to maximise utility, a consumer will adjust their purchases of any two goods until their marginal utilities are proportional to their prices. In other words, the consumer wants the same marginal utility per penny spent on A as on B. So, for example, if a unit of A costs four times as much as a unit of B then the consumer must get four times as much marginal utility from the last unit of A as from the last unit of B.

Using the information we have gained so far, we can now determine how much of a particular good will be demanded at a given price, and we can therefore derive the slope of the demand curve. To summarise the discussion so far, the conditions which we require to hold are:

CONDITION (1): marginal utility falls as quantity consumed rises

CONDITION (2): consumers seek to maximise their utility

CONDITION (3): to maximise utility, consume that level of output where the marginal utility of 1p spent on one good equals the marginal utility of 1p spent on another good

Derivation of the demand curve

We can now see why the demand curve is downward sloping. Keeping all other things constant, suppose the price of good A falls. The consumer restores equilibrium by consuming more of A until its marginal utility falls in the same proportion that its price has fallen.

Algebraically, suppose that from the starting equilibrium as defined by Equation 2.3, the price of good A falls. We now have a situation where:

$$MU \text{ of A } / \text{ Price of A} > MU \text{ of B } / \text{ Price of B} \qquad (2.5)$$

In order to restore the equilibrium, the individual will buy more of good A (and therefore less of good B), thereby reducing the marginal utility of A and increasing the marginal utility of B. The individual will continue to substitute A for B until the equilibrium is achieved.

This therefore demonstrates the relationship between price and quantity demanded. As price falls, so quantity demanded increases so that marginal utility falls to re-establish the equilibrium. As price rises, so quantity demanded falls so that marginal utility increases to re-establish the equilibrium.

We have therefore derived a normal downward-sloping demand curve, as demonstrated in Figure 2.1.

The determinants of demand

There are many factors which affect the level of demand. These include the price of the good, income, the prices of other goods and tastes.

1. Price of the good

As we have already seen, as the price of a good changes, so the quantity of the good demanded changes. When prices change, there is a movement along the demand curve, as characterised in Figure 2.1.

2. Income

Since demand is defined as the quantity of a good that consumers are willing *and able* to buy in a specific time period, it is obvious that there must be a relationship between the demand for a good and an individual's income, since income affects how much of a good people are able to buy. The relationship between income and demand will depend on the type of good considered and the level of income of the consumer. There are two basic types of good: normal goods and inferior goods.

All other things being equal, if the quantity demanded of a good increases as income increases, the good is said to be *normal*.

All other things being equal, if the quantity demanded of a good decreases as income increases, the good is said to be *inferior*.

An example of a normal good might be video cassettes. If income increases and so we have more money to spend, on the whole, we would expect to buy more video cassettes, and so demand increases as income increases. An example of an inferior good might be cotton shirts. As our income increases and so we have more money to spend we might expect to buy fewer cotton shirts since we can now afford to buy silk shirts instead. Therefore, the demand for cotton shirts will fall as income increases.

3. The prices of other goods

The demand for different goods is often interrelated since all goods compete for the limited income of the consumer. The relationship between two goods will depend on their nature, and there may well be no relationship at all. Alternatively, two relationships may be quantified: substitutability and complementarity.

All other things being equal, if a fall in the price of one good causes a fall in the quantity demanded of another good, then the goods are *substitutes*.

All other things being equal, if a fall in the price of one good raises the quantity demanded of another good, then the goods are *complements*.

An example of substitutability is the relationship between butter and margarine. If the price of butter falls, then consumers will buy more butter, and therefore less margarine, and vice versa. An example of complementarity is the relationship between video recorders and video cassettes. If the price of video recorders falls consumers will buy more video recorders, and therefore will need to buy more video cassettes, and vice versa.

4. Tastes

Tastes, habits and customs may be extremely important in determining the demand for a good. A change in tastes in favour of a good, such as if a good becomes more fashionable, will cause an *increase* in demand. A change in tastes away from a good will cause a *decrease* in demand.

A shift in demand

As shown in Figure 2.1, a change in the price of a good will result in a movement *along* the demand curve, either up or down, depending on whether the price increases

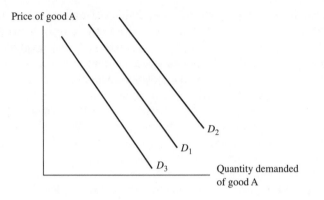

Figure 2.3 A shift in demand.

or decreases, respectively. However, a change in any other factor affecting demand will cause a *shift* in demand, shown by a movement, to the right or left, of the whole demand curve. This is shown in Figure 2.3 above.

Suppose an original demand curve characterised by D_1. The circumstances which might cause an increase in demand and a shift outwards to the right to D_2 are:

1. a rise in income of the consumer if the good is normal;
2. a fall in income of the consumer if the good is inferior;
3. a fall in the price of a complement to good A;
4. a rise in the price of a substitute to good A;
5. a change in tastes in favour of good A.

The circumstances which might cause a decrease in demand and a shift inwards to the left to D_3 are the opposite of these, namely:

1. a fall in income of the consumer if the good is normal;
2. a rise in income of the consumer if the good is inferior;
3. a rise in the price of a complement to good A;
4. a fall in the price of a substitute to good A;
5. a change in tastes away from good A.

Supply

We will now examine the other side of the market, which is supply. The supplier is the basic unit which makes decisions about how many goods to supply or sell. The term supplier may be used interchangeably with the words sellers, producers, firms, businesses and enterprises. In this discussion we will use the term producers to refer to parties or individuals who supply goods. The quantity of goods which are supplied may also be referred to as the output of producers.

By supply we mean the quantity of a good that producers will wish to offer for sale at a particular price per time period. We assume that producers make their decisions with respect to a single objective: profit maximisation. This is analogous to the goal of consumers which is utility maximisation. The producer is said to be in an optimal position when profits are being maximised. Given the goal of the producer, we now wish to ask the question how much of some good will a producer offer for sale? In other words, we wish to know how much of a good will be supplied in any one time period.

Supply and the price of a good

In a similar fashion to the discussion of demand above, we will first concentrate on the single major influence determining supply: the price of the good itself. All other things being equal, a greater quantity will be supplied at a higher price. In other words, the quantity that a producer will supply is positively associated with the price of the good.

The quantity of a good supplied rises when the price of the good rises, and the quantity supplied falls when the price falls. This result has an intuitive appeal for two reasons, which apply first to producers currently supplying the good in question, and secondly to new producers who wish to enter the market and start supplying the good:

1. Producers currently supplying the good in the market

As price increases, the prospects for making profits are greater and therefore there is a greater incentive for current producers in the market to produce more and offer it for sale.

2. Producers who wish to start supplying the good in the market

As price increases, producers who could not profitably supply goods at a lower price would find it possible to do so at the higher price. Therefore, as price increases so more producers will enter the market and the quantity supplied will increase.

Therefore, as price increases so the quantity supplied will increase for these two reasons. The relationship between price and quantity supplied may be demonstrated graphically, by constructing a supply curve (see Figure 2.4).

The supply curve shows the quantity supplied at every price. This curve is upward sloping from left to right and it therefore has a positive slope. At a relatively low price such as P_3 only a relatively low quantity of the good is supplied, Q_3. If price increases, say to P_4, then the quantity supplied also increases, to Q_4.

In the case of the demand curve we were able to derive the downward slope using the theory of diminishing marginal utility, combined with the assumption of utility maximisation. Analogous assumptions may be used to explain the upward-sloping supply curve: increasing marginal cost and profit maximisation. To explain the effects of these concepts, we first need to examine the various costs of production.

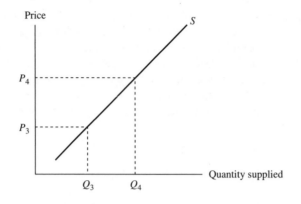

Figure 2.4 The supply curve, *S*.

Costs of production

Each level of output which is supplied by the producer will imply a cost to that producer. It is intuitively obvious that the greater the output of the producer, the greater the costs of production. This is because, for example, to produce a larger output requires more labour and more capital equipment and machinery, all of which must be paid for. To see the exact effect on the costs of production of increasing output we may distinguish between three basic types of cost: total cost; average cost; and marginal cost.

Total cost

Total cost (*TC*) is the cost of all the resources necessary to produce any particular level of output. Total cost always rises with output. For example, suppose a producer wishes to supply chocolate bars. As more chocolate bars are produced so that they may be offered for sale, total costs will increase.

Average cost

Average cost (*AC*) is the total cost divided by the quantity or number of units of the good produced (*Q*), to give the average cost per unit produced. Algebraically,

$$AC = TC \, / \, Q \qquad\qquad (2.6)$$

So, if the total cost of producing three chocolate bars is 30p then the average cost of producing one chocolate bar is 10p.

We may wish to know the rate at which costs rise as output increases. To do so we use the notion of marginal cost, which is analogous to the concept of marginal utility to the consumer.

Marginal cost

Marginal cost (MC) is the cost of producing one unit more or less of a good. It is the increase in total costs from producing an extra unit of output. So, if nine chocolate bars cost 50p to produce, and ten chocolate bars cost 60p to produce, then the marginal cost of producing the tenth chocolate bar is 10p. Algebraically, if the total cost of producing n units of output is TC_n and the total cost of producing $n+1$ units of output is TC_{n+1}, then the marginal cost of the $n+1$th unit (MC_{n+1}) is defined as:

$$MC_{n+1} = TC_{n+1} - TC_n \qquad (2.7)$$

We can use the notion of marginal cost to explain the shape of the supply curve. First, however, we need to examine how marginal cost behaves as output varies. To do this we refer to the Law of Increasing Costs.

The Law of Increasing Costs

This law basically states that the marginal cost of producing extra output rises. Therefore, marginal cost increases as output increases. In other words, each unit produced adds more to total costs than did each preceding unit produced.

So, if nine chocolate bars cost 50p to produce, and ten chocolate bars cost 60p to produce, then the marginal cost of the tenth chocolate bar is 10p. Now suppose that eleven chocolate bars cost 72p to produce, giving the marginal cost of the eleventh chocolate bar at 12p. Thus, marginal cost is increasing as output is increasing.

The intuitive reason for marginal cost to increase as output increases is that production becomes less and less efficient as more output is squeezed from its existing machinery and equipment. This result comes about because overcrowding can occur. For example, suppose there is a machine for making chocolate bars. If one person uses it they can make 1,000 chocolate bars in one day. If two people use it, they will make 1,700 chocolate bars. If three people are on the machine, only 2,100 chocolate bars are produced because the chocolate bar making machine is now overcrowded with three people working on it. Therefore, as the output of the machine is increased, more people are needed in the production process, but then overcrowding will occur and so production is less efficient. The marginal cost of producing chocolate bars rises.

The relationship between quantity, total cost, average cost and marginal cost may be seen clearly using a more extensive numerical example.

Table 2.2 presents a hypothetical example illustrating the relationship between output and the costs of production. It can be seen that as the quantity of chocolate bars produced each day rises so total costs rise also. Note also that up to a certain output marginal costs are falling. However, after producing the third chocolate bar marginal costs begin to rise. After this point, overcrowding occurs, increasing costs set in, and marginal costs rise. Therefore, total costs rise at an increasing rate. For example, the total cost of producing five bars of chocolate is 20p, implying an

Table 2.2 Costs of producing chocolate bars.

Quantity of chocolate bars, Q	Total cost, TC (pence)	Average cost, AC (pence)	Marginal cost, MC (pence)
0	0	0	
1	5	5	5
2	8	4	3
3	9	3	1
4	12	3	3
5	20	4	8
6	30	5	10
7	42	6	12
8	56	7	14
9	72	8	16
10	90	9	18

average cost of 4p, and the total cost of producing six bars of chocolate is 30p. Therefore the marginal cost of the sixth bar of chocolate is 10p. The total cost of producing seven bars of chocolate is 42p, implying a marginal cost of producing the seventh bar of chocolate of 12p. Thus, marginal cost is increasing and total costs are increasing at an increasing rate.

We can use the Law of Increasing Cost to demonstrate the shape of the supply curve. However, in order to determine how much of a good a producer is willing to supply we need to examine in more detail the goal of the producer, which we assume is that of profit maximisation.

Profit maximisation

The single goal of the producer is to make as much profit as possible. Therefore, the producer wishes to produce that level of output which maximises profits. When profits are maximised, the producer is said to be in an optimal position in which they are maximising their utility.

Using the information we have gained so far, we can now determine how much of a particular good will be supplied at a given price, and we can therefore derive the slope of the supply curve. To summarise the discussion so far, the two conditions which we require are:

CONDITION (1): marginal cost rises as output rises
CONDITION (2): producers seek to maximise their profits

The derivation of the supply curve

Given that conditions (1) and (2) above hold, we can predict how much of a good should be supplied: for profit maximisation to occur, that level of output should be supplied at which marginal cost (MC) is equal to price (p):

$$MC = p \qquad\qquad (2.8)$$

For every unit of output produced, the marginal costs are the *outgoings* of the producers, incurred from the production of the good. The price of the good is the *income* or *revenue* to the producer for each good sold, which is received every time one unit of the good is paid for by a consumer.

To explain why the optimum quantity supplied is defined by this point, we can examine what happens if the rule does not hold. Suppose therefore that marginal cost does not equal price. It follows then that one of two situations may arise:

1. marginal cost is less than price, $MC < p$;
2. marginal cost is greater than price, $MC > p$.

We can examine each of these in turn.

Marginal cost is less than price, $MC < p$

Suppose that we are producing a level of output where marginal cost is less than price ($MC < p$). This means that an extra unit of output can be produced at a cost *less* than it can be sold for. Production of the good will add to profits, and therefore it should be produced. Whenever, at the present level of output, marginal cost is less than price, output should therefore be *increased*.

For example, suppose a producer is deciding how many chocolate bars to supply and the marginal cost of producing the fifth bar of chocolate is 8p. If the price of the bar of chocolate is 12p (so that $MC < p$), then the fifth bar of chocolate costs less to produce than it can be sold for. A profit of 4p is made by the producer in this case. Therefore, the producer will wish to produce this chocolate bar since it will add to their profits. The sixth bar of chocolate is produced at a marginal cost of 10p and so, at a price of 12p, production of this will also add to profits (of 2p in this case). Therefore, to maximise their profits, the producer will produce this chocolate bar and will continue to increase output as long as marginal cost is less than price. Note that due to increasing costs, as output increases, so marginal cost also increases and converges on the price of the good.

Marginal cost is greater than price, $MC > p$

Now suppose that at the present level of output, marginal cost exceeds price ($MC > p$). This means that the last unit produced adds more to total cost than it adds to the producer's revenue. In other words, there is a loss being made on producing this last unit of output, and therefore it should not be produced. Whenever, at the present level of output, marginal cost exceeds price, output should be *reduced*.

For example, suppose the price of chocolate bars is again 12p and the marginal cost of producing the eighth chocolate bar is 14p. Therefore, when the eighth chocolate bar is sold the producer incurs a loss of 2p, since this bar costs 14p to produce and the producer only receives 12p from selling it. Wishing to maximise profits, the producer will not supply the eighth chocolate bar. Therefore, to maximise their profits, the producer will decrease output when marginal cost is greater than price.

From these two results, it follows that only when marginal cost equals price is there no incentive to alter output. We can therefore derive the supply curve, with this, the third condition:

CONDITION (3): to maximise profits, produce at that level of output where
$$MC = p$$

Since the profit maximising level of output occurs where marginal cost equals price, the marginal cost curve is the supply curve. Since we have also shown that marginal cost increases as output increases, this explains why supply curves are upward sloping from left to right. As soon as we know the producer's marginal cost we know exactly what level of output should be produced at each price. Therefore, we have seen why there is a positive relationship between price and quantity supplied.

The determinants of supply

Just as the demand curve is influenced by a number of factors, so the amount of a good that a producer will offer for sale in each time period will also be influenced by a number of factors. These include the price of the good, the costs of production and the prices of other goods.

1. Price of the good

As we have already demonstrated, this is a major influence on the quantity supplied of a particular good. When the price of the good changes there is a movement along the supply curve, as characterised in Figure 2.4.

2. Costs of production

Firms will offer goods for sale so long as the marginal cost of producing them exceeds the price. Therefore, all other things being equal, any change in production costs will affect quantity supplied.

The costs of production depend on two variables: the prices of the inputs in the production process (called the factors of production); and the current state of technology.

(a) The prices of the inputs into the production process

All other things being equal, if the price of an input into the production process rises, then the costs of production will rise. If the market price for the good remains unchanged, then less profit is made by the producer from selling the good, and so there will be a *decrease* in supply.

For example, if the price of chocolate used to make chocolate bars increases then the overall costs of production will also increase. Therefore, since marginal cost has increased, less profit will be made from selling chocolate bars, and so fewer will be produced.

A fall in the price of an input into the production process will have the opposite effect, and cause an *increase* in supply.

(b) The state of technology

The costs of production depend not only on the prices of the inputs into the production process but also on the productivity of those inputs. Productivity will be affected by the state of technology. Over time, technology advances, and the productivity of inputs increases. All other things being equal, more goods will be supplied at any given price since they are cheaper to produce. Therefore, the state of technology advances, causing an *increase* in supply.

For example, suppose the state of chocolate bar production improved such that more chocolate bars could be made at a faster rate using more technologically advanced machinery and equipment, then the costs of production would decrease and more chocolate bars would be supplied.

A fall in the productivity of inputs into the production process will have the opposite effect, and cause a *decrease* in supply.

3. Prices of other goods

Prices should be viewed as being relative to one another. When the price of one good falls and the price of another good remains the same, so the first good becomes relatively cheaper, while the second good has become relatively more expensive.

If the price of one good rises it becomes relatively more expensive to consumers wishing to buy the good, and therefore producers will shift production into these goods so they are able to make greater profits at the higher price. Therefore, as the price of a good increases relative to another, there will be an *increase* in supply of the relatively more expensive good.

For example, if the price of chocolate were to rise and the price of bread were to remain the same, there would be a reduction in the desired output of bread accompanied by a rise in the output of chocolate bars, as producers switched to supplying chocolate bars.

Conversely, if the price of chocolate bars were to fall, so producers would switch to supplying bread as more profits could be made supplying that good. Therefore, a fall in the price of a good relative to another will have the opposite effect, and cause a *decrease* in supply.

A shift in supply

As shown in Figure 2.4, a change in the price of a good will result in a movement *along* the supply curve, either up or down, depending on whether prices increase or

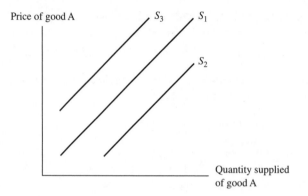

Figure 2.5 A shift in supply.

decrease, respectively. However, a change in the other factors affecting supply will cause a *shift* in supply, shown by a movement, to the right or left, of the whole supply curve. This is shown in Figure 2.5 above.

Suppose an original supply curve characterised by S_1. The circumstances which might cause an increase in supply and a shift outwards to the right to S_2 are as follows:

1. a fall in the price of inputs into the production process;
2. an improvement in the state of technology (or a rise in productivity);
3. a fall in the price of an alternative product.

The circumstances which might cause an increase in supply and a shift inwards to the left to S_3 are the opposite of these:

1. a rise in the price of inputs into the production process;
2. a fall in productivity;
3. a rise in the price of an alternative product.

Market price determination

Previously in this chapter we have examined the two components of a market: supply and demand. Demand is the quantity of a good which is purchased over a specific period of time at a certain price, and all other things being equal, more of a good will be demanded at a lower price. By supply we mean the quantity of a good that producers wish to offer for sale at a particular price. All other things being equal, a greater quantity will be supplied at a higher price.

We can now put these two components together to see how they interact and form a market. A market has been defined as any institutional arrangement in which

Table 2.3 The demand and supply of chocolate bars at various prices.

Price of chocolate bars (pence)	Quantity demanded	Quantity supplied
10	10,000	1,000
20	9,000	1,500
30	7,500	2,500
40	6,000	4,000
50	5,000	5,000
60	4,500	6,000
70	3,500	8,000
80	2,500	10,500
90	1,500	13,000
100	500	16,000

buyers and sellers communicate with each other to buy and sell a good. On the demand side of the market we have consumers, who wish to buy the good, and they do so in such a way so as to maximise their utility. On the supply side of the market we have producers who offer goods for sale, and they do so in such a way so as to maximise their profits. Communication in the market framework is made through the medium of prices.

Given this information, and the importance of price in the market framework, we may now combine our analysis of demand and supply to show how a competitive market price is determined. For the purposes of the analysis, we will use an example of the market for chocolate bars. Table 2.3 presents hypothetical data for the quantity of chocolate bars demanded and supplied in the market, and shows how these quantities vary at different market prices. Note that in this market there are many consumers and producers of chocolate bars, so that no one party is able to influence the market price solely on the basis of their own behaviour.

In this market, at a market price for chocolate bars of 40p, consumers will demand 6,000 chocolate bars in total. Producers will supply 4,000 chocolate bars. Note that the quantity demanded falls as price rises, and that the quantity supplied rises as price rises. These quantities are consistent with the theoretical and intuitive explanations of the demand and supply curves outlined above. We can use this information now to generate an equilibrium price.

The equilibrium price

In the hypothetical market for chocolate bars, consider the price of 50p. At this price the quantity demanded is 5,000, and the quantity supplied is also 5,000. In other words, at the market price of 50p the quantity the consumers wish to demand is exactly the same as the quantity that producers wish to supply. This is the *equilibrium price*. The quantity bought and sold at that price, 5,000 chocolate bars, is the *equilibrium quantity*.

More generally, the equilibrium price is the price at which the wishes of the buyers and sellers coincide. At this price, the quantity that consumers wish to buy is exactly the same as the quantity that producers wish to sell.

Equilibrium therefore occurs when supply and demand are balanced, or when the quantity that producers want to offer for sale is the same as the quantity that consumers want to purchase, so that at this price there are no unsatisfied buyers or sellers.

Diagrammatically, the equilibrium price is defined by the intersection of the demand and supply curves. Superimposing Figures 2.1 and 2.4 on to each other, we can plot and overlap the demand and supply curves for chocolate bars on the same graph, using 'price' and 'quantity' as the axes, as presented in Figure 2.6, where the data from Table 2.3 are displayed. The equilibrium price (50p) and the equilibrium quantity (5,000 chocolate bars) occur at the intersection of the demand and supply curves. At this intersection point, the quantity demanded, which is read off the demand curve, is exactly the same as the quantity supplied, which is read off the supply curve.

In Figure 2.6 the equilibrium price of 50p is denoted by p^*, which is the prevailing price at the intersection of the demand curve D and the supply curve S. The equilibrium quantity corresponding to the equilibrium price is 5,000 chocolate bars

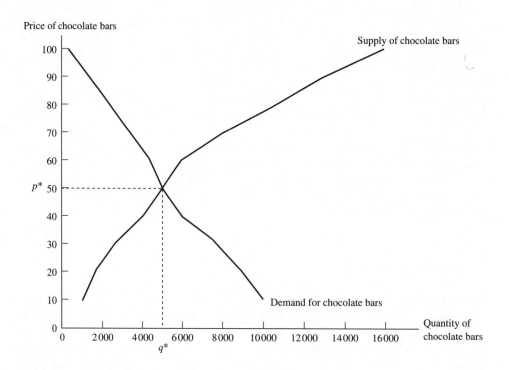

Figure 2.6 Market equilibrium.

and is denoted by q^*. We can therefore say that in this market, the *equilibrium position* is defined by the point p^*q^*.

Disequilibrium prices

The equilibrium price is the price at which demand equals supply and there are no unsatisfied consumers or producers. This may differ from the *market price*. The market price p is the price that is actually used in the market at any one time.

The equilibrium price will not change unless either the demand or supply curves shift, but the actual market price can change all the time. Three situations can arise:

1. the market price may be above the equilibrium price $(p > p^*)$;
2. the market price may be less than the equilibrium price $(p < p^*)$;
3. the market price may equal the equilibrium price $(p = p^*)$.

We can examine the effects of these three situations with reference to Figure 2.7.

Market price is greater than equilibrium price, $p > p^*$

This situation is demonstrated in Figure 2.7(a). The market price, denoted by p_1, is greater than the equilibrium price, p^*. With a market price of p_1 we can ascertain the quantity of the good demanded and supplied: at this price, from the demand curve D, q_1 is the quantity demanded; from the supply curve, q_2 is the quantity supplied. It is the case that q_2 is greater than q_1 and we therefore are in a position of *excess supply*, where quantity supplied is greater than quantity demanded.

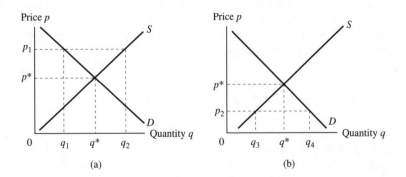

Figure 2.7 Excess supply and excess demand.

Table 2.4 Excess supply and excess demand in the market for chocolate bars.

Price of chocolate bars (pence)	Quantity demanded	Quantity supplied	Market state
10	10,000	1,000	excess demand
20	9,000	1,500	excess demand
30	7,500	2,500	excess demand
40	6,000	4,000	excess demand
50	5,000	5,000	equilibrium
60	4,500	6,000	excess supply
70	3,500	8,000	excess supply
80	2,500	10,500	excess supply
90	1,500	13,000	excess supply
100	500	16,000	excess supply

In a situation of excess supply producers will find themselves unable to sell all they produce. This may be demonstrated using the previous example of the market for chocolate bars (see Table 2.4).

In the hypothetical market for chocolate bars, the equilibrium price is 50p and the equilibrium quantity is 5,000 chocolate bars. If the market price is greater than the equilibrium price then there is excess supply. This is demonstrated at the market price of, say, 70p in Table 2.4. At this price, 8,000 chocolate bars are supplied, but only 3,500 are demanded. Therefore, there is an excess supply of chocolate bars of 4,500.

Market price is less than equilibrium price, $p < p^*$

This situation is demonstrated in Figure 2.7(b). The market price, denoted by p_2, is less than the equilibrium price p^*. With a market price of p_2, q_4 is the quantity demanded, and q_3 is the quantity supplied. q_3 is less than q_4 and the quantity demanded is greater than the quantity supplied. We are therefore in a position of *excess demand*, where quantity demanded is greater than quantity supplied.

From Table 2.4 we can see that excess demand occurs when the market price is below the equilibrium price. For example, at a market price of 30p, 7,500 chocolate bars are demanded but only 2,500 chocolate bars are supplied. There is therefore an excess demand of 5,000 chocolate bars.

Market price equals equilibrium price, $p = p^*$

Only when the market price equals the equilibrium price is there no excess demand or excess supply. When the market price is not the equilibrium price (that is, when $p > p^*$ or $p < p^*$) a number of factors come into play which will affect the market. These factors, which may be called *market forces*, can be used to show that the equilibrium price is self-seeking.

The effects of market forces

When the market price does not equal the equilibrium price then market forces come into play and put pressure on the market price to return it to the equilibrium price. Two situations may arise:

1. $p > p^*$ and there is excess supply;
2. $p < p^*$ and there is excess demand.

$p > p^*$ and there is excess supply

When the market price is greater than the equilibrium price and there is excess supply in the market, producers will not be able to sell all they wish to sell. In this situation, the market price will *fall*. This will occur for two reasons:

1. producers, in an effort to make their goods more attractive to consumers, will ask for lower prices for what they sell;
2. consumers, observing quantities of unsold output, will offer to buy goods at lower prices from producers.

Both of these pressures will push the market price *down*. Therefore, when there is excess supply and the market price is greater than the equilibrium price, market forces come into play and a downward pressure is exerted on the market price.

$p < p^*$ and there is excess demand

When the market price is less than the equilibrium price and there is excess demand in the market, consumers will not be able to buy all they wish to buy. In this situation, the market price will *increase*. This will occur for two reasons:

1. consumers, finding themselves unable to buy as much as they wish, will offer to buy the good at higher prices in an attempt to get more of what is available;
2. producers, finding themselves able to sell easily all of their output, will begin to ask for higher prices for the quantities that they have produced.

Both of these pressures will push the market price *up*. Therefore, when there is excess demand and the market price is less than the equilibrium price, market forces come into play and an upward pressure is exerted on the market price.

The only situation where the market forces do not come into play is when the market price equals the equilibrium price, and the wishes of the buyers and sellers coincide. At this point, where there is no excess demand or excess supply, no pressure, either upward or downward, is exerted by the market. Therefore, the equilibrium position is self-seeking, since the pressures exerted by the existence of excess demand and excess supply cause the market price to tend towards the equilibrium price.

In the discussion so far, we have implicitly assumed that, whilst the market price may be altered through the effects of market forces, the equilibrium price remains constant. We may now relax this assumption and examine the ways in which the equilibrium position may change, and the effects this has on the equilibrium price and quantity. The equilibrium position will change only if there is a shift in either demand, or supply, or both.

Shifts in demand and supply

An equilibrium price is not permanent: it lasts only as long as the demand and supply characteristics which produced it persist. A change or shift in demand or supply will bring about a new equilibrium price. Such a change may be caused by a change in one of the determinants of demand or supply (not the price of the good itself). Diagrammatically, any change in supply or demand will cause the demand and supply curves to shift. This will bring about a new intersection point of the two curves which in turn will imply a new equilibrium position.

If we consider all the possible shifts in demand and supply, it is apparent that only four basic movements are possible: a rise in demand (so the demand curve shifts to the right); a fall in demand (so the demand curve shifts to the left); a rise in supply (so the supply curve shifts to the right); and a fall in supply (so the supply curve shifts to the left). These are demonstrated in Figure 2.8. In all cases, the original equilibrium position is defined by p^*q^* at the intersection of the original demand and supply curves, D_0 and S_0.

1. A rise in demand

With a rise in demand, the demand curve shifts to the right. This is shown in Figure 2.8(a). With a change in the determinants of demand, suppose an increase in consumers' income, this increases the quantity that consumers wish to buy at every price. Therefore, the demand curve D_0 shifts to the right to, say, D_1. There is, therefore, a new equilibrium position brought about by the intersection of the new demand curve and the supply curve. This is position $p_1^*q_1^*$. The new equilibrium price, p_1^*, is greater than p^*, and the new equilibrium quantity, q_1^*, is greater than q^*.

Therefore, a rise in the demand for a good (or a shift to the right in the demand curve) causes an *increase* in the equilibrium price and an *increase* in the equilibrium quantity.

2. A fall in demand

With a fall in demand, the demand curve shifts to the left. This is shown in Figure 2.8(b). With a change in the determinants of demand, suppose a fall in consumers'

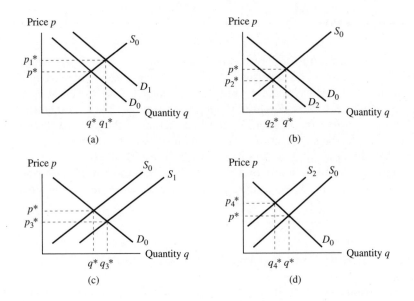

Figure 2.8 Shifts in demand and supply.

income, this decreases the quantity that consumers wish to buy at every price. Therefore, the demand curve D_0 shifts to the left to, say, D_2. The new equilibrium position brought about by the intersection of the new demand curve and the supply curve is $p_2^*q_2^*$. The new equilibrium price, p_2^*, is less than p^*, and the new equilibrium quantity, q_2^*, is less than q^*.

Therefore, a fall in the demand for a good (or a shift to the left in the demand curve) causes a *decrease* in the equilibrium price and a *decrease* in the equilibrium quantity.

3. A rise in supply

With a rise in supply, the supply curve shifts to the right. This is shown in Figure 2.8(c). With a change in the determinants of supply, suppose a decrease in the costs of production, this increases the quantity that producers wish to sell at every price. Therefore, the supply curve S_0 shifts to the right to, say, S_1. There is therefore a new equilibrium position brought about by the intersection of the new supply curve and the demand curve. This is position $p_3^*q_3^*$. The new equilibrium price, p_3^*, is less than p^*, and the new equilibrium quantity, q_3^*, is greater than q^*.

Therefore, a rise in the supply for a good (or a shift to the right in the supply curve) causes a *decrease* in the equilibrium price and an *increase* in the equilibrium quantity.

4. A fall in supply

With a fall in supply, the supply curve shifts to the left. This is shown in Figure 2.8(d). With a change in the determinants of supply, suppose an increase in the costs of production, this decreases the quantity that producers wish to sell at every price. Therefore, the supply curve S_0 shifts to the left to, say, S_2. There is therefore a new equilibrium position brought about by the intersection of the new supply curve and the demand curve. This is position $p_4^*q_4^*$. The new equilibrium price, p_4^*, is greater than p^*, and the new equilibrium quantity, q_4^*, is less than q^*.

Therefore, a fall in the supply of a good (or a shift to the left in the supply curve) causes an *increase* in the equilibrium price and a *decrease* in the equilibrium quantity.

The role of the market in the allocation of resources

In the market situation, consumers aim to maximise their utility and producers aim to maximise their profits. To achieve these goals, consumers and producers adjust the demand and supply of goods in response to signals produced by changing market conditions, influenced by the determinants of demand and supply. The price system responds to a need for change in the allocation of resources, say in a shift in income or tastes. Changing the relative prices signals the need for change to which consumers and producers respond.

Prices in the market therefore provide signals to both consumers and producers. Prices that are high relative to other prices provide an incentive to consumers to buy less of that product via income and substitution effects. On the supply side, high profits attract further resources into production from existing and new producers and thus encourage producers to supply more. Relatively low prices provide opposite incentives: consumers are inclined to buy more; sellers are inclined to produce less and move resources into more profitable undertakings. Therefore, prices of goods adjust, providing information and incentives to ensure that scarce resources are used to produce the goods and services that society demands.

In this chapter we have seen how the market may be used to allocate scarce resources among competing uses. Through the interaction of market forces, the market provides the means for society to solve the questions relating to the basic economic problem: what goods to produce, how to produce them and who to give them to.

1. What goods and services shall be produced?

Through the price system, the market decides which goods and how much of each good should be produced, by finding the price at which the quantity demanded equals the quantity supplied. The equilibrium quantity corresponding to this price defines how much of each good should be demanded and how much of each good should be supplied.

2. How shall these goods and services be produced?

The market also tells us who should produce the good: the good is supplied by those producers willing to supply at the equilibrium price.

3. Who will receive these goods and services?

The market also tells us for whom the goods are being produced: goods are purchased by those consumers who are willing and able to pay the equilibrium price.

Therefore, within the market framework, the goods which will be produced are for those that consumers are willing and able to spend their money on, and those that may be supplied profitably by producers.

Consumers are ultimately in a position to determine the appropriate price level at which supply will equal demand, since they have the knowledge and ability to switch their demands for goods from one producer to another. Consumers examine the costs and benefits of consuming different quantities of goods and make informed decisions, buying only those goods whose benefits are greater than their costs. This dominance of consumers' preferences is known as *consumer sovereignty*, and is a necessary condition for the market to allocate resources efficiently.

Therefore, the intuitive reason for using the market framework to address the issue of scarcity is that markets provide a means of allocating resources which is efficient. Aiming to maximise their utility, consumers will spend the amount of money which will maximise their well-being, resulting in allocative efficiency. At the same time, producers, seeking to maximise profits, will compete for custom by producing goods most highly valued by consumers at least cost, thus behaving in a technically efficient manner.

It might well be the case that society in general does not like the solution to the problem of scarcity that markets provide. For example, markets do not necessarily provide enough food to feed everyone who is hungry or enough health care to treat everyone who is ill. A market will provide only enough health care, for example, for those consumers who are willing and able to pay the equilibrium price. Society may wish to adopt the view that the less well off should be able to enjoy more food and more health care than the market solution provides them with, in which case the market solution may be found to be wanting. This and other possible shortcomings of the market solution are topics for discussion in the following chapters.

The discussion so far has concentrated on examining the demand and supply of all goods in general, and we have seen how, in theoretical terms, the price system may help to determine the optimal production and consumption of a good. In the following chapter an application of the market framework is provided, concentrating on the demand and supply of a specific good, namely, health care.

Suggested further reading

There are a great many economics textbooks available, any of which might be used for further reading on the basic workings of the market system. However, a possible starting point might be any one of the following:

Begg D., Fischer S. and Dornbusch R. (1994) *Economics*. Fourth edition. London: McGraw-Hill, pp. 32–46.
Lipsey R.G. and Chrystal K.A. (1995) *An introduction to positive economics*. Eighth edition. Oxford: Oxford University Press, pp. 62–77.
Parkin M. and King D. (1992) *Economics*. Wokingham: Addison-Wesley, pp. 62–87.

Each of these textbooks has scope for further reading if required.

3   The demand and supply of health care

In Chapter 3 we examine how the basic theory of economics may be applied to health care. An analysis of the supply and demand of health care is provided, and the discussion centres on whether the market framework will provide an efficient method for allocating scarce health care resources. Concentrating on the problems of imperfect knowledge and informational asymmetry, we analyse how conventional economic theory may be modified to accommodate the peculiarities of the health care market.

Summary

1. The problem of scarcity is exceptionally acute in the health care sector. The market framework provides a means of addressing this problem, though the conventional theories of demand and supply may be inadequate.

2. Whilst the assumption that consumers of health care are utility maximisers is plausible, the relationship between demand and price, income, the prices of other goods and tastes is not so straightforward.

3. Similarly, the supply of health care may not behave in the way that economic theory predicts. Whilst there are similarities between the quantity supplied of health care and the quantity supplied of other goods, the supply of health care clearly may not be classified in the same way.

4. The term market failure is used to cover all circumstances in which equilibrium in the market will not achieve an efficient allocation of resources.

5. Conditions required for the ideal market are: certainty; no externalities; perfect knowledge; consumers to act free of self-interested advice from health care providers; and several small suppliers to promote genuine competition. Unfortunately, in the health care market these conditions rarely exist. However, the market may still provide a useful tool for allocating health care resources.

6. The extent to which the conventional theories of economics should be modified will be largely dependent on the nature of health care.

7. The demand for health care is derived from the demand for health, and this in turn is linked to the idea that individuals demand health for both consumption and investment reasons.

8. The demand for a good or service is simply the expression of a need felt by the consumer, though the need for health care may be difficult to define owing to the existence of imperfect knowledge on the part of the consumer.

9. The term clinical iceberg is used to describe the fact that only a proportion of people requiring health care ever reach the medical services.

10. Illness behaviour is the study of the influence of different factors on an individual's perception of and reaction to ill health.

11. Once individuals decide to seek medical advice, asymmetry of information requires that an agency relationship develops between consumers of health care and health care providers, who make available their specialised knowledge of health and health care to the patient.

12. A perfect agent acts in such a way so as to maximise the utility of the consumer. An imperfect agent fails to maximise the utility of the consumer.

13. Imperfect agency might occur for two reasons: health care providers may not have the information required to act as a perfect agent; and the agent may exploit the ignorance of the consumer in order to maximise their own utility.

14. Supplier-induced demand is said to occur when the supplier, acting as an agent for the consumer, brings about a level of demand that is greater than the level that would have been chosen by the consumer had they been fully informed.

15. Conditions favouring demand inducement include: fee-for-service reimbursement; third party payment; limited peer review; infrequent purchase of health care; and the medico-judicial environment.

16. Evidence of a relationship between doctor/population ratios and health service utilisation rates per capita, and evidence of wide variations in health care utilisation between areas in the same country and between countries, suggest the existence of supplier-induced demand. However, ultimately it is extremely difficult to prove the existence of supplier-induced demand since we can never be sure that we have accounted for all the relevant variables.

Scarcity and health care

Because of scarce health care resources, it is often not possible to provide every individual with the full amount of health care which they would like. Because, for instance, there are not enough doctors, nurses, hospitals and hospital beds, it is necessary to make choices, for example, between different methods of treating an individual, or whether to treat one individual as opposed to another. Obviously these choices are not pleasant ones to have to make, and inevitably they will mean that people will suffer by not receiving the benefits of health care which they need. These choices often imply an explicit allocation of health care to one individual rather than to another, and people may be denied the treatment they require. Perhaps an individual denied treatment will even die because of the choice made. However, such choices *are* necessary because of the existence of scarcity, and they do occur all the time in clinical practice, though often only implicitly (for example, through the use of waiting lists).

The existence of scarcity in the health care sector therefore implies that some sort of choice is required in order that limited resources are used in the best possible way. In light of the problem of scarcity, a number of issues arise which correspond roughly with those presented in Chapter 2:

1. What health care interventions or treatments should be made available?
2. How should these treatments be provided?
3. Who should receive these treatments?

In the previous chapter we have seen that in a market situation, consumers and producers adjust the demand and supply of goods in response to signals produced by changing market conditions. Prices in the market therefore provide signals to both consumers and producers, and prices adjust to ensure that scarce resources are used to produce the goods and services that society demands. Under the ideal conditions discussed in Chapter 2, resources will be allocated efficiently.

A health care market thus provides a framework for obtaining a solution to these three questions:

1. What health care interventions or treatments should be available?

Through the price system, the health care market will decide which treatments should be made available, by finding the price for health care at which the quantity demanded equals the quantity supplied. The equilibrium quantity corresponding to this price defines how much of each treatment should be demanded and how much of each treatment should be supplied.

2. How should these treatments be provided?

A health care market also tells us who should provide different treatments, and the form of that provision: health care interventions will be supplied by those providers willing to supply at the equilibrium price.

3. Who should receive these treatments?

A health care market also tells us for whom the treatments are being provided: treatment is purchased by those individuals who are willing and able to pay the equilibrium price.

Therefore, within the framework of a health care market, the treatments which will be produced are those which individuals are willing and able to spend their money on, and those that may be supplied profitably by health care providers.

In its purest form, therefore, a health care market will provide only enough health care for those individuals who are willing and able to pay the equilibrium price. This feature of a health care market may well be deemed undesirable, and consequently, the introduction of a completely free market for health care may well be considered unacceptable.

We shall now examine the feasibility of using a market framework to allocate health care resources, and explore these issues in more detail.

Demand for and supply of health care

In the previous chapter we examined the use of some basic economic tools which may be used to address the problem of scarcity and to allocate limited resources. We have seen how the market can function and how the interaction of demand and supply can generate a market price which is used as a signal by consumers and producers to allocate resources. We shall now examine whether the basic economic theories of demand and supply may be applied to the provision of health care. For instance, are the determinants of the demand for goods such as clothing and food relevant as determinants of the demand for health care? Is it plausible to construct an upward-sloping supply curve for health care?

For the purposes of this analysis we will assume there are individuals who wish to demand health care, and these are called the consumers. There are also suppliers of health care, who are called providers. At this stage we do not wish to apply the market framework to a specific health care system or to a particular country.

Applying the theory of demand to health care

The demand for a particular good has been defined as the quantity that consumers are willing and able to buy in a specific time period. The theory of demand requires that consumers act in such a way so as to maximise their utility, and that there is an inverse relationship between price and quantity demanded. A number of determinants will affect the level of demand such as income, the prices of other goods, and tastes. In order to apply the theory of demand to health care, the plausibility of these assumptions should be addressed. More specifically we are interested in asking whether:

1. consumers of health care are utility maximisers;
2. the quantity of health care demanded is affected by price and, if so, whether there is an inverse relationship;

3. the quantity of health care demanded is affected by income;
4. the quantity of health care demanded is affected by the prices of other goods;
5. the quantity of health care demanded is affected by tastes and trends.

We will now address each of these issues in turn.

Are consumers of health care utility maximisers?

It has been suggested that health care is broadly bad in consumption, since its consumption usually involves some kind of disutility, resulting from the possible pain and anxiety associated with receiving treatment (McGuire *et al.*, 1988). Consequently, there are few people who normally would willingly consume health care purely for the utility they derive from its consumption. Health care will usually be demanded only if it is absolutely necessary. However, since people *do* demand health care, then presumably these consumers trade the short-term disutility derived from the receipt of health care against the long-term advantages of improved health. Therefore, health care may be treated as an investment where short-term costs or disutility may be overshadowed by long-term returns. In this sense, it may be argued that consumers of health care do act in such a way so as to maximise their overall level of utility.

Is there an inverse relationship between the price of health care and the quantity of health care demanded?

It has been argued previously that price is the most important factor in determining the level of demand for a good. Standard economic theory predicts that as the price of a good rises so the quantity of the good demanded will fall, and vice versa. Whilst this may be true for most goods and services, it seems rather odd to say that the demand for health care will behave in this way. The demand for health care is likely to be 'lumpy', particularly in the treatment of acute illnesses and conditions, where often only a single one-off intervention is required. To say that an individual will purchase more health care if it is cheaper will clearly be wrong in the majority of cases, since individuals will not be willing to consume health care that is unnecessary. To this extent, it could well be argued that within the constraint imposed by the income of the consumer, the demand for health care may well not be affected by price at all. Nevertheless, in order to examine the effects of changes in price on the quantity of health care demanded it is worthwhile to examine each of the two possible price changes separately.

1. A rise in the price of health care

To the extent that price acts as a constraint against the quantity of health care that a consumer is able to buy, then as the price of health care increases, so the quantity of health care demanded will decrease, since there will come a point when the consumer simply cannot afford to buy further treatment on a limited income. However, if the price rises, so long as it does not rise above this income level, the consumer may not necessarily buy less health care. If health care is considered an absolute necessity, the consumer may be prepared to buy treatment whatever its price: a consumer might well pay any price for the treatment of an urgent and life-threatening condition. For example, suppose the price of treatment for acute myocardial infarction increased from £1,500 to £2,000. Consumers requiring this treatment are unlikely to buy any less care following the price increase.

2. A fall in the price of health care

If the price of health care falls then we would not necessarily consume any more, since the consumption of health care may well involve disutility, and it would be frivolous and unnecessary to continue consumption beyond a certain point. It seems rather odd to say that we would demand more health care if it were cheaper. For instance, if the price of a hip replacement fell from £2,500 to £2,000 then, as individual consumers, we would not buy more hip replacements in the same way that we would buy more, say, chocolate bars.

Is the quantity of health care demanded affected by the level of income?

When income rises, the demand for most goods and services often increases and typically consumers will buy more of everything. The majority of goods are normal and exhibit this relationship. When income increases, the demand for some goods falls, and these are called inferior goods. Provided that income does not act as a constraint to the desired level of demand for health care, it is unlikely that an individual would purchase more or less health care if her income increased, and therefore the demand for health care would remain largely unaffected by income.

To what extent is the quantity of health care demanded affected by the prices of other goods?

The general health of an individual will be affected by a number of factors, of which health care is only one. These other factors include diet, level of exercise, living conditions and lifestyle. Therefore, there are other factors which may be improved to augment health. However, it is difficult to think of a good which will directly affect the demand for health care. We have seen previously that the relationship between two related goods may be one of either complementarity or substitutability. Whilst there are a number of goods or activities which improve health in addition to health care, it is difficult to imagine a complement for health care in the strict economic sense. Similarly, it is difficult to imagine anything which may be used as a substitute for health care.

Is the amount of health care demanded affected by tastes and trends?

The tastes and preferences of consumers are affected by convenience, custom and social attitudes. For example, a trend towards growing long hair will cause the demand for haircuts to fall. Emphasis in society on health and fitness will increase the demand for exercise equipment, more healthy foods and sports facilities, at the same time reducing the demand for unhealthy foods and cigarettes. These are examples of how tastes and trends may well affect the overall health of the population, and thus ultimately the demand for health care. However, to say that there might be a direct trend towards or away from health care which will affect the quantity demanded, in the same way that clothes might go out of fashion, is clearly inaccurate.

Therefore, whilst there may be some similarities between the demand for health care and the demand for other goods, the demand for health care may not be classified in the same way. The relationship between the demand for health care and the various determinants of demand is not as clear and straightforward as basic economic theory predicts.

Applying the theory of supply to health care

The theory of supply is concerned with the quantities of a good or service that producers wish to offer for sale per period of time. This theory requires that producers are profit maximisers, that there is a positive relationship between price and quantity supplied, and that supply will be affected by a number of determinants including the costs of production and the state of medical technology. For the theory of supply to be strictly applicable to health care, the plausibility of these assumptions and issues should be addressed. More specifically we are interested in asking whether:

1. health care providers are profit maximisers;
2. the quantity of health care supplied is affected by price and, if so, whether there is a positive relationship;
3. the costs of production have an impact on the supply of health care;
4. changes in technology affect the quantity of health care supplied;
5. the quantity of health care supplied is affected by the prices of other goods.

We will now address each of these issues in turn.

Are health care providers profit maximisers?

It is difficult to ascertain the goals of health care providers. In a world of unlimited resources, a purely benevolent health care provider would aim solely to maximise the welfare of patients, regardless of the costs incurred or the size of profits desired. However, we live in a world of scarcity. Whilst it is extremely difficult to ascertain the goals of health care providers, it would clearly be incorrect to argue that all health care providers aim solely to maximise their profits. It is more appropriate to argue that the goals of providing health care are centred much more on improving the health of patients. However, the profit and income of providers is clearly an important factor in determining the level of health care provision, since providing treatment to patients is not possible without incurring a cost. Whilst it may be argued that individual providers such as doctors and nurses do not aim solely to maximise their profits or income, the same may not necessarily be true of institutions such as hospitals which need to make money in order to employ doctors and nurses and provide health care services.

Is there a positive relationship between the price of health care and the quantity of health care supplied?

If the relationship between price and quantity supplied predicted by economic theory were applicable to the market for health care, then at low prices only the best providers would be able to make profits supplying health care. As prices rise, providers who could not previously compete will find that they can now make a profit in the market and will wish to provide health care. Also, previously existing providers may be able to expand output to levels which were not justified at the lower price.

It seems plausible to suggest that there is a positive relationship between the price and the quantity supplied of health care. However, it is worthwhile examining each possible price change separately.

1. A rise in the price of health care

An increase in price might well cause existing providers of health care to provide a greater quantity of services, since the revenue of providers will be increased and this may be used to increase supply. However, the upward-sloping supply curve is also partially explained by the fact that as prices increase, so more producers enter the market. Whilst this might be a plausible assumption in the market for some goods, it is not realistic in the market for health care, since the initial costs to providers on entering the market are high (for example, it is very expensive to build a new hospital).

2. A fall in the price of health care

As the price of health care falls, providers will supply less health care. This is because they will receive less money for the health care services which they provide. Therefore, they will be unable to maintain a constant level of provision. This might well cause providers of health care to leave the industry (for example, hospitals might close).

What impact do the costs of production have on the supply of health care?

Clearly the costs of provision are extremely important in determining the quantity of health care supplied. The provision of health care is not costless, and the costs of production will affect the level of supply. The extent of health care provision is limited by the size of the budget allocated to a provider for expenditure on treatment and care. This budget is not unlimited and will be fixed. Therefore, any change in the costs of supplying health care will affect the health care budget, which will in turn directly affect the quantity of health care supplied. For example, one obvious input into the health care production process is nursing labour. If the costs of nursing labour were to rise through an increase in wages, then because health care budgets are fixed, fewer nursing staff would be employed and so the supply of health care would decrease. Therefore, as costs increase, less health care is supplied. Conversely, if the costs of inputs into the production process were to fall then the quantity of health care supplied is likely to rise.

How do changes in technology affect the quantity of health care supplied?

An improvement in technology will enable producers to supply larger and better quantities of goods and services. Medical technology is continually changing and improving, with new therapies constantly being found for previously untreatable conditions, and existing treatments being substituted with improved ones. As medical technology improves, so the standard of health care rises and treatments become more effective in improving the quality and length of life of patients. Similarly, the shift to better medical technologies often enables more patients to be treated. For example, the introduction of minimally invasive surgery techniques in recent years has led to a decrease in the length of time patients are required to stay in hospital after treatment. Procedures such as hysteroscopies which previously required in-patient admission to hospital may now be provided on a day case or even an outpatient basis. This allows more patients to be treated since the number of cases is not constrained by limited inpatient bed availability. Therefore, as medical technology improves, so the quantity of health care supplied will increase.

To what extent is the quantity of health care supplied affected by the prices of other goods?

If the price of one good rises it becomes relatively more expensive to consumers wishing to buy that good. Therefore, producers will shift production into that good so they are able to make greater profits at the higher price. Hence, as the price of a good increases relative to another, there will be an increase in supply of the relatively more expensive good. Whilst this hypothesis is realistic for most goods, it is implausible when applied to the supply of health care. The initial costs incurred by a provider wishing to supply health care are likely to be extremely high. For instance, building a new hospital requires a great deal of initial capital. Furthermore, whilst buildings and people might be put to alternative uses, medical equipment may often only be used in the task for which it is designed. This implies that it would be difficult for health care providers to switch production to an alternative good or service which appears to be more lucrative. Nevertheless, health care is a diverse good which comes in many forms, and providers may switch production to other types of health care should the need arise. For example, a provider specialising in obstetric procedures may decide to concentrate more on gynaecological procedures should they appear more financially attractive. In this case, the supply of one component of health care might be affected by the price of another.

Is price important in health care?

In our analysis so far we have examined the application of demand and supply to health care. Whilst the usefulness of the theories of supply and demand is obvious in the provision of most goods, we have seen that health care may not behave in the same way that economic theory predicts. Most notably, the importance of the market price in determining the level of demand and supply is questionable.

We may use demand and supply curves to generate an equilibrium price which may be used to allocate scarce resources. Communication in the market framework is therefore made using the medium of prices. However, in the market for health care, prices seem to have less significance. On the demand side of the market, health care is consumed by patients only if it is necessary, and it results in short-term disutility and long-term benefits. If the price of health care rises or falls, consumers are unlikely either to increase or to decrease the quantity demanded. On the supply side, price is important since providers need to receive revenue for the services they produce since the provision of health care is not costless. However, other factors, such as the desire to improve the quality and length of life of patients, may be equally or more important in determining the level of health care provision than price.

It is therefore unlikely that the demand and supply of health care will behave in the way that basic economic theory requires for the formation of a perfect market. However, this is not to say that the market solution has nothing to contribute to the problem of scarce health care resources. The health care resource allocation problem

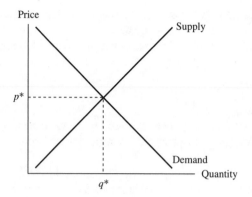

Figure 3.1 The market equilibrium.

may still be addressed using markets. Indeed, as we shall see in Chapter 7, the application of markets to the health care sector provides the basis for health care provision in the UK National Health Service. Therefore, it is worthwhile examining the application of the market solution to health care in greater detail.

Applying the market solution to health care

We have previously seen how the market can function and how the interaction of demand and supply can generate a market equilibrium, such as that presented in Figure 3.1 at p^*q^*.

Market signals in the form of prices and quantities ensure that the optimum solution of cleared markets is found. If this model is applied to health care it means that fully informed consumers weigh up the costs and benefits of health care relative to other goods, and they will spend on health care that amount of money that maximises their well-being. Health care providers, wishing to maximise profits, will compete for the custom of consumers and supply those types of health care most highly valued by consumers at least cost. Therefore the well-being of consumers is maximised at the least cost to society, resulting in an efficient allocation of scarce resources. Unfortunately, as we have already seen, owing to the nature of health care, markets may not function perfectly, resulting in market failure.

Market failure

In Chapter 2 we discussed how a freely competitive market could achieve efficiency in the allocation of resources. The term *market failure* is used to cover all circumstances in which equilibrium in the market will not achieve an efficient allocation.

It is worth considering the existence of market failure in the health care sector. Donaldson and Gerard (1993) address this exact issue and state that for a health care market to be desirable a number of conditions are required, namely:

1. certainty;
2. no externalities;
3. perfect knowledge;
4. consumers to act free of self-interested advice from health care providers;
5. several small suppliers to promote genuine competition.

We shall address each condition in turn and examine why these conditions are required in the market for health care. We shall then see whether these conditions are likely to be met in reality.

Certainty

The assumption of certainty requires that consumers know exactly what goods and services they wish to consume, that they know when they want to consume them, and how they can obtain them.

Certainty is required in a market since for a market solution to be feasible, consumers must know the quantity of health care they would like to demand. Similarly, producers need to know the quantity of health care to provide. Therefore, under conditions of certainty, the demand and supply of goods may be planned. Under conditions of uncertainty a market is unable to function properly since consumers and producers do not know how much of a good to demand and supply. There may be certainty in a number of markets for goods and services. For instance, in the market for chocolate bars, individuals know which items they would like to purchase. Also it is possible for individuals to predict when they would like to buy chocolate bars and how they can obtain them.

The assumption of certainty may also hold for certain aspects of health care. For example, pregnancies may be planned and it is possible to predict the timing of a birth and the cost of health care services. Therefore, consumers of maternity services will know how much health care to demand, and providers know how much health care to supply. Consequently, the use of maternity services may be planned. However, the consumption of the majority of health care items obviously cannot be planned in this way. This is because illness and deteriorations in health are often sudden and unexpected. Therefore, there is uncertainty in the market and the demand for health care cannot be predicted in advance. In certain situations, health care expenditure may be 'catastrophic' if individuals are unable to afford treatment for sudden and unexpected ill health. In this way the market fails as a means of allocating resources.

Whilst the uncertainty surrounding the demand for health care certainly implies that markets may not allocate health care resources efficiently, the market does not become redundant as a tool for resource allocation. The problem of uncertainty may be solved with the introduction of an insurance market. Insurance markets usually develop in the face of uncertainty, and generally entail the development of an insurance contract between insurance companies and individuals considered at risk. These insurance contracts usually operate in terms of an agreement by the insurance company to make a payout to the insured party in the event that a particular outcome occurs, in exchange for the payment of an insurance premium.

In the health care sector, the demand for health care is uncertain and individuals are unable to plan their demand for health care services, leaving them at risk from the unexpected nature of ill health and the possibility of incurring large catastrophic expenditures for treatment. Hence, health insurance markets are likely to develop to counter the financial burdens of the uncertain effects of ill health. The subject of health insurance and the various effects insurance has on the demand and supply for health care services will be discussed in greater detail in Chapter 5.

No externalities

Externalities are spillovers from other people's production or consumption of goods that affect an individual in either a positive or a negative way. An externality exists when the production or consumption of a good affects producers or consumers not directly involved with the good, and those spillover effects are not reflected in market prices. The costs and benefits of such spillovers cannot be accounted for in market transactions, since consumers and producers consider only the costs and benefits to themselves. Therefore, if externalities exist, an incorrect quantity of a good will be provided in a market, since the equilibrium price determined by the intersection of the supply and demand curves will not reflect all the costs and benefits to society. Rather, the demand and supply curves will be formed without accounting for the full value of marginal utility and marginal cost derived from consumption and production. For this reason, the condition of no externalities is required for a market to function perfectly.

The classic example of an externality is pollution. A factory producing chemicals might disperse the waste into the atmosphere, thus polluting the environment and adversely affecting the population of the surrounding area. These adverse effects represent costs to society and so should be reflected in the price of chemicals produced by the factory. However, these costs may not be incorporated into the market price, and therefore the market for chemicals will understate the marginal cost to society, and the factory will overprovide chemicals.

There are many manifestations of externalities in health care because one individual may often benefit from the consumption of health care by another. An obvious example is the decision to seek medical advice when suffering from a contagious disease. Individuals may weigh up the costs and benefits to themselves from receiving medical attention and decide against seeking help. However, by only including the costs and benefits to themselves, individuals have not included the greater costs to others, incurred by the spread of the disease. If a market does not account for the effects of these externalities then this may lead to the wrong level of health care being provided, since the equilibrium quantity defined by the market solution may not be the true quantity desired by society. Other examples of externalities in health care might be the decision by an individual not to receive a vaccination, or the decision not to use a condom in a random heterosexual encounter.

Perfect knowledge

Unless consumers and producers are well informed, they may take actions that are not in their best interests. Unless decisions are based on good information, markets will not work well as tools for allocating resources. In a situation of imperfect knowledge, consumers will not have the information to achieve their goal of utility maximisation, and producers will not have the information to achieve their goal of profit maximisation. Therefore, perfect knowledge in the market is necessary to achieve an efficient allocation of resources.

The assumption of perfect knowledge on the part of consumers means that they are aware of their health status and of all the options open to them to maintain or improve it. Although this may be the case with minor ailments, this is clearly not the case with the majority of illnesses. Therefore, the market for health care is characterised by imperfect knowledge. Unfortunately, perfect knowledge is especially important in the market for health care since making the wrong decision may have much more serious consequences than the decision of whether or not to, say, consume a chocolate bar.

The majority of individuals clearly have very little or no knowledge regarding health status and health care. However, this does not necessarily undermine the usefulness of markets because individuals are able to seek the help of a suitably qualified and knowledgeable individual whose job is to provide expert advice on health and health care: health care providers are (it is hoped) available to provide the information which individuals need in order to formulate health care consumption decisions.

Consumers act free of self-interested advice from health care providers

In the market for health care, consumers, aiming to maximise their utility, will spend the amount of money which will maximise their well-being. At the same time, providers, seeking to maximise profits, will compete for custom by producing goods most highly valued by consumers at least cost, thus behaving in a technically efficient manner. However, if imperfect knowledge exists in the market on the part of consumers, then providers may be able to manipulate the demand for goods and services by consumers to meet their own goal of profit maximisation. This may lead to the wrong level of health care provision in the market.

Due to the lack of perfect knowledge in health care, health care providers find themselves placed in the position of offering expert advice to consumers about health care. However, it is these very health care providers who also supply health care and who receive revenue from the services they provide. Therefore, the supplier of health care is in a position to substantially influence the demand for health care, and thus for their own services, which may in turn affect their income. Consumers of health care may be unable to act free of self-interested advice from health care providers, and the market may fail to provide an efficient level of health care. Issues surrounding the existence and consequences of this problem are discussed in greater detail later in this chapter.

Several small suppliers to promote genuine competition

The use of markets as a means of allocating scarce resources depends upon there being competition between suppliers. This, coupled with the assumptions of self-interest in the form of utility and profit maximisation on the part of consumers and producers, leads to an optimum allocation of resources. The market will not function properly if there is not free competition.

In a perfect market, producers are small and numerous so that they do not have any market power and they are unable to influence the price of the good. Producers compete only on the basis of price. Therefore, in order to attract customers, producers have an incentive to keep prices as low as possible. This results in an optimal allocation of resources because producers will provide high-quality goods and services as cheaply as possible.

A monopoly exists when there is only one producer of a good or service. A monopoly producer is able to influence the price of that good, thus allowing the monopoly considerable opportunity to exploit its position and to discriminate in such a way so as to make large amounts of profit at the expense of the consumer. In this situation, the market will fail to allocate resources efficiently since the costs of producing any given output will not be minimised and the benefits of that output will not be maximised.

Geographical and occupational monopolies exist in health care. Geographical monopolies exist because it is usual for there to be only a single provider of health care in any one geographical area. Occupational monopolies exist because some health care providers specialise in providing certain medical services in which they have developed expertise (one example of this might be a hospital which specialises in treating sick children). Therefore, monopolies do exist in health care, and providers are able to influence the market price so that the allocation of resources may not be efficient.

Are markets useful in the allocation of health care resources?

We have seen how markets for health care would work under idealised conditions. Unfortunately, in reality these conditions rarely exist. This is not to say that markets are of no use in the allocation of health care resources. Whilst perfect markets may not exist, the basic market structure may be modified to allow for imperfections. For instance, market imperfections may well warrant some form of government inter-vention in which the market is not left to its own devices but where action by governments seeks to reduce the impact of market failure and to achieve an efficient allocation of resources.

Therefore, two main issues arise from the failure of health care markets to allocate resources optimally:

1. If the basic economic theories of demand, supply and markets cannot be directly applied to health care, how may they be modified to allow for the peculiarities of this good?
2. What should be done in reaction to the imperfections in the health care market?

The first question is the discussed in the remainder of this chapter. The second is addressed in following chapters.

The nature of health care

The discussion so far suggests that the application of the conventional theories of demand and supply to health care may well be questionable. Health care markets are often characterised by uncertainty, externalities, imperfect knowledge, exploitation by health care providers and monopoly power, which have a detrimental effect on the application of market forces to the health care sector. The existence of market failure will influence the ability of the demand and supply of health care to function as basic economic theory predicts.

However, the market is still useful and relevant as a tool for allocating health care resources, though the traditional market framework requires some modification. The extent of the modification required is dependent upon the nature of health care, which is therefore worth examining in more detail.

The household production function

Central to any economic analysis of health care is a clear distinction between health (as an output of health care) and health care (as one of the many inputs used to produce health). Of key importance to the demand for health is the household production function.

It has been suggested that the way in which we view health should be as a durable capital asset which is a basic fundamental good, underpinning the consumption of many other goods (Grossman, 1972). The relationship between health and health care may be defined using the household production function, where individuals combine marketed goods and non-marketed goods together with time to produce health stock,

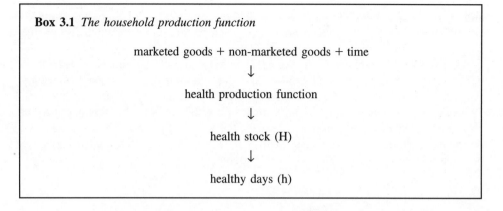

Box 3.1 *The household production function*

marketed goods + non-marketed goods + time

↓

health production function

↓

health stock (H)

↓

healthy days (h)

H, which is transformed into healthy days, h (see Box 3.1). Marketed goods include items such as food and clothing, and non-marketed goods include items such as health care and environmental and social factors.

Since health care is one input into the production function which produces health, the demand for health care is said to be a derived demand.

Derived demand

Using the principles of the household production function, a major feature of the demand for health care is that the basic demand by the consumer is for health and not health care directly. In other words, the demand for health care is a *derived demand*: the demand for health care is derived from the demand for health. Because the consumption of health care usually involves some kind of disutility, we do not demand health care for its own sake, but because we want to be healthy.

It has also been argued that the demand for health is also a derived demand (Grossman, 1972). Grossman argues that individuals demand health (and therefore health care) for two reasons: consumption benefits and investment benefits.

1. Consumption benefits

These are derived from the things that we can do when we are healthy (for example, taking a walk in the park, or eating a cake).

2. Investment benefits

These are derived from the income that can be produced when health is combined with time. Therefore, by being healthy, an individual decreases the time that they will have to spend off work through ill health.

There is therefore both an investment and a consumption motive for demanding health, and so also for demanding health care.

In summary, the demand for health care is linked to the demand for health, and this in turn is linked to the idea that individuals demand health for both consumption and investment reasons. Consequently, the demand for health care is extremely complicated. These complexities are exacerbated by the lack of knowledge on the part of the consumer.

As discussed in Chapter 2, in the ideal market situation, resource allocation is dominated by consumers' preferences, and the situation of consumer sovereignty prevails. It is thus assumed that consumers are the best judge of their own interests. This assumption does not hold in the context of health care because there is imperfect knowledge on the part of patients. Therefore, the ability of patients to make their own decisions is impaired. More specifically, health care providers are placed in a position to determine the *needs* of their patients.

Need

The demand for a good or service is simply the expression of a need felt by the consumer. Therefore, every demand is a declaration of need by someone for something. Consumers exercise their sovereignty by making explicit demands for goods and services on the basis of their needs. In the health care sector, it is important to make the distinction between demand and need since the existence of imperfect knowledge implies that consumers are unable to act according to their needs, in which case there may be *unmet* need.

Therefore, the level of need for health care required is difficult for the consumer to ascertain. An individual's need for health care will therefore normally depend upon identification of that need by a clinical examination carried out by a health care provider. However, if an individual is unsure if they are ill, then they may not know to go and seek medical advice in the first place.

Various studies have shown that the number of individuals presenting themselves for treatment may be far less than the number estimated to have treatable illnesses. This therefore leads us to two important issues: the so-called 'clinical iceberg' and the factors affecting illness behaviour.

The clinical iceberg

It is often assumed that all those in need of health care will visit a health care provider in order to receive medical attention. It is not often questioned whether individuals know whether they need medical care in the first place. The process of becoming ill is often thought to be a clear-cut situation, since the majority of people perceive that they are healthy, and a minority are equally aware that they are ill because they are able to perceive their symptoms and appreciate their significance.

During the 1950s, community surveys began to discover unreported levels of illness in the general population. The term *clinical iceberg* was used to describe this phenomenon because it was thought that only a small proportion of the population (the tip of the iceberg) actually reach the health care services.

Wadsworth *et al.* (1971) examine a sample of 2,153 people from the London boroughs of Bermondsey and Southwark. During a 14-day period, only 5 per cent

Box 3.2 *The 14-day incidence of symptoms and subsequent illness behaviour of 2,153 randomly selected individuals in two London boroughs* (source: *Adapted from Wadsworth, Butterfield and Blaney, 1971*).

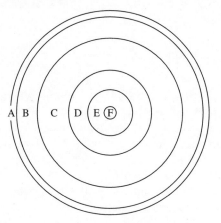

A.   105 individuals (4.9%) with no symptoms
B.   405 individuals (18.8%) with symptoms taking no action
C.   1211 individuals (56.2%) with symptoms taking non-health service action
D.   361 GP patients (16.8%)
E.   61 outpatients (2.8%)
F.   10 inpatients (0.5%)

reported no health problems. Self-medication was resorted to by approximately 60 per cent of the sample (see Box 3.2).

One explanation of the clinical iceberg could be that only serious complaints are taken to the general practitioner (GP). However, numerous studies have indicated that serious and treatable illnesses do go unreported. For example, Williamson *et al.* (1964) examined the elderly patients of one GP practice: 25 per cent of respondents with chronic bronchitis and 33 per cent of respondents with heart disease had not contacted their GP. The clinical iceberg is a notoriously common phenomenon for mentally ill individuals. For example, a survey of a sample of elderly patients attending GP surgeries found that nearly one third were depressed (MacDonald, 1986). Despite this high prevalence, only 10 per cent of sufferers were receiving treatment.

The problem of the clinical iceberg has obvious ramifications for the allocation of health care resources. Individuals demand goods and services on the basis of their needs. However, in the context of health care individuals may not know what their needs are and so they go to see a health care provider who makes available their specialised knowledge to advise patients what health care to demand. Unfortunately, individuals may not know to go and seek medical advice in the first place. Such individuals do not communicate their needs and so will not be able to demand health care at all. The provision of health care in the market will then not reflect the needs of the consumers.

The decision to seek medical advice is therefore important in the allocation of resources. This leads us to examine the factors which do influence the decision by an individual to seek health care.

Illness behaviour

The study of illness behaviour is the study of the influence of different factors on an individual's perception of and reaction to ill health. Whilst more of a sociological issue than an economic one, illness behaviour has obvious repercussions for the allocation of health care resources and the utilisation of medical services. It therefore warrants further discussion here.

Mechanic (1968) describes illness behaviour as 'the way in which symptoms are perceived, evaluated, and acted upon by a person who recognizes some pain, discomfort, or other signs of organic malfunction'.

Factors affecting illness behaviour

There are many factors which affect the way individuals react to perceived symptoms of ill health. Mechanic lists ten key variables associated with seeking medical advice (see Box 3.3). Each of these factors will, to a greater or lesser extent, determine whether an individual will initiate a visit to see a health care provider.

Even if we assume that an individual does seek medical advice, other problems arise from the existence of imperfect knowledge. Owing to patients' ignorance of health and health care, an individual's demand for health care will normally depend upon identification of need by a clinical examination carried out by a health care provider. We have discussed the factors influencing whether the individual will initiate an examination, but equally important is what actually happens in the clinical

---

Box 3.3 *Factors associated with seeking medical advice.*

1. the visibility and recognisability of symptoms;
2. the extent to which the symptoms are perceived as serious;
3. the extent to which symptoms disrupt family, work and other social activities;
4. the frequency and persistence of the appearance of symptoms;
5. the tolerance threshold of those who are exposed to and evaluate symptoms;
6. available information, knowledge and cultural assumptions to the evaluater;
7. the needs competing with illness responses;
8. the possible competing interpretations that can be assigned to the symptoms once they are recognised;
9. the availability of treatment resources;
10. the monetary costs of taking action.

setting. In this situation, imperfect knowledge on the part of patients is offset by the specialised knowledge of health care providers. However, whilst the availability of such specialised knowledge may potentially alleviate the problem of ignorance associated with the general population, the unique position in which health care providers then find themselves may lead to alternative problems arising from the existence of asymmetry of information.

Asymmetry of information

One feature of the health care market is imperfect knowledge, characterised by the fact that generally consumers have little or no knowledge regarding health and health care. Whilst this potentially weakens the power of the market as a tool for resource allocation, this problem is overcome by the existence of health care providers who make available their specialised knowledge to consumers so that they might demand health care in such a way so as to maximise their utility. The existence of the medical and nursing professions can be partially explained by imperfect knowledge on the part of consumers.

Imperfect knowledge is therefore not, in itself, a problem. However, complications arise in health care markets not through lack of information but through *asymmetry* of information.

Asymmetry of information arises because the suppliers of health care, including doctors and nurses, know more about health and health care than the consumers of health care, the patients. Generally, potential consumers of health care are in a poor position to judge if they are ill. Furthermore, they usually have no idea about what action to take even if they are ill. If they do know what action to take they still do not know whether or not it has been successful. On the other hand, health care providers (it is hoped) know the answers to all these questions. There is therefore asymmetry of information since the suppliers of health care are better informed than the consumers of health care.

Patients often acquire some limited knowledge of health and health care through use of medical services. However, detailed knowledge about health status and health care from experience is limited by the infrequency of health care consumption, and the huge range of illnesses to which we are prone. Also, information on health and health care is costly to acquire, since it is very difficult, time-consuming and expensive to become, for example, a nurse.

Therefore, it is difficult to acquire medical and nursing knowledge, and because it is hard for the consumers of health care to judge the quality of health status and health care, consumers and producers in the health care market usually initiate what is called an *agency relationship*.

The agency relationship

One way in which demand and need may be reconciled is through the agency relationship in which health care providers act as agents for ill-informed consumers.

The specialised medical knowledge of providers is made available to patients, and they therefore act as agents for the patient.

The different types of information that a patient lacks and therefore requires will usually fall into one of three categories:

1. information about health status;
2. information about available treatments;
3. information about the effectiveness of treatment.

The relationship between health care providers and patients works in the same way that there is an agency relationship between a consumer and a car mechanic: because the majority of individuals know nothing about the functioning of a car, we ask the mechanic to act on our behalf, and thus an agency relationship develops.

Concerns regarding imperfect knowledge in the market for health care may be partly dispelled through the introduction of agency. However, the relationship between health care providers and their patients will not necessarily be ideal. An agent may act perfectly or imperfectly, as follows:

1. a perfect agent acts in such a way so as to maximise the utility of the consumer;
2. an imperfect agent fails to maximise the utility of the consumer.

In the market for health care, imperfect agency might occur for two reasons:

1. health care providers may not have the information required to act as a perfect agent;
2. health care providers may exploit the ignorance of consumers in order to maximise their own utility.

We shall examine each of these problems in turn.

Health care providers may not have the information required to act as a perfect agent

For the agency relationship to operate efficiently, Mooney (1992) argues that three sets of information are required:

1. medical knowledge;
2. knowledge of the patient's circumstances;
3. knowledge of the patient's individual preferences.

Therefore, assuming health care providers are suitably qualified, one of the difficulties in developing a perfect agency relationship is that this is likely to vary according to the individual patient. For instance, each patient will place a different amount of utility on receiving information and delegating treatment decisions to health care providers. Furthermore, for each patient this level of utility will vary according to the individual health care provider and the particular health condition involved.

In this regard, then, the perfect agency relationship is clearly difficult to obtain. The task of the health care provider is to aid the utility-maximising behaviour of the consumer. This requires full knowledge of the patient's relevant tastes, preferences and income.

Health care providers may exploit the ignorance of consumers in order to maximise their own utility

An alternative method by which an imperfect agency relationship may develop is when the agent exploits the ignorance of the consumer in order to maximise their own utility.

An example of an imperfect agency relationship is supplier-induced demand, in which patients are encouraged to consume health care that is of little or no benefit on the recommendation of health care providers, who then receive a fee. If such health care is of little or no value to patients then supplier-induced demand constitutes an inefficient use of resources, since these resources could be used elsewhere in the health care sector.

Supplier-induced demand

Supplier-induced demand is said to occur when the supplier, acting as an agent for the consumer, brings about a level of demand that is greater than the level that would have been chosen by the consumer had they been fully informed. Supplier-induced demand is therefore the amount of demand which exists beyond what would have occurred in a market where consumers have perfect knowledge. If consumers are fully informed, the demand for health care would be less.

The existence of supplier-induced demand may be interpreted as a demonstration of exploitation by the health care sector. It is a display of monopoly power; health care providers have a monopoly in information about health and health care, and supplier-induced demand is one situation where this monopoly power is used to its fullest potential in order to maximise the utility of health care providers rather than patients.

Supplier-induced demand has been linked to the hypothesis that health care providers aim to maximise their income. This is characterised by the observation that an individual's consumption of health care tends to rise with increases in the doctor/ population ratio. Using standard demand and supply analysis, this phenomenon is demonstrated by a shift in the demand curve, induced by supply conditions. For example, the effect of an increase in the supply of health care providers is a shift in the supply curve to the right. If supplier-induced demand occurs, then as the supply curve shifts, demand increases, and so the demand curve will also shift to the right.

Price of health care p

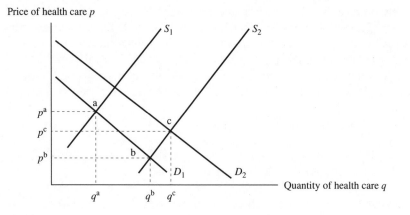

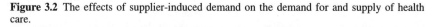

Figure 3.2 The effects of supplier-induced demand on the demand for and supply of health care.

Therefore, the major implication of supplier-induced demand is that demand and supply are no longer independent.

For example, suppose the supply of health care providers does increase. In Figure 3.2 this is shown by an rightward shift in the supply curve from S_1 to S_2. Thus the equilibrium position now shifts from a to b, from $p^a q^a$ to $p^b q^b$. If there were demand inducement, then as supply increases, so too would demand increase, from D1 to D2. Therefore, a new equilibrium would be reached at c, defined by $p^c q^c$.

Conditions favouring demand inducement

The health care sector will not wish to or have the opportunity to induce the demand for health care in every situation. For suppliers to be able to induce demand, a number of conditions may be present. These include the following:

1. fee-for-service reimbursement;
2. third party payment;
3. limited peer review;
4. infrequent purchase of health care;
5. medico-judicial environment.

We shall now briefly discuss each of these in turn.

Fee-for-service reimbursement

There are three basic methods by which any health care provider can be paid: by salary; by capitation; and by fee for service (see Chapter 6 for a detailed discussion of each). If health care providers are paid on a fee-for-service basis then they receive payment for each individual item of service provided. The greater the number of items provided, the greater the income of the provider. Remuneration on this basis will provide an opportunity and a financial incentive to induce demand and thus increase income.

Third party payment

In the basic market scenario, only two parties are involved: buyers and sellers. As we have previously discussed, owing to uncertainty in the health care market and the possibility for patients encountering catastrophic health care expenditure, it is usual for some form of insurance system to develop. Therefore, a third party is introduced into the market such as a government or private insurance firm, which is responsible for financing health care in return for an insurance premium. However, if a third party payer is financing the provision of health care rather than the patient, then health care providers will have few incentives to moderate the amount of health care that they supply.

Limited peer review

In an effort to maintain high clinical standards and good practice, health care providers may wish to subject themselves to peer review. Giving health care providers information regarding their own practice and the practice of others will encourage the provision of high-quality medical care. If there is limited peer review then the actions and decisions made by the health care providers are not open to scrutiny and so there is more opportunity to induce demand.

Infrequent purchase of health care

Patients may acquire some limited knowledge of health and health care through use of medical services. However, detailed knowledge about health status and health care from experience is limited by the infrequency of health care consumption. If consumers do not often consult a health care provider about a particular condition then they will have little knowledge of the medical matters involved, in which case they are more open to exploitation.

Medico-judicial environment

The medico-judicial environment will be an important factor in the utilisation of health care services. If there is a strong possibility that a health care provider will be sued if they make an incorrect decision which may cause them to lose income, then there may be an incentive to induce demand for unnecessary services so that all clinical possibilities are entertained and there is less chance of making a mistake. This offers a reason for health care providers to bring about a level of demand that is greater than the level that would have been chosen by the consumer had they been fully informed.

We have discussed the theory of supplier-induced demand, and examined the conditions under which it may exist. We shall now examine some of the empirical evidence for the existence of supplier-induced demand.

Evidence of demand inducement

Evidence of supplier-induced demand is of two basic types:

1. evidence of a relationship between doctor/population ratios and health service utilisation rates per capita;
2. evidence of wide variations in utilisation between areas in the same country and between countries.

We shall examine each of these in turn, paying specific attention to the type of evidence collected. For a more thorough and complete review of empirical findings on the existence of supplier-induced demand see Donaldson and Gerard (1993).

Evidence of a relationship between doctor/population ratios and health service utilisation rates per capita

The demand for health care may be characterised by the utilisation of medical services. The existence of supplier-induced demand may be linked to the observation that per capita consumption (that is, consumption per person) of the services that health care providers provide tends to rise roughly in line with increases in the doctor to population ratio. This means that as the number of health care providers increases, so the amount of health care demanded by consumers also increases. If supplier-induced demand did not exist then this should not be the case, since the number of ill individuals seeking medical care should not depend on the number of health care providers: just because there are more health care providers this does not mean that there are more ill people.

Therefore as the concentration of health care providers in a given population or geographical area increases we would expect the quantity of health care demanded to remain constant. If utilisation of medical services were to increase, this would be consistent with the notion of supplier-induced demand.

If the number of health care providers in any one area increases then each health care provider will presumably see fewer patients. If these health care providers receive payment for each item of service they provide then, because they are caring for fewer patients, they will receive less income. To raise their income to the desired level, each health care provider could induce their patients to demand more health care. So, in response to an increase in the supply and in order to maintain their income, health care providers may encourage patients to use more services.

Cromwell and Mitchell (1986) examine physician-induced demand for various surgical procedures in the US. They conducted an analysis of supplier-induced demand covering the time period 1969 to 1976. The quantity of health care services consumed over time in certain geographical areas in the US was compared with the number of physicians. Specifically, they counted the number of surgeons per 1,000 individuals in the population. The results provided by Cromwell and Mitchell show statistically significant demand inducement for surgical procedures: overall rates of surgery increase by about 0.08 per cent for each 1 per cent increase in surgeon supply.

Evidence of wide variation in health care utilisation rates between areas in the same country and between countries

Generally we would expect health care utilisation rates to be similar between areas in the same country. We would also generally expect health care utilisation rates between developed countries to be broadly similar. If utilisation rates are different then this may indicate the existence of supplier-induced demand, since relatively high utilisation rates in some areas may be explained by health care providers inducing patients to demand more health care.

For this form of evidence to be reliable we must allow for any other differences in the nature of health care and its provision between geographical areas which might explain differences in utilisation rates.

McPherson (1990) provides evidence on health care utilisation rates between areas in the state of Maine in the US from 1980 to 1982. The demand for health care, characterised by health care utilisation rates, is defined by hospital rates of admission for various medical procedures. There was a significant variation in the utilisation rates of particular hospitals for a number of medical procedures. For instance, there was a greater than 8.5-fold variation between hospitals in the number of admissions for tonsillectomies, treatment of hypertension, treatment of atherosclerosis, and transurethral operations (that is, the hospital with the highest admission rates for patients requiring a tonsillectomy had 850 per cent more admissions than the hospital with the lowest). In such a relatively geographically small area we would not expect there to be such a vast variation in the demand for health care. One explanation for this difference could be supplier-induced demand.

Information is also available on health care utilisation rates between countries (see Table 3.1). For instance, McPherson (1990) found that in 1980, the number of admissions in Japan for coronary artery bypass grafts (CABGs) was 1 per 1,000 individuals in the population. In the US at the same time the number of admissions for the same procedure was 61 per 1,000 individuals in the population.

Therefore, on the basis of initial evidence from doctor/population ratios and from geographical variations in health care utilisation rates, there may well be cause to

Table 3.1 Number of admissions per 1,000 individuals in the population for various medical procedures in 1980.

Country	Tonsillectomy	CABG	Cholecystectomy	Inguinal hernia repair	Hysterectomy	Operation on lens	Appendectomy
Australia	115	32	145	202	405	101	340
Canada	89	26	219	224	479	139	143
Ireland	256	4	91	100	123	64	245
Japan	61	1	2	67	90	35	244
Netherlands	421	5	131	175	381	68	149
New Zealand	102	2	99	211	431	95	169
UK	26	6	78	154	250	98	131
US	205	61	203	238	557	294	130

Source: Adapted from McPherson (1990).

argue that supplier-induced demand is a very real problem in the market for health care. However, considerable caution must be exercised in analysing the results of this empirical research. Most notably, difficulties arise since there may be other possible explanations of the data, that is, there may be omitted variables.

Omitted variables

The problem with all studies which form the basis of any judgement on the existence of supplier-induced demand is that other relevant factors or variables may have been omitted from the analysis. These omitted variables may explain why hospital admission rates increase as the doctor/population ratio increases and why there are such large geographical variations in admission rates for certain medical procedures. In other words, there are explanations other than supplier-induced demand which may be used to explain the observed differences in utilisation rates. Possible alternative explanatory factors are as follows:

1. size of the population;
2. health status of the population;
3. artefactual errors;
4. method of hospital admission;
5. costs to patients of consumption;
6. supply and availability of resources and unmet need;
7. clinical uncertainty.

Size of the population

When comparing geographical variations in the quantity of health care demanded, it is important to allow for differences in the size of the populations under considera- tion. For example, when comparing the admission rates for tonsillectomies between the Netherlands and the US we would expect the overall number of admissions to be much higher in the US since the population is much larger. Therefore, figures should be standardised so that a uniform population size is compared. In Table 3.1 the number of admissions are standardised and presented *per 1,000 individuals in the population.*

Health status of the population

The overall level of health in the population will obviously be extremely important in determining the demand for health care. Variations in utilisation rates, rather than providing evidence for supplier-induced demand, may in fact simply be displaying differences in underlying levels of morbidity. If there is a difference in the level of health care between two geographical areas then hospital admission rates are likely to differ. Thus, the large difference in admissions between the UK and the US for cholecystectomies presented in Table 3.1 may simply be due to the fact that there are more ill people requiring this procedure in the US.

Artefactual errors

Other causes of variation may be artefactual: mistakes may have been made in the calculation of the various statistics that are compared, or there may be incomplete recording in some geographical areas by, for instance, failing to account for individuals receiving treatment in private or religious health care facilities. Furthermore, institutions may have alternative methods for recording the demand for services. In other words, care must be exercised when comparing figures to ensure that like is being compared with like.

Method of hospital admission

Another important consideration is the way in which patients are admitted to hospital. In a referral-based system, all decisions to admit patients into hospital are the outcome of several screening processes. This is the case in the UK National Health Service (NHS), where patients first have to decide to obtain advice from their GP who in turn has to decide to refer them to hospital. In the US individuals may often refer themselves directly to hospital and this is likely to result in higher utilisation rates.

Costs to patients of consumption

Whilst there is a cost to the health service for each individual patient treated, patients and their families also incur costs when receiving health care. These costs include costs from time spent travelling to and from the health care provider, and loss of earnings incurred from taking time off work. In some cases these costs may be considerable and may affect the decision of an individual to seek medical advice initially. If the number of health care providers in any one geographical area is high, then this will be associated with lower costs of consumption to the patient resulting from reduced waiting and travel time, reduced financial costs of travelling and reduced loss of earnings from time off work. In this case, utilisation of health care services will be higher even without supplier-induced demand.

Supply and availability of resources and unmet need

The size and availability of health care resources will affect the use of health care services. In those areas with high levels of expenditure on health care per person, utilisation rates will generally be higher anyway. Conversely, in those areas where practically nothing is spent on health care, utilisation rates will obviously be low. Therefore, increases in hospital admissions associated with increases in the doctor/population ratio may be explained by the existence of unmet need subsequently being met by the increase in the availability of health care resources.

For example, it would clearly be wrong to examine differences in health care utilisation rates between a developed country and a developing country and conclude that such differences were caused by supplier-induced demand. Rather, these differences are more likely to be caused by the lack of health care resources in the developing country.

Clinical uncertainty

There may be clinical uncertainty regarding the appropriate treatment for a particular diagnosis. If there is a link between clinical certainty and a low variation in utilisation, this implies that clinical uncertainty might be the cause of the variation. If there is no one procedure wholly accepted to be correct for a particular illness, then clinical uncertainty could explain any differences in demand: if health care providers are unsure of the correct treatment for a specific illness then there will be variation in admission rates between geographical areas.

It is difficult to prove the existence of supplier-induced demand since we can never be sure of the extent to which we have accounted for all the relevant influencing variables. This discussion has presented only a few, and there are likely to be many others which should also be accounted for. The general conclusion of this discussion must therefore be that, whilst there is some supporting evidence, it is possible to dispute the existence of supplier-induced demand. Nevertheless, there is a limited body of evidence which indicates that providers in the health care market in the UK National Health Service do exploit the asymmetry of information between themselves and consumers.

Evidence of supplier-induced demand in the NHS

In the NHS, a mechanism has been devised to allow for flexibility of referral by general practitioners and to allow for patients needing treatment when they are away from home. These extra-contractual referrals, whilst unpredictable in terms of their quantity and their cost, are income-generating for the health care provider, since non-local patients are financed on a fee-for-service basis using a cost-per-case contract. Therefore, the greater the number of patients treated as extra-contractual referrals, the greater the additional income for the provider.

Ghodse and Rawaf (1991) examined all extra-contractual referrals received by Merton and Sutton Health Authority in London from 1 April to 30 June in 1991, and raised concerns that it is not possible to establish whether emergency extra-contractual referral admissions to hospital are necessary or whether they could be dealt with equally effectively in Accident and Emergency departments (in which case the provider will not receive any additional income).

An indication as to whether these concerns are realistic is provided by an anonymous Director of Purchasing of an NHS Trust, who reports on a number of allegedly common practices (Anonymous, 1992). In an effort to maximise their income, health care providers are reported to:

1. ensure that patients are always recorded as having a non-local address, since more income will be generated as non-local patients are financed as extra-contractual referrals;
2. deliver patients deliberately to the wrong hospital ward, so that the health care purchaser (the third party payer of health care) can be charged for two separate admissions for the patient, one for admission to the 'wrong' ward and another for readmission to the 'right' ward;
3. discharge patients before the conclusion of treatment in order to save on expenditure;
4. discretely plan readmissions, so that the health care purchaser may then be charged for two admissions.

This evidence suggests that exploitation by health care providers does occur.

Conclusion

This chapter has considered how the conventional analyses of demand and supply may be applied to health care, and to what extent the basic theories may require modification. The basic assumptions of economic theory may have to be modified in order to cope with the peculiarities of the health care market. Specifically, the demand and supply of health care may not behave in the way that theory predicts and that is normal for most other goods. Furthermore, health care markets may fail as an efficient method of allocating health care resources since the conditions required for an efficient market solution do not hold.

Particular importance has been placed on the assumption of perfect knowledge and it has been emphasised how the demand for health care is heavily influenced by the suppliers of health care since there is asymmetry of information in the health care market. It is normal for an agency relationship to develop between patients and health care providers in which the specialised knowledge of health care providers is made available. Unfortunately, owing to the financial incentives provided by this informational asymmetry, health care providers are in a position to exploit their knowledge of health status and health care. Whilst evidence proving the existence of supplier-induced demand may always be refuted owing to the problem of omitted variables, what limited evidence there is suggests that demand inducement should be a source of some concern in the NHS.

Now that we have seen the extent to which imperfections exist in the health care market, our discussion will continue to examine what should be done in reaction to these imperfections. Of particular importance are the structure of health care finance and whether the health care market will provide a fair allocation of resources. It is to this second topic which we shall now turn.

References

Anonymous (1992) Gain without pain. *Health Services Journal* 30 January: 25.
Cromwell J. and Mitchell B. (1986) Physician-induced demand for surgery. *Journal of Health Economics* 5: 293–313.
Donaldson C. and Gerard K. (1993) *Economics of health care financing: the visible hand.* Basingstoke: Macmillan.
Ghodse B. and Rawaf S. (1991) Extra-contractual referrals in first three months of NHS Reforms. *British Medical Journal* 303: 497–9.
Grossman M. (1972) *The demand for health: a theoretical and empirical investigation.* New York: Bureau of Economic Research.
MacDonald A.J. (1986) Do general practitioners miss depression in elderly patients? *British Medical Journal* 292: 1365–7.
McGuire A.J., Henderson J. and Mooney G. (1988) *The economics of health care.* London: Routledge.
McPherson K. (1990) International differences in medical practices. In: *Health care systems in transition.* Paris: OECD.
Mechanic D. (1968) *Medical sociology: a selective view.* New York: Free Press, pp. 115–57.
Mooney G. (1992) *Economics, medicine and health care.* Hemel Hempstead: Harvester Wheatsheaf.
Wadsworth M.E., Butterfield W.J. and Blaney R. (1971) *Health and sickness: the choice of treatment.* London: Tavistock, pp. 32–43.
Williamson J. (1964) Old people at home: their unreported needs. *Lancet* 1: 1117–20.

Suggested further reading

For an introduction to the demand and supply of health care see:

Donaldson C. and Gerard K. (1993) *Economics of health care financing: the visible hand.* Basingstoke: Macmillan, pp. 12–26.
Mooney G. (1992) *Economics, medicine and health care.* Hemel Hempstead: Harvester Wheatsheaf, pp. 21–33.

A discussion of the difference between health care markets and standard competitive markets is presented by:

Stiglitz J.E. (1988) *Economics of the public sector.* New York: Norton, pp. 287–96.

For a discussion of market failure in health care see:

Donaldson C. and Gerard K. (1993) *Economics of health care financing: the visible hand.* Basingstoke: Macmillan, pp. 19–48.

For a detailed discussion of the factors affecting illness behaviour see:

Mechanic D. (1968) *Medical sociology: a selective view.* New York: Free Press, pp. 115–57.

An analysis of need and the agency relationship is provided by:

Mooney G. (1992) *Economics, medicine and health care.* Hemel Hempstead: Harvester Wheatsheaf, pp. 67–82.
Mooney G. (1994) *Key issues in health economics.* Hemel Hempstead: Harvester Wheatsheaf, pp. 87–112.

For a discussion of supplier-induced demand and a review of empirical findings see:

Donaldson C. and Gerard K. (1993) *Economics of health care financing: the visible hand.* Basingstoke: Macmillan, pp. 103–7.
McGuire A.J., Henderson J. and Mooney G. (1988) *The economics of health care.* London: Routledge, pp. 150–66.

4 Equity in the finance and distribution of health care

In Chapter 4 we address issues surrounding equity, or fairness, in the finance and distribution of health care. The discussion centres on the various issues which might be used in order to establish the existence of equity in the health care sector. The analysis then concentrates on evidence which may be used to determine the existence of equity in the UK NHS.

Summary

1. Another word for equity is fairness. Whilst the desire to achieve equity prevails within any society, what is meant by equity clearly may differ between individuals.

2. There are two main areas of health care in which issues surrounding equity are likely to arise: the finance of health care and the distribution of health care.

3. Evidence is available on both social and geographical inequalities in health.

4. There are two main areas of inquiry which we may wish to address in order to examine whether a health care system is successful in achieving an equitable basis for the finance of health care: the burden of finance and the extent of protection from catastrophic expenditure.

5. The system of paying for and financing health care may be progressive, regressive or proportional.

6. Health care expenditure may be catastrophic if it is necessary for poorer individuals to spend large amounts of income on health care as a result of unforeseen or unexpected illness.

7. The main source of finance for the UK NHS is general taxation. The bulk of this money is raised by income tax, which is progressive.

8. In the NHS, the tax payment covers all basic health care finance so that the consumer is able to use health care services at zero price. This provides protection to

individuals from unexpected ill health and possible catastrophic health care expenditure.

9. Pareto efficiency is achieved if it is not possible to move to an alternative distribution which would make someone better off without making anyone else worse off.

10. The number of possible definitions which may be used to signify an equitable distribution of health care is infinite. These include: utilitarianism; equality of health; equality of expenditure; equality of use for equal need; equality of access for equal need; and Rawlsian maximin.

11. There are two main areas of inquiry which we may wish to address in order to examine whether a health care system is successful in achieving equity in the distribution of health care: the distribution of health care by social class and income and the distribution of health care by geographical region.

12. Only a limited amount of research has been conducted examining the relationship between the distribution of illness and the distribution of health care expenditure by social class and income.

13. The limited evidence which is available seems to indicate that there is an unequal distribution of health care expenditure across social classes and income groups. Furthermore, this unequal distribution cannot be accounted for by the distribution of illness.

14. Health care resources are distributed to geographical regions in the form of NHS Health Authorities by the Department of Health according to a weighted capitation formula based on the size, age and health of the resident population. Also, an allowance is made for the higher costs of providing services in the Thames regions.

15. There is considerable variation across geographical regions not only of illness but also of total health care expenditure. The unequal distribution of health care expenditure cannot be wholly explained by geographical variation in illness, since there are differences between the proportion of expenditure which a region receives and the proportion of illness incurred by that region.

Equity

In preceding chapters we have examined the economic problem of scarcity and a response to this problem, namely, the market solution. Our analysis has concentrated on the demand and supply of health care, in order to examine the application of economics to the health care sector and its empirical relevance and validity. We have seen how the basic economic problem of scarcity is exceptionally acute in health care, since the need and demand for health care far exceeds the resources available. The three basic problems which we are interested in as health economists are as follows:

1. What health care services shall we provide?
2. How shall we provide these services?
3. Who will receive these services?

In this chapter we seek largely to address this third question. Because of the problem of scarcity, individuals may not be able to obtain all the health care which ideally they would like. Therefore, it will be necessary to develop some method for dividing up these limited health care services among all individuals in society. Inevitably this will lead to some discussion of whether this division is a 'fair' one.

Another word for fairness is *equity*, and whilst the desire to achieve equity prevails within any society, what is meant by the word equity clearly may differ between individuals. The precise meaning and importance of equity will depend mainly upon subjective factors such as cultural beliefs and attitudes.

Within any health care sector there usually exists in some form or other concerns regarding equity. There are two main areas of health care in which issues surrounding equity are likely to arise. First, issues of equity and fairness may arise regarding the finance of health care. For example, is the way in which health care is paid for fair? Do certain individuals in society, such as the poor, pay more for health care than they ought to? Secondly, issues of equity and fairness may arise regarding the distribution of health care. For example, is the way in which health care is distributed fair? Do those individuals who have most need for health care, the most ill individuals in society, receive the health care which they ought to?

In this chapter we shall explore issues of equity arising from both these areas. As a starting point we shall first examine the distribution of ill health and evidence on social and geographical inequalities in health.

Evidence on social inequalities in health

Measures of social inequality identify groups in the population which differ in a variety of charcteristics, including:

1. social status;
2. income and economic resources;
3. living and working conditions;
4. attitudes and behaviour.

These differences may then be associated with differences in health and health care utilisation. Measures of social inequality may therefore contribute to an understanding of the causes and spread of illness, by examining the relationship between a factor such as income and the distribution of ill health. Furthermore, identification of social inequality may assist in the identification of target groups for health care services within a population.

Table 4.1 Classifications of social class.

Social class	Description
Social class I	Professional occupations (for example, economists, university academic staff, medical practitioners, dental practitioners and lawyers)
Social class II	Managerial and technical occupations (for example, nurse administrators, nurses, medical technicians, dental auxiliaries, physiotherapists, police officers and teachers)
Social class IIIN	Non-manual skilled occupations (for example, clerks and shop assistants)
Social class IIIM	Manual skilled occupations (for example, bricklayers and coal miners)
Social class IV	Partly skilled occupations (for example, bus conductors and postmen)
Social class V	Unskilled occupations (for example, porters and labourers)

Source: OPCS (1980).

The basis of social inequality is occupation, which gives rise to the formulation of social classes, where the population may be grouped according to occupation. Numerous occupational classification systems have been developed. The earliest and one of the more widely used in the UK is the Registrar General's social class classification. This system is utilised in this chapter, and the 1980 *Classification of occupations* (OPCS, 1980) is used to define social class. The various social class categories are presented in Table 4.1.

Using this classification system, evidence is available on the distribution of ill health in England and Wales with respect to social class. This evidence shows that, generally, those individuals earning lower incomes (those in social classes IV and V) are more ill than those individuals earning higher incomes (those in social classes I and II).

Any number of indicators might be used to examine the distribution of ill health. Two indicators presented here are infant mortality and all-cause death rates. Figure 4.1 shows the number of stillbirths and infant deaths by social class in England and Wales in 1992. Both stillbirths and infant deaths are more common in social classes IV and V. For example, in social class I, for every 1,000 live births, approximately three live births will result in infant deaths, compared with approximately five per 1,000 live births in social class V.

With regards to the death rates from all causes for males aged 20 to 64 years in 1981, a gap exists between those individuals in social class I and those in social class V (see Figure 4.2). For example, in social class I, approximately 1.3 per cent of males aged 20 to 64 years died, compared to 4.3 per cent of males aged 20 to 64 years in social class V. Similar trends regarding deaths from all causes exist for females and for other age groups in this and subsequent years (Delamothe, 1991).

Evidence on geographical inequalities in health

Evidence also exists on geographical inequalities in health. Just as measures of social inequality may contribute to an understanding of the relationship between the causes

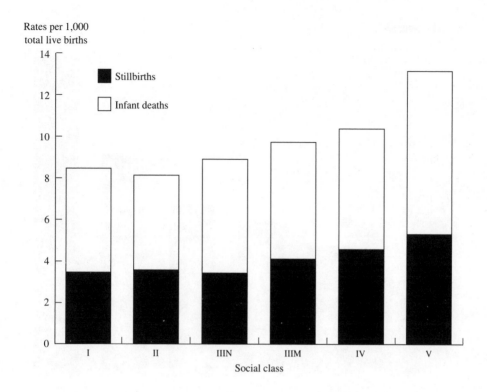

Figure 4.1 Stillbirths and infant deaths per 1,000 total live births by social class (*source*: OPCS, 1995a).

and spread of illness and social factors such as income and occupation, so evidence of geographical inequality may be used to examine the nature of ill health across geographical regions. This information may also be used to provide an understanding of the possible causes and spread of disease, and to target more effectively the use of health care services.

Evidence suggests that geographical inequalities do exist. In Table 4.2, England is geographically divided into regions. A number of indicators are presented relating to stillbirths and infant deaths in 1992, and each displays some geographical variation in the number of deaths per 1,000 total or live births. For example, in the West Midlands there were 7.0 infant deaths per 1,000 live births compared to 4.1 infant deaths per 1,000 live births in East Anglia.

Differences also exist in average life expectancy across regions in England and Wales. For example, in 1992, the average life expectancy at birth for males in the North Western region was 72.3 years. In East Anglia the average life expectancy was 75.4 years (see Table 4.3). Similar trends exist for females.

Therefore, evidence exists of inequalities in health, both in terms of social class and geographical area. Whilst health care will clearly play an important role in this

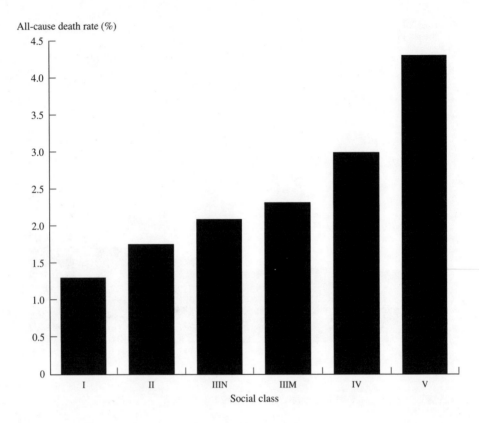

All-cause death rate (%)

Figure 4.2 Deaths from all causes for males aged 20–64 years, by social class (*source*: OPCS, 1986).

distribution of ill health, other factors are also important. These other factors include:

1. education;
2. diet;
3. income;
4. working conditions;
5. living environments;
6. lifestyle (for example, consumption of cigarettes and alcohol).

It may well be the case that we do not believe social and geographical inequalities in health to be equitable. For example, is it fair that, on the whole, individuals in social classes IV and V are more ill than those in social classes I and II? Is it fair that the incidence and prevalence of ill health is higher in certain geographical regions than in others?

Table 4.2 Stillbirths and infant deaths per 1,000 total live births by region.

Region	Stillbirths	Perinatal deaths	Neonatal deaths	Postneonatal deaths	Infant deaths
Northern	3.6	6.9	4.3	1.8	6.1
Yorkshire	4.1	7.0	4.1	2.4	6.5
Trent	4.3	7.9	4.3	7.1	5.9
East Anglia	3.9	5.9	2.6	1.5	4.1
North West Thames	4.0	6.5	3.1	1.6	4.6
North East Thames	4.0	6.5	3.1	1.6	4.6
South East Thames	4.5	7.4	3.9	1.6	5.5
South West Thames	3.6	6.1	3.2	1.7	4.9
Wessex	4.1	6.2	2.6	1.9	4.5
Oxford	3.0	5.9	3.7	1.6	5.3
South Western	3.9	6.4	3.3	1.5	4.9
West Midlands	4.1	8.3	5.2	1.8	7.0
Mersey	3.2	5.7	3.1	1.9	4.9
North Western	4.4	7.9	4.6	2.3	6.9

Source: OPCS (1995a).

Table 4.3 Average expectation of life at birth in 1992 by region.

Region	Males	Females
Northern	72.4	77.7
Yorkshire	73.6	78.8
Trent	73.6	78.9
East Anglia	75.4	80.3
North West Thames	74.5	80.1
North East Thames	73.8	79.5
South East Thames	74.0	79.6
South West Thames	75.2	80.3
Wessex	75.0	80.3
Oxford	74.9	79.6
South Western	74.9	80.3
West Midlands	73.4	78.7
Mersey	72.9	78.2
Wales	73.5	78.9
North Western	72.3	77.6

Source: OPCS (1996).

Whilst the answers to these individual questions may well be clear cut, they pose another, much more problematic yet fundamental question: what do we actually mean by equity in health care? From a policy perspective, this is a crucial question since it is important to specify precisely what is meant by equity in order to devise appropriate policies for pursuing equity goals. Unfortunately, as we shall see, there is no uniquely right definition of equity in health care, and the correctness of any possible definition is subjective and may differ across individuals, across populations and across societies.

There are two areas of health care in which issues surrounding equity are likely to emerge:

1. The finance of health care. For example, is the way in which health care is paid for fair? Do certain individuals in society, such as the poor, pay more for health care than they ought to?
2. The distribution of health care. For example, is the way in which health care is distributed fair? Do those individuals who have most need for health care, the most ill individuals in society, receive the health care which they ought to?

We shall now consider each of these areas in turn, and, whilst no firm conclusions may be drawn, it is possible to provide evidence which may be used to judge subjectively whether there is equity in the finance and distribution of health care in the UK.

Equity in the finance of health care

There are two main areas of inquiry which we may wish to address in order to examine whether a health care system is successful in achieving an equitable basis for the finance of health care:

1. The burden of finance. Do richer members of society finance a greater share of health care expenditure than poorer members?
2. Protection from catastrophic expenditure. Is there adequate protection for all members of society from unplanned expenditure arising from unexpected ill health?

We shall now examine both of these in turn.

Equity in the finance of health care: the burden of finance

Some conclusions may be drawn as to whether a health care system is financed in an equitable way by examining the burden of financing health care on individuals in the population. For example, is it the case that those individuals earning higher incomes pay more or less for health care than those individuals earning lower incomes?

In order to ascertain whether richer members of society finance a disproportionately greater or lesser share of health care expenditure than poorer members, we need to look more closely at the distribution of income and health care finance contributions.

The system of paying for and financing health care may be *progressive*, *regressive* or *proportional*.

(a) Progressive financing system

Under a progressive financing system, the proportion of income which individuals use to pay for health care *rises* as income rises. Therefore, progressive payments absorb a higher proportion of income as income rises.

(b) Regressive financing system

Under a regressive financing system, the proportion of income which individuals use to pay for health care *falls* as income rises. Therefore, regressive payments take a lower proportion of income as income rises.

(c) Proportional financing system

A proportional financing system would exist if the proportion of income paid *does not vary* with the level of income.

These three methods of health care financing may be differentiated more clearly with reference to the example in Table 4.4.

Column 1 displays the income deciles of a hypothetical population of individuals. The first decile shows, for instance, the income and amount spent financing health care of the lowest 10 per cent of income recipients (that is, the poorest 10 per cent of the population). The second income decile shows the income and amount spent financing health care of the second lowest 10 per cent of income recipients (the second poorest 10 per cent of the population), and so on.

Column 2 shows the average annual income of each income decile. This shows, for example, that the poorest 10 per cent of individuals (income decile 1) earn an average annual income of £2,000. In comparison, the richest 10 per cent of individuals (income decile 10) earn an average annual income of £100,000.

Columns 3–5 show three hypothetical scenarios examining the amount which each income decile spends financing health care, and, in brackets, the proportion of income which is spent financing health care. For example, in Column 3, income decile 1 spend on average £160 per annum financing health care, or 8 per cent of income. By comparison, income decile 10 spend £17,000 per annum financing health

Table 4.4 Amount and proportion of income spent financing health care, by income decile.

1 Income decile	2 Average annual income (£)	3 Annual amount spent financing health care (%)	4 Annual amount spent financing health care (%)	5 Annual amount spent financing health care (%)
1	2,000	160 (8)	340 (17)	240 (12)
2	5,000	450 (9)	800 (16)	600 (12)
3	9,000	900 (10)	1,350 (15)	1,080 (12)
4	14,000	1,540 (11)	1,960 (14)	1,680 (12)
5	20,000	2,400 (12)	2,600 (13)	2,400 (12)
6	27,000	3,510 (13)	3,240 (12)	3,240 (12)
7	35,000	4,900 (14)	3,850 (11)	4,200 (12)
8	45,000	6,750 (15)	4,500 (10)	5,400 (12)
9	65,000	10,400 (16)	5,850 (9)	7,800 (12)
10	100,000	17,000 (17)	8,000 (8)	12,000 (12)

care, or 17 per cent of income. Column 3 thus portrays a *progressive* financing system, because the proportion of income which is spent financing health care rises as income rises.

Column 4 portrays a *regressive* financing system because the proportion of income which is spent financing health care falls as income rises. For example, income decile 1 spend 17 per cent of income financing health care, whereas income decile 10 spend only 8 per cent. Note that even though this is a regressive system, the rich still pay more than the poor. However, they pay a *smaller proportion* of income than the poor.

Column 5 portrays a *proportional* financing system, because the proportion of income which is spent financing health care is the same across all income deciles (12 per cent of income). Note again that the rich still pay more overall than the poor, but the proportion of income which is spent financing health care is the same across all income groups.

Equity in the finance of health care: protection from catastrophic expenditure

As we have seen in the previous chapter, the incidence of ill health is uncertain in the sense that individuals do not know when they are going to be ill. Depending on the way in which health care is financed, this uncertain nature of ill health may have serious consequences for the amount of health care which certain individuals in the population are able to receive. Health care expenditure may be catastrophic if it is necessary for poorer individuals to spend large amounts of income on health care as a result of unforeseen or unexpected illness.

The ability of individuals to cope with catastrophic health care expenditure may help to provide some evidence as to whether a health care system is financed in a fair and equitable way. By examining the sources of health care finance, it is possible to examine, for example, the extent to which poorer individuals in society can cope with catastrophic expenditure.

Equity in the finance of health care in the UK National Health Service

The burden of finance in the UK National Health Service

In 1995, total National Health Service (NHS) expenditure in the UK was £41,517 million (OHE, 1995). Of this total, 84.2 per cent was raised from general taxation, 12.7 per cent was raised from NHS contributions and 3.1 per cent was raised from patient payments such as prescription charges (OHE, 1995). Therefore, the main source of finance for the NHS is general taxation. The bulk of funds from general taxation are obtained from income tax. Therefore, income tax provides the

Table 4.5 Rates of income tax and National Insurance contributions.

Bracket	Slice of income per annum (£)	Rate (%)
Income tax		
Personal allowance	1–4,049	0
Lower rate	4,050–8,149	20
Basic rate	8,150–30,149	23
Higher rate	30,150+	40
National Insurance		
Lower rate	1–3,224	2
Basic rate	3,225+	10

Source: Inland Revenue (1997).

main source of funds for the NHS. NHS contributions paid by employers and employees via the National Insurance scheme may also be regarded as a form of taxation on earned income. Therefore, taxation accounts for 96.9 per cent of total NHS finance, where the contribution of an individual to the NHS is part of their total tax payment.

Table 4.5 presents the rates of income tax and National Insurance contributions in the UK. It is evident that the income tax rate increases at higher income levels. For example, any income earned between £8,150 and £30,149 per annum is taxed at a rate of 23 per cent (that is, for every £1.00 of income earned between £8,150 and £30,149 per annum, £0.23 is paid in income tax). At higher income levels, a greater income tax rate is incurred. For example, any income of £30,150 or more per annum is taxed at a rate of 40 per cent (that is, for every £1.00 of income earned over £30,149 per annum, £0.40 is paid in income tax). Similarly, the National Insurance contribution rate also increases at higher income levels.

Using the taxonomy outlined earlier, this indicates that the method of financing the NHS is *progressive*, because not only do those individuals earning higher incomes pay more income tax and more National Insurance, they also pay a greater proportion of their earned income. Therefore, the proportion of income which individuals use to pay for health care rises as income rises.

In recent years, only a limited amount of research has been conducted examining the relationship between income distribution and the distribution of health care finance. A comparison of the distribution of total health care expenditure and post-tax income in the UK, by income decile, is presented in Figure 4.3 (adapted from Donaldson and Gerard, 1993). This indicates, for example, that the lowest income decile, income decile 1, receives approximately 3 per cent of income in the UK and pays approximately 2 per cent of NHS finance. Conversely, the highest income decile, income decile 10, receives approximately 24 per cent of income in the UK and pays approximately 26 per cent of NHS finance. As Figure 4.3 indicates, across all income deciles, there is a close match between the level of post-tax income and the level of health care finance.

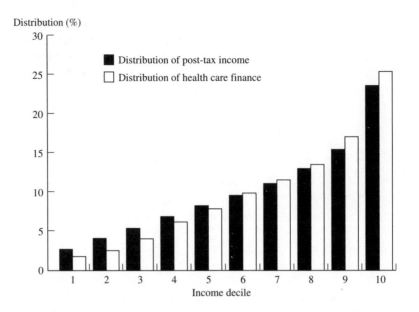

Figure 4.3 Comparison of the distribution of total health care expenditure and post-tax income by income decile (*source*: Donaldson and Gerard, 1993).

Protection from catastrophic expenditure in the UK National Health Service

In the NHS, the income tax payments and National Insurance contributions made by the population cover the finance of all basic health care so that individuals are able to use health care services at a zero price. No maximum quantity of health care services which an individual is able to use is stipulated, and therefore individuals have unlimited access to health care.

This method of finance therefore does provide protection to individuals from unexpected ill health and possible catastrophic health care expenditure: should an individual require a significant amount of health care arising from an unforeseen illness then, whatever their income, they will be able to receive the medical services they require.

Equity in the distribution of health care

In addition to equity in the finance of health care, there usually exists within most societies a concern that health care is also *distributed* in some fair or just way. Therefore, interest exists with equity not only in the finance of health care, but also in the distribution of health care.

The desire to achieve an equitable distribution of health care prevails within any society. However, what exactly is meant by an equitable distribution of health care may differ between societies. Problems arise in defining what is meant by equity in the distribution of health care. The extent of these problems may be more clearly highlighted by comparing the notions of equity and Pareto efficiency.

Equity and Pareto efficiency

Figure 4.4 shows a hypothetical society with only two individuals, A and B, between whom a good, X, is to be distributed. The initial distribution at point p_1 gives individual A an allocation of Q^A and individual B an allocation of Q^B. We would like to examine whether p_1 is an *efficient* distribution of good X. In other words, we wish to examine whether resources are being wasted with this specific distribution.

Let us suppose that it is possible to reorganise the distribution of good X with a distribution defined by point p_2. If individuals assess their utility on the basis of the quantity of good X which they receive, and it is assumed that more of good X is preferred to less, p_2 is a better distribution of good X than p_1 since both individuals A and B get more. Similarly, a shift from p_1 to point p_3 makes both individuals A and B worse off.

In each of these cases, whether society is better or worse off is clear. Society must be better off with a shift from p_1 to p_2 since both individuals get *more* of the good. Conversely, society must be worse off with a shift from p_1 to p_3 since both individuals get *less* of the good.

Suppose now a redistribution of good X from p_1 to either point p_4 or p_5. With either of these shifts, one individual gains and the other individual loses (for instance, with a shift from p_1 to p_4, individual A gains by receiving more of good X and individual B loses by receiving less of good X).

How we judge a change from p_1 to p_4 or p_5 depends on how we value the utility of individual A compared to individual B. For example, if we value the utility of individual A more than the utility of individual B then we may well consider a shift from p_1 to p_4 to be a good thing. However, the decision about whether this move is a good thing is no longer objective. Rather it depends upon our subjective views and value judgements.

This example has shown the difference between the distribution of a hypothetical good on an efficiency basis, and the distribution of a hypothetical good on an equity basis. Economics uses the idea of *Pareto efficiency* to assess whether a distribution of a good or service is efficient: Pareto efficiency is achieved if it is not possible to move to another distribution which would make someone better off without making anyone else worse off.

In terms of Figure 4.4, a move from p_1 to p_2 is a *Pareto gain*, since individual A is better off and individual B is no worse off. Therefore, if it is possible to distribute good X at point p_2, p_1 is *Pareto inefficient*, and the shift in the distribution of good X to p_2 should be made on efficiency grounds. Conversely, a shift in distribution from p_1 to p_3 is a *Pareto loss* and should not be made on efficiency grounds.

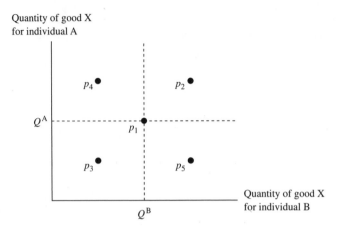

Figure 4.4 Distribution of good X between two individuals, A and B.

Therefore, the concept of Pareto efficiency provides a decision-making criterion which may be used to distribute goods and services.

However, this *Pareto criterion* is not all-encompassing as a decision-making tool. For instance, the Pareto efficiency criterion is unhelpful regarding a change from p_1 to p_4 or p_5, since one individual is being made worse off and another is being made better off. A move from p_1 to p_4 will make individual A better off, and individual B worse off. A move from p_1 to p_5 will make individual B better off, and individual A worse off. Without bringing in a subjective judgement about the relative importance of the utility of individual A compared to individual B, we are unable to evaluate these changes.

Therefore, the Pareto criterion has only a limited use in assessing the distribution of a good on efficiency grounds. From Figure 4.4, the Pareto criterion only allows us to evaluate shifts in the distribution of a good to the north-east or the south-west quadrants. It is unhelpful regarding changes to the north-west or south-east quadrants, since then we become entangled with considerations of equity.

These considerations are seen more clearly with reference to Figure 4.5, which displays an *efficiency frontier*.

An efficiency frontier displays all distributions of a good which are efficient. Suppose that by all the possible reorganisations of production of good X in society, an economy can produce anywhere inside or on the frontier FF. Therefore, it is possible to distribute good X between individuals A and B in such a way that the combination of quantities of good X received by each individual is either within or on the frontier FF in Figure 4.5. From any distribution of good X inside the frontier, such as q_0, it is always possible to achieve a Pareto gain by moving to the north-east on to the frontier to, say, q_1. Therefore, any distribution inside the frontier, such as q_0, must be Pareto inefficient since it is possible to make someone better off without making anyone else worse off. Allocation q_1, on the frontier, is Pareto efficient. Any

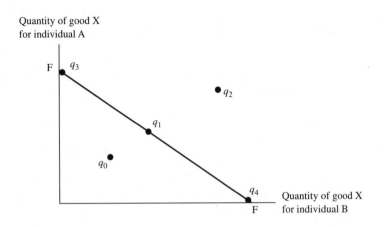

Figure 4.5 An efficiency frontier.

distribution outside the frontier, such as q_2, is unfeasible and not possible given the constraints imposed by scarce resources.

Therefore, all points on the frontier, such as q_1, are Pareto efficient, since it is not possible to make a Pareto gain because it is not possible to make one individual better off without making another individual worse off. However, since all points on the frontier are Pareto efficient, then, on efficiency grounds, the distribution of good X defined at point q_1 is as efficient as that defined by points q_3 or q_4, which are also on the frontier. It is unclear which Pareto efficient point on the frontier is most desirable, since this decision will ultimately depend upon a value judgement regarding the relative importance of the utility of individual A and individual B. This decision is purely a judgement about equity.

Whilst the discussion so far has concentrated on the distribution of a generic good X, the concepts which have been examined have a clear application to health care. The discussion so far indicates that the real conflict in the distribution of health care lies not so much between equity and efficiency, but between rival concepts of equity.

Concepts of equity in the distribution of health care

The number of possible definitions which may be used to signify an equitable distribution of health care is infinite. The following list provides perhaps some of the more feasible possibilities:

1. utilitarianism;
2. equality of health;
3. equality of expenditure;
4. equality of use for equal need;

5. equality of access for equal need;
6. Rawlsian maximin.

We shall now look in closer detail at each of these concepts in turn and examine the difficulties involved with implementing each as an equity goal.

Utilitarianism

The principle of utilitarianism was first formally stated by Jeremy Bentham in 1789. The basic principle behind utilitarianism is to act always in such a manner so as to maximise the utility or welfare of society.

This is consistent with the discussion of economic theory in Chapter 2, where it was assumed that the consumers of a good are utility maximisers and that the producers of that good are profit maximisers. Restated, a policy of strict utilitarianism will ultimately seek to distribute health care in such a manner that the greatest good will be achieved for the greatest number of individuals.

Possible problems with utilitarianism

In principle, a policy of utilitarianism may be perfectly acceptable. In practice, it may lead to distributions of health care which are considered unsavoury by society. Health care is one example of a good where the main goal perhaps should not be that of maximising the welfare of society because whilst this policy would be beneficial for the majority of individuals, it will inevitably mean that certain individuals lose out in some way. That is, a few individuals lose out for the good of the rest of society. To concentrate on utilitarianism may therefore create a distribution of health care which discriminates against certain members of society, such as the poor, those in the lower social classes and the seriously ill, so that the rest of society may benefit.

Therefore, whilst utilitarianism might do the greatest good for the greatest number of individuals it may well result in unacceptable levels of health care for a few unlucky individuals.

Equality of health

Using this definition of equity, the distribution of health care is fair if it results in every individual obtaining the same level of health. This does not necessarily mean equality of health across all age and sex groups, since this would be biologically impossible. However, within age and sex groups, equality of health means just that: equal or the same health for all.

Possible problems with equality of health

As argued by Donaldson and Gerard (1993), controversy exists regarding exactly what is meant by the terms 'health' and 'good health'. If we are unsure of what we mean by 'health' then it becomes very difficult to formulate and implement a workable policy of equality of health into the distribution of health care.

Health is affected by a number of factors, such as diet, lifestyle, education and housing, and not just health care. Indeed, the actual effects of health care may often be quite limited. Moreover, it is hard to quantify the relationship that each factor has with the health status of the population. However, these other factors need to be included in any distribution of health care aiming to equalise health. Clearly this will be very difficult.

Equality of health within age and gender groups will invariably not be possible because of the current state of technology. Some illnesses are currently incurable (such as AIDS), and therefore a policy aimed at improving the health of some individuals to bring about equality of health would be unsuccessful.

Furthermore, given the current limitations of health care technology, in order to achieve equality of health, the health of some individuals will need to improve and the health of other individuals will need to deteriorate. Therefore, it would be necessary to pursue a policy where the health status of some individuals (the most healthy) will deliberately be made worse.

Attempting to achieve equal health implies that certain individuals in society may be prevented from choosing their own preferred level of health should it fall below the level of equality. For example, an individual may not wish to give up smoking, but would be required to do so in order to achieve equality of health.

These are just some of the problems which would be encountered when attempting to distribute health care in such a way so as to achieve equality of health. Therefore, whilst a policy of equality of health might be desirable, it would be very difficult, if not impossible, to fulfil.

Equality of expenditure

A distribution of health care which concentrates on equality of expenditure would be relatively easy to achieve, because at its most simple all it would require is that each individual receives the same distribution of health care.

Possible problems with equality of expenditure

The health status of individuals differs widely across society, and the incidence of ill health is much higher for some individuals than others. Therefore, certain individuals obviously require more health care than others. If health care is provided in such a way that expenditure on each individual is the same, then no recognition is given of the differences in health care needs across society: if all individuals receive the same health care expenditure then no account is made of the effects of health care on overall health status. Clearly, this may result in a situation where certain health care resources are underutilised, but where there is a need for them elsewhere. Therefore, whilst it might be possible to provide each individual with the same expenditure on health care, it may not be acceptable because it takes no account of need.

Equality of use for equal need

A more plausible definition of equity might be equality of use. It would clearly be wrong to concentrate on equal use on its own, since the health care that each individual requires is different because everyone has a different level of health. Resources would undoubtedly be wasted if all individuals were given equal use of health services. This equity goal may therefore be modified to become equal use for equal need.

Using the definition of equal use for equal need, if two individuals have the same condition that requires the same treatment, then their use or consumption of health care services should be the same.

Possible problems with equal use for equal need

A distribution of health care which assumes equal use for equal need presupposes that individuals have the same attitudes not only to health but also to health care. It is necessary that uptake and compliance with health care services be equal for all individuals with the same health care needs. Clearly this is an inaccurate assumption since it ignores the fact that variations occur in preferences for both health and health care. For example, two individuals may have exactly the same condition that requires exactly the same treatment, but their preferences for health and health care are different and so they will not want equal use of the services available. The process of consuming health care involves different levels of utility or disutility for different individuals (for example, some individuals have a greater fear of dentists than others), yet equal use for equal need as a definition of equity requires that such variations are not taken into account when distributing health care.

Equal use for equal need requires that medical practices for treating conditions are standardised across health care providers. Whilst treatment regimes may be similar within geographical regions, the way in which individuals are treated is unlikely to be identical across all geographical regions.

Equality of access for equal need

It may be preferable to distribute health care in such a way that there is equal access to health care for everyone. Equal access on its own is not an appropriate objective if taken irrespective of other characteristics: clearly it would be wrong to concentrate solely on equal access, since the health care requirements of each individual are different. Therefore, as above, this equity goal may be modified to become equal access for equal need.

Equal access for equal need simply means that individuals are provided with the same opportunity to use needed health care services. This definition of equity has advantages over equality of use for equal need, since it may legitimately lead to different patterns of health care utilisation arising from different preferences of individuals towards health and health care. What is important is not that individuals with the same need for health care use the same health care services, but rather that they have the same *opportunity* to use, or the same access to, the same health care services.

A usable definition of equality of access is difficult to formulate. However, one possibility may be that two individuals have equal access if the costs to them in using a particular health care service are valued the same. Using this formulation, equality of access implies that every individual faces the same costs in utilising the facilities of a health care provider. Note that the costs involved include travel costs and time costs as well as monetary costs arising directly for health care. This then defines equality of access in terms of geographical as well as financial equality.

Possible problems with equal access for equal need

As with most possible definitions of equity, equality of access for equal need becomes difficult to achieve within the constraints imposed by scarce resources. For example, pursuit of equal access to health care for equal need would require that health care be provided equally in sparsely populated rural areas and in densely populated urban areas. For example, it should be just as quick and easy to travel to hospital for treatment in isolated farmland in Yorkshire as it is in, say, London. Obviously, equality of access for equal need will be extremely difficult to achieve, and it would impose a very large burden on limited health care resources. Donaldson and Gerard (1993) argue that for two communities to face equality of access to health care, the following factors which affect access to health care services will need to be the same:

1. geographical factors (for example, travel distances and the travel times);
2. availability of transport;
3. communication facilities;
4. waiting times for treatment;
5. information known by patients.

Clearly, as a workable definition of equity in the distribution of health care, equal access for equal need will be very difficult to achieve.

Rawlsian maximin

Rawls (1972) provides a slightly different approach to social and ethical decision-making, and defines equity in terms of justice. Rawls identified equitable behaviour as that which would be chosen by individuals if they were placed under what he called a 'veil of ignorance'. Under this veil of ignorance, every individual is ignorant of the position which they will have in society. There is therefore uncertainty as to the future position which an individual will take in society. For example, an individual will not know if they will be rich or poor, and they will not know if they will be healthy or unhealthy. Placed in this situation, Rawls argued that individuals would adopt what is called a *maximin* decision rule with regards to the distribution of resources. This means that individuals will advocate those policies that will maximise the welfare of the worst-off individuals in society.

If this were our definition of equity in the distribution of health care, then this would mean that health care would be distributed in such a manner so as to maximise the health of the most ill individuals in society.

Possible problems with Rawlsian maximin

Whilst it would be possible to concentrate solely on providing health care to the most ill individuals in society, it would undoubtedly be an extremely costly rule to follow, both financially and in terms of health gains from scarce health care resources. Given the current state of technology and the fact that there are numerous illnesses which are currently incurable, a policy of Rawlsian maximin would concentrate the distribution of health care on individuals who may never regain full health, and who may only ever be extremely ill. Whatever quantity of health care that is distributed to treating such individuals will not prevent them from remaining the most ill individuals in society. In this situation, health care would never be distributed to the treatment of less ill, but perhaps still very sick, individuals.

It is also open to criticism whether the foundations of the maximin rule are sound anyway. For example, under a veil of ignorance it is not certain that an individual would choose to maximise the health of the most ill people in society. This maximin rule partly arises from the fact that in a state of ignorance as to our future circumstances and position in society, we would take an overtly pessimistic view and assume that we would be the worst-off individuals, which is why we would choose to distribute health care to these individuals. However, it is not necessarily the case that we would take such a view, in which case the foundations of the Rawlsian maximin distribution rule become invalid.

This list of concepts of equity in the distribution of health care is by no means exhaustive, and there are many other possibilities which could be added. However, this serves to highlight the problems surrounding equity in the distribution of health care. We may all agree that equity is an important goal, but we may not agree on what we actually mean by equity. There is no uniquely correct way of defining equity: it is dependent upon a subjective value judgement.

Equity in the distribution of health care in the UK National Health Service

Whichever equity goal is chosen for the distribution of health care, this goal may be applied across income groups or social classes and across geographical regions. There are therefore two main areas of inquiry which we may wish to address in order to examine whether a health care system is successful in achieving an equitable basis for the distribution of health care:

1. the distribution of health care by social class and income (for example, do richer members of society or those in the higher social classes receive a greater share of health care than poorer members or those in the lower social classes?);
2. the distribution of health care by geographical region (for example, do individuals in certain geographical areas receive a greater share of health care than those in other geographical areas?).

We shall now examine each of these issues in the context of the NHS. The distribution of health care by social class and income is assessed in terms of the utilisation of health care services. The distribution of health care by geographical region is assessed in terms of the allocation of total NHS expenditure.

Distribution of health care by social class and income in the UK National Health Service

In recent years, only a limited amount of research has been conducted examining the relationship between the distribution of illness and the distribution of health care expenditure by social class. A comparison of the distribution of total health care expenditure and illness in England and Wales, by social class, is presented in Figure 4.6 (adapted from Le Grand, 1978). This indicates, for example, that social classes IV and V receive approximately 27 per cent of health care expenditure in England and Wales, and incur approximately 32 per cent of illness. Social classes I and II receive approximately 17 per cent of health care expenditure in England and Wales, and incur approximately 14 per cent of illness. Figure 4.6 indicates, therefore, that across social classes, some divergence exists between the distribution of illness and the distribution of health care expenditure.

Figure 4.7 (adapted from Wagstaff et al., 1993) presents a comparison of the distribution of total health care expenditure and illness in England and Wales, by income decile. This shows, for example, that the lowest income decile, income decile 1 (that is, the lowest 10 per cent of income recipients or the poorest 10 per cent of the population), receives approximately 18 per cent of NHS expenditure, and incurs approximately 12 per cent of illness. Conversely, the highest income decile, income decile 10, receives approximately 8 per cent of NHS expenditure, and incurs approximately 5 per cent of illness. Across all income deciles, Figure 4.7 also

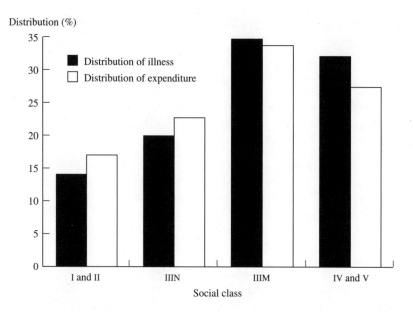

Figure 4.6 Comparison of the distribution of illness and total health care expenditure by social class (*source*: Le Grand, 1978).

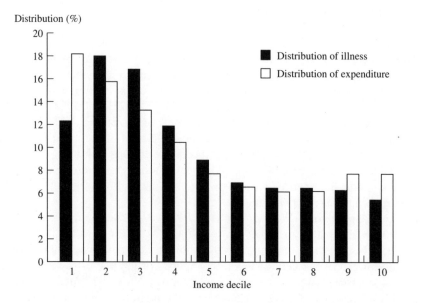

Figure 4.7 Comparison of the distribution of illness and total health care expenditure by income decile (*source*: Wagstaff *et al.*, 1993).

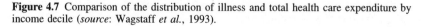

indicates some divergence between the distribution of illness and the distribution of health care expenditure.

This limited evidence therefore indicates that there is an unequal distribution of health care expenditure across social classes and income groups in England and Wales. Furthermore, this unequal distribution cannot be accounted for by the distribution of illness.

Distribution of health care by geographical region in the UK National Health Service

Health care resources for hospital and community health services are distributed geographically according to a weighted capitation formula based on the size, age and health of the resident population (HFMA/CIPFA, 1995). An allowance is also made for the higher costs of providing services in London.

Key variables in the current funding formula for the geographical distribution of health care are as follows (HFMA/CIPFA, 1995):

1. Population. Estimates of the population of each geographical region are estimated, and this forms the basis of the weighted capitation formula.
2. Age. Population data is weighted to reflect the extent to which each age group utilises health care services.
3. Need. Population data is also weighted to reflect the fact that healthier individuals require less use of health care services. Need is determined by calculating, within any one geographical area, data on: the number of individuals with long-term illness, health problem or handicap which limits daily activity; the number of deaths; the number of individuals of pensionable age living alone; and the number of individuals who are permanently sick.
4. Market forces. Finally, population data is weighted to reflect the fact that the cost of providing health care services varies across the UK (for example, staff costs are likely to be higher in London and the South East than in the rest of England).

It is possible to compare the distribution of health care expenditure in England with the distribution of illness. In Figure 4.8 England is divided into geographical regions. Using data from the 1993 General Household Survey (OPCS, 1995b), the figure shows the prevalence of illness in these regions in 1992. These data are compared with total health care expenditure (Central Statistical Office, 1995).

Figure 4.8 therefore presents a comparison of the distribution of total health care expenditure and illness in England, by geographical region. This shows considerable variation across geographical region not only of illness but also of total health care expenditure. Furthermore, this also suggests that the unequal distribution of health care expenditure cannot be wholly explained by geographical variation in illness, since there are differences between the proportion of expenditure which a region receives and the proportion of illness incurred by that region. For example, North

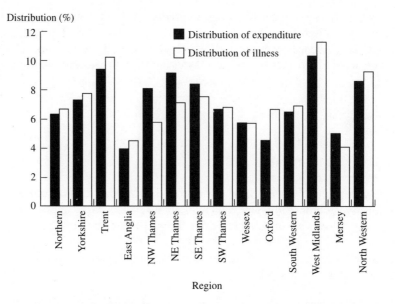

Figure 4.8 Comparison of the distribution of illness and total health care expenditure by region (*source*: OPCS, 1995b; Central Statistical Office, 1995).

West Thames incurs approximately 5 per cent of all illness, yet receives approximately 8 per cent of total health care expenditure.

Equity in the finance and distribution of health care in the UK National Health Service

Evidence from four sources might be used in order to establish the existence of equity in the finance and distribution of health care in the NHS:

1. the burden of finance;
2. protection of individuals from catastrophic expenditure;
3. the distribution of health care by social class and income;
4. the distribution of health care by geographical region.

Clearly it is difficult to decide whether the NHS is equitable without some suggestion of the equity goals which are to be achieved. This illustrates the problem surrounding any judgements regarding the relative merits of one health care system over another in terms of equity criteria: whilst the desire to achieve equity prevails within any society, what is meant by the word equity is likely to differ between individuals and between populations.

With regard to equity in the finance of health care in the NHS, if we believe that the most acceptable distribution of health care finance is achieved with a progressive financing system rather than a regressive or proportional system, then it may be argued that the NHS is equitable: the bulk of expenditure by the NHS is derived from income tax payments and National Insurance contributions which are progressive, with those individuals earning higher incomes paying a greater portion of their income.

If a health care financing system is considered to be more equitable if those individuals earning lower incomes are given protection from catastrophic health care expenditure arising from unexpected illness, then the NHS may be deemed equitable. This is because the tax payment covers all basic health care so that individuals are able to use the NHS at zero price. No maximum quantity of health care services is stipulated, and individuals have unlimited access to health care services.

With regard to equity in the distribution of health care, the concept of equity which is most often associated with the distribution of health care in the NHS is that of equal access for equal need (see, for example, Carr-Hill, 1990; HFMA/CIPFA, 1995). This applies across social classes and income groups and geographical regions. Unfortunately, data on equal access for equal need are extremely limited. The evidence which does exist seems to suggest there is an unequal distribution of health care expenditure across social classes and income groups and that this unequal distribution cannot be accounted for by the distribution of illness. Furthermore, the unequal distribution of health care expenditure across geographical regions cannot be explained by geographical variations in illness, since there are differences between the proportion of expenditure which a region receives and the proportion of illness incurred by that region. This seems to indicate that the goal of equal access for equal need has yet to be achieved. However, from a policy perspective the crucial issue of determining what we mean by equity in the health care sector appears to have been answered. Clearly this makes it much easier to devise appropriate policies for pursuing equity goals.

In this chapter we have examined various methods for financing health care and for distributing limited health care services among individuals in society. The analysis has concentrated on various equity goals which may be pursued, and we have examined the importance of equity considerations in the provision of health care in the NHS. In the following chapter, another issue arising from the provision of health care is discussed which is equally important and fundamental to the structure of any health care system: health insurance.

References

Carr-Hill R. (1990) RAWP is dead: long live RAWP. In: Culyer A.J., Maynard A.K. and Posnett J.W. *Competition in health care: reforming the NHS*. Hong Kong; Macmillan.

Central Statistical Office (1995) *Regional trends*. London: HMSO.

Delamothe T. (1991) Social inequalities in health. *British Medical Journal* 303: 1046–50.

Donaldson C. and Gerard K. (1993) *Economics of health care financing: the visible hand*. Basingstoke: Macmillan.

HFMA/CIPFA (1995) *Introductory guide to NHS finance in the UK*. Third edition. London: HFMA.

Inland Revenue (1997) *Taxable pay tables*. London: HMSO.

Le Grand J. (1978) The distribution of public expenditure: the case of health care. *Economica* 45: 125–42.

Office of Health Economics (OHE) (1995) *Compendium of health statistics*. London: OHE.

OPCS (1980) *Classification of occupations, 1980*. London: HMSO.

OPCS (1986) *Occupational mortality*. London: HMSO.

OPCS (1995a) *Mortality statistics: perinatal and infant*. London: HMSO.

OPCS (1995b) *General household survey 1993*. London: HMSO.

OPCS (1996) *Population trends*. London: HMSO.

Rawls J. (1971) *A theory of justice*. Cambridge MA: Harvard University Press.

Wagstaff A., van Doorslaer E. and Paci P. (1991) Equity in the finance and delivery of health care: some tentative cross-country comparisons. In: McGuire A., Fenn P. and Mayhew K. (eds.) *Providing health care: the economics of alternative systems of finance and delivery*. Oxford: Oxford University Press.

Suggested further reading

For a discussion of social inequalities in health see:

Delamothe T. (1991) Social inequalities in health. *British Medical Journal* 303: 1046–50.

For an exposition of alternative concepts of equity in the distribution of health care see:

Mooney G. (1992) *Economics, medicine and health care*. Hemel Hempstead: Harvester Wheatsheaf, pp. 102–20.

For a detailed review of the evidence of equity in the finance and distribution of health care in the UK (and also other countries) see:

Donaldson C. and Gerard K. (1993) *Economics of health care financing: the visible hand*. Basingstoke: Macmillan, pp. 143–64.

For a concise guide to resource allocation in the UK NHS see:

HFMA/CIPFA (1995) *Introductory guide to NHS finance in the UK*. Third edition. London: HFMA, pp. 5–18.

5   Health insurance

In this chapter we examine the effects of uncertainty on the market for health care, and a possible solution to this problem, namely, the introduction of health insurance. A basic framework for the formation of a health insurance market is established which lays the foundation for the discussion of the following chapters. The analysis concentrates on the demand and supply of health insurance and the derivation of the insurance premium at which health insurance may be bought and sold. Problems generated by health insurance are discussed.

Summary

1. Within the market framework, consumers of health care face uncertainty regarding both the timing of health care expenditure and the amount of expenditure on health care which is required.

2. Because of this uncertainty, individuals are at risk from the unexpected nature of ill health and the possibility of incurring large unplanned catastrophic expenditures for treatment which they are unable to afford.

3. Problems arising from the existence of uncertainty may be addressed with the introduction of health insurance.

4. Health insurance involves the development of an insurance contract between insurance companies and individuals who consider themselves to be at risk of ill health. When an individual buys health insurance, they enter into an agreement with an insurance company to pay an agreed price, called an insurance premium, in exchange for a payout to be made to the individual by the insurance company should some specific event occur, such as their becoming ill.

5. Individuals choose to buy health insurance because they are risk averse. Insurance companies are able to supply health insurance because they can pool risks across a large number of insured individuals.

6. Just as a market may be used for the distribution of goods and services such as chocolate bars and health care, so there may also be a market for health insurance, where buyers and sellers meet and demand and supply insurance contracts.

7. The fair premium is defined as an insurance premium charged by an insurance company for health insurance which is equal to the amount of expenditure on health care that the individual will incur on average if they are not insured.

8. A risk premium is a sum of money which an individual is prepared to pay over and above the fair premium so that risk and uncertainty might be reduced.

9. When there is a difference between the fair premium and the actual insurance premium charged by an insurance company it is called loading the premium, and a loading factor is added to the fair premium.

10. If the risk premium is greater than the loading factor then the extra amount of money which a risk-averse individual is prepared to pay in order to reduce uncertainty is greater than the amount of money which an insurance company is prepared to offer in order to make a profit. In this case, a market for health insurance will exist.

11. Adverse selection may be defined as the situation in which exactly the wrong individuals from the point of view of the insurance company choose to buy health insurance. This condition arises due to informational asymmetry. Adverse selection may result in a situation where the insurance market will fail to provide health insurance for low-risk individuals. The problem of adverse selection may be solved with the introduction of experience rating.

12. The existence of moral hazard implies an excessive use of health care resources. This problem affects both the consumers and providers of health care. Moral hazard exists because the effect of health insurance is to make health care, in effect, free to consumers, and so more health care expenditure will be incurred by an insurance company on behalf of an individual with insurance than would be incurred by that same individual without insurance. The problem of moral hazard may be addressed with the introduction of coinsurance and deductibles.

13. Since health care is, in effect, free with health insurance, patients will choose the health care provider where they receive treatment not on the basis of price but, instead, on the basis of other non-price factors. Therefore, non-price competition will emerge, where health care providers must compete for the custom of patients on the basis of factors such as comfort, the pleasantness of surroundings and the quality of the food, rather than price. This will result in a situation where costs will increase in the health care market.

14. Whilst health insurance protects individuals from expenditure arising from the unpredictable nature of illness it still relies on individuals being able to afford health

insurance premiums in the first place. Some individuals in the population, such as those earning low incomes, or those at very high risk of illness, would find it difficult to afford health insurance, even if it were charged at only the fair premium rate with no additional loading factor.

Uncertainty and health care

Uncertainty

Within the framework of a perfect health care market, the treatments which will be made available are those which individuals are willing and able to spend their money on, and those that may be supplied profitably by health care providers. In its purest form, therefore, a health care market will provide only enough health care for those individuals who are willing and able to pay the market price.

In order to achieve an efficient allocation of resources in this way, a health care market requires a number of conditions to hold. These are: certainty; no externalities; perfect knowledge; consumers to act free of self-interested suppliers; and several suppliers to promote genuine competition. In this chapter we shall examine one of these assumptions in greater detail, namely, the existence of *certainty*. In Chapter 3 we saw how the assumption of certainty is unlikely to hold in the health care market and how health care expenditure may be catastrophic if individuals are unable to afford treatment for sudden and unexpected ill health. In this chapter we shall explore the effects of this uncertainty on the provision of health care in more detail.

In a generic market situation, the assumption of certainty requires that consumers know exactly what goods and services they wish to consume. Furthermore, they should know when they want to consume them, how they can obtain them and at what cost. Therefore, certainty is required with regards to both the timing and the size of expenditure on the consumption of goods. With this knowledge, expenditure on consumption is known in advance and may be planned so that individuals are able to pay the market price for those goods and services which they wish to consume. Conversely, under conditions of uncertainty, consumers have little or no knowledge regarding the timing and size of expenditure on consumption. This may result in a situation where individuals are unable to afford those goods and services which they wish to consume.

Uncertainty in the market for health care

In the market for health care, demand is contingent upon the incidence of ill health, which is generally unpredictable. This means that certainty does not exist in the demand for health care. Instead, consumers of health care face a position of *uncertainty*. More specifically, within the market framework, consumers of health care face uncertainty regarding two key issues:

1. the *timing* of health care expenditure;
2. the *amount* of expenditure on health care which is required.

The demand for health care is therefore uncertain and individuals are unable to plan their consumption of health care services. Because of this, individuals are at risk from the unexpected nature of ill health and the possibility of incurring large unplanned expenditures for treatment. In the previous chapter we saw how health care expenditure may be 'catastrophic' if it is necessary for individuals to spend large amounts of income on health care as a result of unforeseen or unexpected illness. Ultimately, this catastrophic expenditure may result in a situation where individuals are unable to afford the health care which they need.

Uncertainty surrounding the demand for health care implies that markets may not allocate health care resources efficiently. However, this does not mean that the market becomes redundant as a tool for resource allocation. Problems arising from the existence of uncertainty may be addressed with the introduction of *health insurance*.

Health insurance generally entails the development of an *insurance contract* between insurance companies and individuals considered to be at risk of ill health. These insurance contracts usually operate in terms of an agreement, by the insurance company, to make a payout to the insured individual in the event that a particular outcome occurs (for example, the individual becomes ill), in exchange for the payment of an *insurance premium*.

Therefore, just as there may be a market for health care services, so there may also be a market for health insurance, where buyers and sellers meet and demand and supply insurance contracts. In the market for health insurance, individuals, as the consumers of insurance, choose whether to buy insurance, and insurance companies, as the providers of insurance, choose whether to sell insurance.

Since the assumption of certainty does not hold in the market for health care we must develop a more general understanding of how individuals respond to uncertainty, and, in particular, we need to develop a model of health insurance which may explain individuals' actions. Before we may proceed with a closer examination of the market for health insurance, clarification of certain fundamental concepts is required.

Key concepts

It is necessary to be familiar with the following concepts for a full understanding of how individuals respond to uncertainty:

1. uncertainty;
2. states of the world;
3. probability;
4. payoffs;

5. contingency matrices;
6. expected value.

We shall now examine each of these concepts in turn.

Uncertainty

Parkin and King (1995) define uncertainty as 'a state in which more than one event may occur, but we don't know which one'. Therefore, a situation is uncertain when any one of a number of states of the world may occur, though it is unclear as to which. Uncertainty arises in the market for health care because, since the incidence of ill health is unpredictable, it is generally impossible to anticipate future health states.

EXAMPLE _____

A 50-year-old male with hypertension who smokes is uncertain as to his future health (for example, this individual may or may not develop coronary heart disease [CHD] in the next five years).

States of the world

The states of the world that an individual faces are the set of different outcomes which may result from the condition creating the uncertainty.

EXAMPLE _____

Two states of the world which may occur for a 50-year-old male with hypertension who smokes are, firstly, that he develops CHD and, secondly, that he does not develop CHD.

Probability

To describe uncertainty we use the concept of probability. The probability of a state of the world is a number between zero and one that measures the chance of that state occurring. A probability of zero means that the state of the world will not occur. A probability of one means that the state of the world will occur for sure, or with certainty. Therefore, the probability of a given state of the world is a measure of the likelihood that it will occur.

EXAMPLE _____

The probability that a 50-year-old male with hypertension who smokes will develop CHD in the next five years is 1/20, or 0.05. This means that there are 5 chances in 100, or a 5 per cent chance that this individual will develop CHD.

For any uncertain situation, the probabilities of all the separate states of the world occurring must add up to one, because what is certain is that one of the possible states of the world will occur. In other words, if there are only two possible states of the world, and the probability of the first state occurring is p, then the probability of the second state of the world occurring is $(1 - p)$.

EXAMPLE

Because the probability that a 50-year-old male with hypertension who smokes will develop CHD in the next five years is 1/20, the probability that this individual will not develop CHD is 19/20, or 0.95 (that is, $1 - 1/20$).

Payoffs

Another basic concept to be introduced is the payoff in each possible state of the world. This is the outcome which will be obtained if a particular state of the world is realised. Each possible state of the world has a corresponding payoff. Payoffs are often defined in monetary terms, though they need not necessarily be defined in this way.

EXAMPLE

If a 50-year-old male with hypertension who smokes does develop CHD in the next five years, then he has a life expectancy of 60 years. However, if the same individual does not develop CHD in the next five years, then he has a life expectancy of 70 years.

Contingency matrices

Once data are available on the probabilities and payoffs associated with all the possible states of the world relevant to an uncertain situation, it is possible to construct a *contingency matrix*, which is a summary table of the possible payoffs arising from each state of the world.

EXAMPLE

A contingency matrix for a 50-year-old male with hypertension and who smokes is presented in Table 5.1.

Table 5.1 Contingency matrix for 50-year-old male with hypertension and who smokes.

State of the world (disease state)	CHD	Not CHD
Payoff (life expectancy)	60	70
Probability	1/20	19/20

Expected value

The notion of expected value is a general one that arises whenever we are evaluating the possibility of the occurrence of uncertain states of the world. The expected value is the value that occurs *on average*. To find the expected value of an uncertain situation, simply weight the payoff in each state of the world by the probability of that state of the world occurring.

EXAMPLE

The life expectancy of a 50-year-old male with hypertension who smokes depends on what the life expectancy of the individual will be in each state of the world, weighted by the probabilities of each of the different states of the world occurring. In this case, there is a 5 per cent chance that the individual will develop CHD in the next five years, in which case he will have a life expectancy of 60 years, and there is a 95 per cent chance that the individual will not develop CHD in the next five years, in which case he will have a life expectancy of 70 years. Therefore, the average life expectancy of a 50-year-old male with hypertension who smokes is $69\frac{1}{2}$ years (that is, $[60 \times 1/20] + [70 \times 19/20] = 69\frac{1}{2}$)

For a more detailed and general exposition of the notion of expected value, see Appendix 5.1.

Using these key concepts, we may now examine the effects of uncertainty on the market for health care in greater detail. We shall begin by examining the concept of risk.

Risk

In economics, a risky situation is one in which more than one outcome may occur, and the probability of each possible outcome occurring can be estimated.

EXAMPLE

Whether or not a 50-year-old male with hypertension and who smokes will develop CHD in the next five years may be defined as a risky situation.

More generally, in the context of health and health care, individuals often find themselves in situations where the future state of the world is less than perfectly certain, but a probability may be attached to each of the possible outcomes. These situations are therefore risky. In particular, individuals are at risk from incurring large unplanned expenditures on treatment for unexpected illness, which they may not be able to afford.

In the following sections we shall address two key issues related to the problem of uncertainty in the consumption of health care:

1. how individuals may deal with the uncertain nature of ill health;
2. how the presence of uncertainty affects the actions of individuals, and, in particular, how it affects attitudes towards health, ill health and the consumption of health care.

In order to examine how the presence of risk affects our actions and how we deal with the uncertain environment in which we live, it is necessary first to describe an individual's attitude to risk.

Attitudes towards risk

An individual may be classified into one of three groups, which defines their attitude towards risk: they may either be *risk averse*, *risk neutral* or *risk loving*. These attitudes to risk may be described as follows:

1. Risk aversion. A risk averse individual dislikes risk and uncertainty, and will often pay sums of money in order to avoid risky situations.
2. Risk neutrality. A risk neutral individual neither likes nor dislikes risk and uncertainty, but is indifferent to it.
3. Risk loving. A risk loving individual likes risk and uncertainty, and may even pay sums of money in order to enter into risky situations.

Strictly speaking, an individual's attitude towards risk will depend crucially on whether the individual will accept what is known as a *fair gamble*. For a more detailed and general exposition of this notion and of the different attitudes towards risk, see Appendix 5.2.

It is generally assumed that individuals are risk averse. In the context of health and health care, this means that individuals will generally pay money so that their ability to cope with ill health and their ability to afford health care is more certain. We shall see in this and subsequent chapters that these concepts allow us to explain the existence of the National Health Service in the UK where, in return for the payment of a sum of money, individuals are allowed free access to health care services as and when they are required, thus reducing their uncertainty.

Owing to the unexpected nature of ill health it is clearly impossible to entirely remove the uncertainty surrounding future health states. However, it is possible to remove the uncertainty surrounding an individual's ability to cope with future ill health and their ability to pay for health care, should the need for it arise. This may be accomplished with the introduction of *health insurance*.

Health insurance

Uncertainty and risk surrounding the ability of an individual to afford health care may be reduced with the purchase of health insurance.

The nature of health insurance

Health insurance involves the development of an *insurance contract* between insurance companies and individuals who consider themselves to be at risk of ill health. When individuals buy health insurance, they enter into an agreement with an insurance company to pay an agreed price, called an *insurance premium*, in exchange for a payout to be made to the individual by the insurance company should some specific event occur, such as their becoming ill.

Therefore, individuals pay a sum of money to an insurance company on the understanding that if the individuals become ill the insurance company will pay for the treatment that they require. This removes an element of uncertainty arising from the unpredictable nature of ill health, because now individuals are able to afford the health care which they need: whatever the timing of health care expenditure and whatever the amount of expenditure on health care which is required, the individual will be able to afford it, via the insurance company.

Individuals choose to buy insurance because they are risk averse. However, whilst the existence of risk aversion explains why individuals would choose to pay insurance premiums to insurance companies in order to reduce risk, it does not explain why insurance companies choose to sell insurance to individuals. In order to explain this, we use the notion of *risk pooling*.

Risk pooling

Insurance companies are able to offer insurance to individuals who are risk averse by pooling risks across a large number of individuals so that they may confidently predict the number of individuals who will become ill and require health care.

EXAMPLE _____

On average, the probability of a 50-year-old male with hypertension who smokes developing CHD in the next five years is 1/20, or 0.05. Therefore, throughout the entire population, 5 per cent of 50-year-old males with hypertension who smoke will develop CHD in the next five years. However, suppose we randomly choose 100 such males. In this small sample we would expect *on average* that 5 individuals will develop CHD (that is 5 per cent of 100), but *in reality* the actual number may differ from this and may be 4, or 6, or more, or less. The larger we take our sample, the more likely it is that 5 per cent will develop CHD in the next five years. So, with one million 50-year-old males with hypertension who smoke, we may be reasonably confident that around 5 per cent (or 50,000 in this case) would develop CHD.

Therefore, by adding more and more individuals to the sample it is possible to reduce the *spread* or *dispersion* of the average state of the world.

By accepting insurance premiums from large numbers of individuals, an insurance company can thus pool the risks of a large population of individuals becoming ill. In this way the insurance company is able to predict the incidence of ill health and it may be relatively certain of the size of health care expenditure which will be required. The insurance company may then share the costs of health care across all insured individuals. It can do this by collecting insurance premiums from all individuals in a population and paying out benefits only to those who require health care. Therefore, in essence, an insurance company collects a small amount of money from everyone and pays out a large sum of money only to those few individuals who become ill. To do this, the insurance company must collect at least as much money in insurance premiums as it pays out in health care expenditure.

EXAMPLE

Suppose that one million 50-year-old males with hypertension and who smoke would like to be insured against the health care costs which will be incurred should they develop CHD in the next five years. If an individual does develop CHD, the cost of treatment will be £5,000. Each individual pays an insurance premium of £250 giving a total amount of money paid to the insurance company of £250,000,000 (that is, 1,000,000 individuals × £250 each). This sum is to be shared out by the insurance company among those individuals who develop CHD. In this large sample of individuals, let us suppose that the average number do in fact develop CHD, and therefore 50,000 individuals require health care (that is 5 per cent of 1,000,000 individuals). The insurance company distributes the total amount received in insurance premiums among all those individuals who develop CHD in order to pay for their treatment. Therefore, each individual receives £5,000 (that is, £250,000,000/50,000 individuals). This payment covers the cost of treatment for CHD. Therefore, individuals who consider themselves to be at risk of illness can pay a relatively small sum of money (in this case, £250) so that if they do become ill they will receive a much larger sum of money from the insurance company to pay for their treatment (in this case, £5,000).

In summary, health insurance companies accept relatively small insurance premium payments in exchange for a promise to pay a larger sum of money to insured individuals should they require health care. The insurance company can make this promise with a high degree of certainty since it pools its risks over a large number of individuals.

The provision of health insurance is thus determined through the interaction of individuals who wish to buy insurance and insurance companies who wish to sell insurance. Individuals choose to buy insurance because they are risk averse, and insurance companies are able to sell insurance because they are able to pool risks. In this way, health insurance is provided through an *insurance market*.

Just as a market may be used for the distribution of goods and services such as chocolate bars and health care, so there may also be a market for health insurance, where buyers and sellers meet and demand and supply health insurance. In the market for health insurance, individuals, as the consumers, choose whether to buy insurance, and insurance companies, as the providers, choose whether to sell insurance.

As discussed in Chapter 2, the basis of any market is price, and this will define the quantity of a good that is bought and sold. This is also true of insurance markets, where a market price for insurance is derived as the result of the interaction between the demand for and supply of insurance. We shall now examine the interaction of demand and supply and explore the derivation of a market price for health insurance.

In a similar fashion to our general discussion of demand and supply in Chapter 2, we shall examine the demand for health insurance and the supply of health insurance separately. In the following discussion we shall use the term insurance premium to refer to the price of health insurance. Consistent with the assumptions made in Chapter 2, we shall assume that the consumers, individuals who buy health insurance, seek to maximise their total utility, and that the providers, health insurance companies, aim to maximise profit.

Demand for health insurance

To use the general definition of demand provided in Chapter 2, the demand for health insurance is defined as the quantity of health insurance that consumers are willing and able to buy in a specific time period. The demand for health insurance is dependent upon many variables, though the most important factor which will affect the amount of insurance which an individual chooses to buy is the size of the insurance premium.

Using the key concepts outlined above, we shall now calculate the size of the insurance premium that an individual would be willing to pay in order to be insured against treatment costs arising from ill health. To do this, we must first construct a contingency matrix displaying the probabilities and payoffs associated with all the possible states of the world with which an individual might be faced due to the unpredictable nature of ill health (Table 5.2).

Table 5.2 Contingency matrix with and without insurance.

State of the world (disease state)	Not ill	Ill
Payoff if not insured (£)	W	$W - C$
Payoff if insured (£)	$W - R$	$W - R$
Probability	$(1 - p)$	p

An individual has an initial level of wealth, W, which is measured in monetary terms. The probability that the individual will become ill is p, and therefore, the probability that the individual will not become ill is $(1 - p)$.

If individuals decide not to insure against the cost of health care then, should they become ill, individuals will have to pay for their treatment themselves at a cost, C. Therefore, if they are not insured and they become ill the wealth of the individuals will fall to $W - C$. If they are not insured and they do not become ill, then their wealth remains unchanged at W, since they need not incur the costs of treatment.

If individuals decide to take out health insurance, they must pay an insurance premium of size R to the insurance company, so that the insurance company will pay for their health care should they become ill. Therefore, if they are insured and they become ill, individuals will have a level of wealth $W - R$. Similarly, if individuals are insured and do not become ill, they will also have a level of wealth $W - R$, since the insurance premium is paid to the insurance company regardless of whether the individuals become ill.

Therefore, with the introduction of health insurance, individuals have the same level of wealth, $W - R$, regardless of which state of the world occurs (that is, whether or not they become ill). The introduction of health insurance implies not only that the wealth of the individuals is certain because it is the same across all states of the world, but also that there is less risk regarding the ability of individuals to pay for health care.

Using the information from this contingency matrix we can now calculate the insurance premium that an individual would be willing to pay in order to obtain health insurance. In order to do this we use the notion of expected value, as described earlier.

If individuals are not insured then the expected value of their wealth (or their average wealth or expected wealth), $EV(W)$, is defined by weighting the payoff in each state of the world by the probability of that state of the world occurring. Therefore, the expected value of wealth of individuals who are not insured is calculated by weighting the level of wealth if they become ill or not, by the probability of becoming ill or not. This may be calculated using the following formula:

$$EV(W) = [p \times (W - C)] + [(1 - p) \times W] \qquad (5.1)$$

where $p \times (W - C)$ is the probability of becoming ill multiplied by the wealth of individuals if they are not insured and they become ill, and $(1 - p) \times W$ is the probability of individuals not becoming ill multiplied by the wealth of the individual if they are not insured and they do not become ill. This is the level of wealth that the individual will have, on average, if they are not insured.

Equation 5.1 may be rearranged to:

$$EV(W) = [p \times W] - [p \times C] + [W] - [p \times W] \qquad (5.2)$$

Which in turn may be rearranged to:

$$EV(W) = [W] - [p \times C] \qquad (5.3)$$

In this situation, $p \times C$ may be defined as the *expected loss* to individuals if they are not insured. Therefore, $p \times C$ is the amount of health care costs which the individual will pay *on average*. $p \times C$ is also called the *fair premium*.

The fair premium

The fair premium is defined as an insurance premium charged by an insurance company for health insurance which is equal to the amount of wealth that individuals will lose, on average, if they are not insured. The size of the fair premium is denoted by R^F, so that:

$$R^F = p \times C \qquad (5.4)$$

If an individual were to pay the fair premium for health insurance then they would pay an insurance premium exactly equal to the amount which they would lose, on average, if they were not insured. In reality, however, individuals are generally willing to pay more than the fair premium for health insurance because they are risk averse.

Because individuals are risk averse they do not like uncertainty and they are willing to pay for it to be reduced. Risk-averse individuals are therefore often prepared to pay more than the fair premium in order to maximise their utility in this way. On top of the fair premium, risk-averse individuals will also pay what is called a *risk premium*.

The risk premium

A risk premium is defined as a sum of money which individuals are prepared to pay over and above the fair premium so that their risk might be reduced.

Let us suppose that the risk premium which an individual is prepared to pay is some amount of money, denoted by R^R.

Therefore, the total insurance premium which an individual is prepared to pay for health insurance is given by the fair premium plus the risk premium, or:

$$R^F + R^R \qquad (5.5)$$

This defines the amount of money which an individual is prepared to pay for health insurance.

Table 5.3 Contingency matrix with and without insurance for a 50-year-old male with hypertension and who smokes.

State of the world (disease state)	Does not develop CHD	Develops CHD
Payoff if not insured (£)	20,000	15,000
Probability	19/20	1/20

EXAMPLE

Table 5.3 presents a contingency matrix displaying the probabilities and payoffs associated with the states of the world faced by a 50-year-old male with hypertension who smokes. Such an individual has a probability of 1/20, or 0.05, of developing CHD in the next five years, and an initial level of wealth of £20,000. If the individual does develop CHD, then the health care which he requires costs £5,000. Therefore, if this individual does develop CHD and is not insured, his level of wealth will fall to £15,000 (that is £20,000 initial wealth − £5,000 health care costs). If the individual is not insured and does not develop CHD then his level of wealth remains constant at the initial level of £20,000.

Because of the uncertainty surrounding his future level of wealth and whether or not he may have to pay for expensive health care, the individual decides to buy health insurance. Without insurance, the expected loss to the individual is calculated using Equation 5.3, and will be £250 (that is, $p \times C = 0.05 \times £5,000 = £250$), which is the size of health care costs which the individual will pay on average without insurance. From Equation 5.4, we can see that this is the fair premium.

If this were the insurance premium charged by the insurance company, then the individual would pay exactly what his expected loss would be. In fact, the individual would actually be willing to pay more than £250 for health insurance because he is risk averse. In this case, the individual would actually be willing to pay an extra £100 as a risk premium in order to avoid uncertainty. Therefore, from Equation 5.5, the individual would be willing to pay a total of £350 for health insurance (that is, £250 fair premium + £100 risk premium = £350).

We have therefore determined the size of insurance premium that an individual would be willing to pay for health insurance. Now we shall examine the size of the insurance premium that an insurance company would be prepared to offer.

Supply of health insurance

We shall now examine the other side of the health insurance market, which is the supply of health insurance by insurance companies. Using the general definition of supply provided in Chapter 2, the supply of health insurance is the quantity of health insurance that insurance companies wish to offer for sale at a particular insurance premium per time period.

Once individuals are insured, it is the responsibility of the insurance company to pay for their health care should they become ill. Therefore, the total health care expenditure of all individuals who are insured and who become ill is paid by the insurance company. The insurance company is able to do this by risk pooling and estimating the total health care expenditure across all individuals who are insured (that is, by estimating the *total expected health care expenditure*) and then calculating the *average expected health care expenditure per insured individual*. This average expected expenditure per insured individual forms the basis of the insurance premium offered by the insurance company. In summary, the insurance company will supply health insurance at an insurance premium which is determined by spreading the total expected health care expenditure from all individuals who are insured and become ill across the insurance premiums of all individuals who buy insurance.

Let us suppose that the insurance company insures a large number of individuals, *n*. In this case, the total expected health care expenditure by the insurance company on insured individuals who become ill is calculated by multiplying the average health care costs incurred per person by the number of people who are insured. Average health care costs incurred by an individual are $p \times C$ (from Equation 5.3). Therefore, total expected health care expenditure by the insurance company, E, is calculated as follows:

$$E = n \times p \times C \tag{5.6}$$

However, $p{*}C$ is the fair premium (from Equation 5.4). Therefore, Equation 5.6 becomes:

$$E = n \times R^{\mathrm{F}} \tag{5.7}$$

In order to spread this total expected health care expenditure across all individuals who buy insurance, the size of the insurance premium offered to each individual is the total expected health care expenditure paid by the insurance company divided by the total number of individuals who are insured. This is calculated by rearranging Equation 5.7, as follows:

$$E/n = R^{\mathrm{F}} \tag{5.8}$$

E/n is the insurance premium offered by the insurance company, and is, in fact, the fair premium, R^{F}. Therefore, the insurance premium offered by the insurance company is the fair premium.

However, in order to maximise profits, in reality, the insurance company is likely to offer an insurance premium that is higher than this. This is because if the insurance company were to charge only the fair premium for insurance cover then they would make no profit: the insurance company would spend on the health care of insured individuals who become ill exactly the amount of money it receives in insurance premiums from all individuals who are insured. With the assumption of profit maximisation, the insurance company wishes to receive more money from insurance premiums than it spends on health care, and therefore it will actually charge an insurance premium that is higher than the fair premium.

The loading factor

When there is a difference between the fair premium and the actual insurance premium charged by an insurance company it is called *loading* the premium, and a *loading factor* is added to the fair premium.

Let us suppose that the loading factor which an insurance company places on top of the fair premium is some amount of money, L.

The insurance premium which an insurance company is prepared to offer for health insurance is the fair premium plus the loading factor, or:

$$R^F + L \tag{5.9}$$

This is the amount of money which an insurance company is prepared to accept for providing health insurance.

EXAMPLE

Suppose that one million 50-year-old males with hypertension who smoke would like to insure themselves against health care costs which will be incurred if they develop CHD. If an individual does develop CHD, the cost of treatment will be £5,000. The insurance company knows that the probability of one of these individuals developing CHD in the next five years is 0.05 and therefore calculates that the average health care costs incurred by each individual who is insured will be £250 (that is, $0.05 \times £5,000$). For the one million individuals who wish to be insured, the total expected health care expenditure will therefore be £250,000,000 (that is, $£250 \times 1,000,000$ individuals). This amount may be divided across all insured individuals so that each individual pays an insurance premium of £250 (that is, £250,000,000/1,000,000, which is the same as the average expected health care cost per person). From Equation 5.8 we can see that this is the fair premium.

If this were the insurance premium offered by the insurance company, then it would receive in insurance premiums exactly what it expects to pay in total health care expenditure on those insured individuals who develop CHD. In order to maximise profit, the insurance company will therefore actually charge an insurance premium which is greater than this amount. In this case, the insurance company will add an extra £50 as a loading factor. Therefore, from Equation 5.9, the insurance company will offer to provide health insurance for a total of £300 (that is, £250 fair premium + £50 loading factor = £300).

Once the amount of money which an individual is prepared to pay for health insurance and the amount of money which an insurance company is prepared to accept for providing health insurance have been determined, we can incorporate these components together to form a health insurance market.

The market for health insurance

Using the general definition of a market provided in Chapter 2, a health insurance market may be defined as an arrangement in which individuals and insurance companies communicate with each other to buy and sell health insurance. On the demand side of the market there are individuals who wish to buy health insurance, and they do so in such a way so as to maximise their utility. On the supply side of the market there are insurance companies who wish to sell health insurance, and they do so in such a way so as to maximise their profits. Communication in the market for health insurance is made through the medium of insurance premiums.

We may now combine our analyses of the demand and supply of health insurance to show how a market insurance premium is determined. To do this, we use two general results from the analysis of the demand and supply of health insurance above:

1. A risk averse individual will pay a maximum insurance premium of $R^F + R^R$ in order to buy health insurance, where R^F is the fair premium and R^R is the risk premium (Equation 5.5).
2. A profit-maximising insurance company will offer a minimum insurance premium of $R^F + L$ in order to sell health insurance, where R^F is the fair premium and L is the loading factor (Equation 5.9).

Using this information we can see that an insurance contract will develop as long as the amount of money which an individual is prepared to pay on health insurance is equal to or greater than the amount of money which an insurance company is prepared to accept for providing health insurance:

$$(R^F + R^R) \geq (R^F + L) \tag{5.10}$$

In other words, from Equation 5.10 we can see that a contract for health insurance will develop provided the risk premium is greater than or equal to the loading factor:

$$R^R \geq L \tag{5.11}$$

If Equation 5.11 holds, then a health insurance market will exist. This is because if the risk premium is greater than the loading factor then the extra amount of money which a risk-averse individual is prepared to pay in order to reduce uncertainty is greater than the amount of money which an insurance company is prepared to accept in order to make a profit.

In this situation, the individual is willing and able to pay the insurance premium offered by the insurance company, and the insurance company wishes to offer health insurance at an insurance premium which the individual is prepared to pay.

EXAMPLE

A 50-year-old male with hypertension who smokes wishes to buy health insurance to cover the costs of health care should he develop CHD in the next five years. In order to do this he is prepared to pay an insurance premium of up to £350, comprising £250 expected health care costs (the fair premium) and a risk premium of £100.

In order to provide health insurance for 50-year-old males with hypertension who smoke to cover the costs of health care should they develop CHD, an insurance company is prepared to accept a minimum insurance premium of £300, comprising £250 expected health care costs per insured individual (the fair premium) and a loading factor of £50.

The risk premium that individuals are prepared to pay is greater than the loading factor which individuals are prepared to accept (that is, £100 risk premium > £50 loading factor). Therefore, the total amount of money which an individual is prepared to pay for health insurance is greater than the total amount which an insurance company is prepared to accept (that is, £350 > £300). Therefore, a market for health insurance will exist with the development of an insurance contract between the individual and the insurance company.

This analysis shows that there are grounds for an insurance market to exist. Whilst uncertainty might exist in the market for health care, thus reducing the ability of the market to allocate health care resources efficiently, this problem may be addressed with the introduction of health insurance. Unfortunately, a number of problems arise with the introduction of insurance markets in practice which may limit their success in adequately dealing with uncertainty. More specifically, the following problems may be encountered with the introduction of health insurance:

1. adverse selection;
2. moral hazard;
3. non-price competition;
4. affordability of health insurance.

We shall now address each of these issues in turn.

Adverse selection

The problem of adverse selection

In an insurance market, adverse selection may be defined as the phenomenon under which exactly the wrong individuals from the point of view of the insurance company choose to buy insurance. That is, the insurance company gets an *adverse selection* of individuals choosing to buy insurance. In the market for health insurance, adverse selection arises because only individuals with a high risk of illness will choose to buy health insurance.

Only individuals who become ill will gain financially from health insurance. These individuals pay a relatively small insurance premium so that when they become ill the insurance company pays out a much larger sum of money for their health care. Only those individuals at high risk of illness are likely to reap the financial benefits of being insured, since only these individuals will receive money from the insurance company.

Therefore, only individuals with a high risk of illness have a financial incentive to buy health insurance. However, from the perspective of the insurance company, this is exactly the wrong sort of individual to whom the insurance company wishes to supply insurance. Adverse selection therefore arises because only those individuals who expect to benefit from health insurance (that is, those at high risk of illness) will choose to buy insurance.

If individuals have a low risk of illness and believe they will not become ill then they may refrain from buying health insurance because they believe they are unlikely to need health care and so are also unlikely to need money from an insurance company to pay for their treatment.

Adverse selection arises because of the *asymmetry of information* between individuals who wish to buy insurance, who often know whether they are at high risk of becoming ill, and the insurance company, who do not know the risk a specific individual has of becoming ill.

Adverse selection and community rating

Insurance companies pool risks across large numbers of insured individuals. The problem of adverse selection arises because insurance companies base their assessment of the risk of an individual becoming ill on the broad experience of the whole population, which includes both high-risk and low-risk individuals. This is known as *community rating*, where insurance premiums are calculated on the basis of average expected health care expenditure across large numbers of the population. Therefore, any individual who feels that the probability of their needing health care is greater than that on which the insurance company is assessing them (that is, individuals with a high risk of illness) will have an added incentive to insure.

The problem of adverse selection may mean that insurance companies are unable to provide health insurance to all individuals who would otherwise wish to buy it.

Suppose a population consisting of a total number of n individuals. This population is divided into two groups. One group of individuals has a high risk of illness, and the other group has a low risk of illness. The number of individuals in the high-risk group is n^H, and the number of individuals in the low-risk group is n^L, and all individuals in the population fall into one of these two groups (that is, $n = n^L + n^H$).

All individuals in the population consider whether to buy health insurance. Each risk group has an insurance premium associated with it which is the maximum amount that individuals in that group are willing to pay for health insurance. The insurance premium which high-risk individuals are willing to pay is R^H, and the insurance premium which low-risk individuals are willing to pay is R^L. It is the case that R^H is greater than R^L (that is, $R^H > R^L$).

Whilst each individual knows which group they are in (that is, whether they are high or low risk), the insurance company does not and is unable to ascertain the risk group of any particular individual. However, what the insurance company does know is the *number* of individuals in each risk group.

Given this limited information, the insurance company will use a system of community rating to derive the insurance premium to be offered to each individual in the population. Because of the information which the insurance company lacks regarding the risk of individuals in the population, the same insurance premium will be offered to both high-risk and low-risk groups.

The insurance premium offered by the insurance company using community rating, R^C, is calculated as follows:

$$R^C = [(n^H / n) \times R^H] + [(n^L / n) \times R^L] \tag{5.12}$$

Using Equation 5.12, the insurance premium calculated using community rating is *greater than* the insurance premium which low-risk individuals are willing to pay, but *less than* the insurance premium which high-risk individuals are willing to pay (that is, $R^H > R^C > R^L$). Therefore, high-risk individuals must pay less than the insurance premium they are willing to pay (since $R^C < R^H$), and low-risk individuals must pay more than the insurance premium they are willing to pay (since $R^C > R^L$). Therefore, if the insurance company supplies health insurance at an insurance premium R^C, individuals in the low-risk group will *not buy* health insurance since the premium asked for by the insurance company is greater than that which they are willing to pay.

In other words, individuals in the low-risk group will choose not to buy insurance at the community rate insurance premium, R^C. The community rate insurance premium is attractive *only* to high-risk individuals.

So, the only people who are willing to buy insurance in this case are those at high risk. These are exactly the individuals that the insurance company does not want to sell health insurance to, since, because they are at high risk, these individuals are likely to become ill and so require the insurance company to pay for their health care. This is the problem of adverse selection, where, from the perspective of the insurance company, exactly the wrong individuals choose to buy health insurance.

If individuals at low risk of illness choose not to buy health insurance then the insurance company will no longer be able to afford to pay for the health care of those individuals who are insured and become ill. This is because the insurance company calculates the community rate insurance premium on the assumption that both high-risk and low-risk individuals will purchase insurance.

Therefore, the community rate insurance premium must be altered to allow for this change in circumstances. This will mean that R^C will increase. However, this will have the consequence that even more people will choose not to buy insurance, because the new community rate premium will be more than they are willing to pay. Thus, R^C will have to rise again so that the insurance company will cover its costs once more. This process will continue until the community rate converges on the premium acceptable only to high-risk groups (that is, when $R^C = R^H$).

This will ultimately result in a situation where the insurance company will provide health insurance at a premium of R^H, which is acceptable only to those individuals at high risk of illness The insurance market will fail to provide health insurance for low-risk individuals.

EXAMPLE _____

Suppose a population of one hundred 50-year-old males who wish to insure themselves against the health care costs which will be incurred should they develop CHD in the next five years. If an individual does develop CHD, the cost of treatment will be £5,000.

Fifty of these 50-year-old males have hypertension and smoke, and the probability of these individuals developing CHD in the next five years is 1/20, or 0.05. These individuals would be willing to pay £250 for health insurance. The other fifty individuals do not have hypertension and do not smoke, and so the probability of these individuals developing CHD in the next five years is much less at 1/100, or 0.01. These individuals would be willing to pay only £50 for health insurance.

The insurance company offers an insurance premium to these individuals calculated on the basis of community rating. Using Equation 5.12 this community rate is calculated to be £150 (that is, $[(50/100) \times £250] + [(50/100) \times £50] = [\frac{1}{2} \times £250] + [\frac{1}{2} \times £50] = [£125] + [£25] = £150$).

An insurance premium of £150 will seem excessive to those individuals who do not have hypertension and who do not smoke and who are only willing to pay £50 for health insurance. These individuals will therefore not buy health insurance, and the insurance company is left with only those individuals with hypertension who smoke willing to pay the insurance premium.

However, the average expected health care expenditure on those individuals at high risk is the probability of illness multiplied by the cost of treatment, which is £250 (that is, $0.05 \times £5,000$). Therefore, for every individual who buys insurance, the insurance company expects to pay an average of £250 on health care, but the insurance company only receives £150 in insurance premiums at the community rate. Therefore, the insurance company will lose money. The insurance premium will therefore be increased, thus making it unacceptable to individuals at lower risks of developing CHD.

Adverse selection and experience rating

Rather than basing insurance premiums on community rating, the problem of adverse selection may be solved if the insurance company is able to employ a system of *experience rating*. Experience rating occurs when the insurance company is able to identify different risk groups so that it can set a different insurance premium for each.

Adverse selection arises because of the *asymmetry of information* between individuals who wish to buy insurance, who often know whether they are at high risk of becoming ill, and the insurance company, who do not know the risk a specific individual has of becoming ill. Because of this informational asymmetry, the insurance company must employ a system of community rating where an insurance premium is offered equally to all individuals. If this problem of informational asymmetry may be overcome so that the insurance company is able to determine the risk status of an individual wishing to buy health insurance, then experience rating is possible.

Again suppose a population divided into two groups, one of which has a high risk of illness, and another which has a low risk of illness. The maximum insurance premium which high-risk individuals are willing to pay is R^H, and the maximum insurance premium which low-risk individuals are willing to pay is R^L. With a system of experience rating, the insurance company is able to maximise profits by setting an insurance premium of R^H for individuals in the high-risk group, and an insurance premium of R^L is set for individuals in the low-risk group. In this case, all individuals will choose to buy health insurance, though they are paying the maximum they are willing to pay.

EXAMPLE

A population of 50-year-old males may be divided into those with hypertension who smoke and those who do not have hypertension and who do not smoke. Both of these two groups of individuals wish to insure themselves against the health care costs which will be incurred should they develop CHD in the next five years.

For 50-year-old males with hypertension who smoke, the probability of developing CHD in the next five years is 1/20, or 0.05. These individuals would be willing to pay £250 for health insurance. For 50-year-old males without hypertension and who do not smoke, the probability of developing CHD in the next five years is 1/100, or 0.01. These individuals would be willing to pay £50 for health insurance.

The insurance company is able to distinguish between high-risk and low-risk individuals and subsequently offers a different insurance premium to each: to 50-year-old males with hypertension who smoke the insurance company offers an insurance premium of £250, and to 50-year-old males without hypertension who do not smoke the insurance company offers an insurance premium of £50.

All individuals choose to buy health insurance.

Moral hazard

The problem of moral hazard

Health insurance changes the economic incentives facing both the consumers and providers of health care. One manifestation of these changes is the existence of *moral hazard*, which is a problem of *excess use*. Applied to health care, the existence of moral hazard implies an excessive use of limited health care resources. This problem affects both the consumers and providers of health care.

Consumer moral hazard

The effect of health insurance is to reduce the price of health care to the individual from the market price to zero. Having paid the insurance premium, the individual receives all services covered by the insurance contract at zero cost, at the expense of the insurance company. This introduces a problem of excess use, where each individual has an incentive to obtain as much health care as possible, or at least not to limit their consumption in any way.

Therefore, consumer moral hazard exists because individuals who buy insurance have an incentive to bring about additional benefits to themselves at the expense of the insurance company. Therefore, more health care expenditure will be incurred by an insurance company on behalf of an individual with insurance than would be incurred by that same individual without insurance.

The problem of consumer moral hazard arises because, as we have seen on examination of the theory of demand in Chapter 2, it is perfectly rational for individuals to increase consumption in response to a lower price. This is exactly the temptation perceived by those individuals who purchase health insurance.

Whether the problem of consumer moral hazard will be observed in practice is uncertain since it seems unlikely that, given the intrinsic unpleasantness of illness and treatment of illness, an individual would choose either to put themselves at greater risk of illness or obtain more health care just because any treatment they required would be paid for by a health insurance company. Nevertheless, for some minor ailments an individual may choose to obtain health care which they would not have sought had they been uninsured. In this way, use of health care may be deemed frivolous or unnecessary. An example might be an individual who experiences muscle pain consequent to long periods of exercise. Normally the individual would not think to see a physiotherapist since the financial cost would be high and so not worthwhile. However, if physiotherapy were available via a health insurance scheme the individual might choose to obtain treatment.

Producer moral hazard

As we have seen in Chapter 3, under certain circumstances, providers of health care may seek to bring about a level of demand for their services which is greater than the level that would be demanded if consumers of health care were fully informed. This situation, known as supplier-induced demand, is a form of moral hazard and may arise if an insurance company is financing the provision of health care rather than the patient, because providers then have little incentive to moderate the amount of health care they supply. In the knowledge that its patients are insured, a health care provider may buy expensive medical equipment, and use medical and nursing staff inefficiently, and get reimbursed for these unnecessary expenses by the insurance company. This is an example of producer moral hazard.

Therefore, the introduction of health insurance leaves health care providers without the usual mechanism of consumer demand as a cost control.

Deductibles and coinsurance

Two methods which may be used to address the problem of moral hazard are the use of *deductibles* (or user charges) and *coinsurance* (or copayment):

1. A deductible requires an individual to pay for a certain amount of health care received before the insurance comes into effect. This is designed to deter reliance on insurance for the payment of minor illnesses. A deductible of £100 would mean that whenever an individual requires health care, the first £100 worth of treatment would be paid by the individual. The remainder of the expenditure on any required treatment which costs more than £100 would be paid by the insurance company.
2. Coinsurance requires the individual to pay a certain fraction of each £1 spent on their health care by the insurance company, with the insurance company paying the remainder. A coinsurance rate of 25 per cent would mean that for every £1 which is spent on an individual's health care, the individual pays £0.25 and the insurance company pays £0.75.

The introduction of both deductibles and coinsurance is likely to reduce the problem of moral hazard. However, both of these measures also increase the cost of health care to the individual. Left unchecked, the introduction of these measures may limit the extent to which individuals earning lower incomes are able to obtain the health care they need.

Non-price competition

The introduction of a market for health insurance may have a perverse effect on the market for health care. The picture we have been building of the health care market as a means of allocating scarce resources depends upon there being competition between providers, who compete on the basis of price in order to attract the custom of patients. In Chapter 3 we saw that for a market to allocate health care resources efficiently, health care providers, wishing to maximise profits, must compete for the custom of consumers and supply the health care that is most highly valued by consumers *at least cost*. In this way, the well-being of consumers is maximised at the least cost to society, and health care resources are allocated efficiently.

However, with the introduction of health insurance it is unlikely that providers would supply health care at least cost, nor is there any incentive for them to do so. This is because price is no longer important to patients. The effect of health insurance is to reduce the price of health care to the individual from the market price to zero. Therefore, having paid the insurance premium, the individual receives all services covered by the insurance contract at zero cost, at the expense of the insurance company.

Since health care is then in effect free, patients will choose the health care provider from whom they receive treatment *not* on the basis of price but, instead, on the basis of other non-price factors. Therefore, *non-price competition* will emerge, where health care providers must compete for the custom of patients on the basis of factors such as comfort, the pleasantness of surroundings and the quality of the food, rather than price. This will result in a situation where costs will *increase* in the health care market rather than decrease as standard economic theory predicts. Inevitably, resources will not be allocated efficiently since scarce money will be used to pay for, for example, colour televisions for patients rather than nurses.

Affordability of health insurance

The effect of health insurance is to reduce the price of health care to the individual from the market price to zero. Having paid the insurance premium, the individual receives all services covered by the insurance contract at no cost, at the expense of the insurance company. Whilst this protects individuals from catastrophic expenditure arising from the unpredictable nature of illness it still relies on individuals being able to afford health insurance premiums in the first place.

Some individuals in the population would find it difficult to afford health insurance, even if it were charged at only the fair premium rate with no additional loading factor. Specifically, such groups might include:

1. individuals earning low incomes, who do not earn enough money to be able to afford the fair premium;
2. individuals at very high risk of illness, for whom either no health insurance cover is available or the probability of illness approaches one and so the fair premium equals the full cost of treatment, which is unaffordable. (From Equation 5.4, for individuals at very high risk of illness, the probability of illness p tends towards one [that is, $p = 1$]. Therefore, $p \times C$ equals the cost of treatment C [that is, $p \times C = 1 \times C = C$], and the fair premium R^F becomes equal to the cost of treatment [that is, $R^F = C$], which is unaffordable.)

Indeed, certain individuals in society often earn only low incomes and also have a very high risk of illness, which exacerbates the problem. Such a group of individuals might include the elderly who may receive only a limited pension and yet have a very high probability of illness. For these individuals, health insurance may not be an affordable option.

The role of health insurance

In this chapter we have addressed two key issues relating to the problem of uncertainty in the consumption of health care:

1. how individuals may deal with the uncertain nature of ill health;
2. how the presence of uncertainty affects the actions of individuals, and, in particular, how it affects attitudes towards health, ill health and the consumption of health care.

First, we have seen how individuals deal with uncertainty surrounding both the timing of health care expenditure and the amount of expenditure on health care which is required. Health insurance markets develop between individuals and insurance companies where, in return for an insurance premium, the insurance company agrees to pay for the health care of the insured individual should they become ill. This allows the individual to cope financially with unexpected illness and potentially catastrophic health care expenditure.

Secondly, we have seen how the presence of risk and uncertainty affects the actions of individuals, and how they affect the consumption of health care. Attitudes towards risk affect the quantity of health insurance which an individual chooses to buy, and risk-averse individuals will be willing to pay extra sums of money so that their uncertainty might be reduced. Having paid an insurance premium, the individual receives all services covered by the insurance contract at zero cost, at the expense of the insurance company. Whilst the benefits of free health care are clear, this also introduces a number of potential problems such as adverse selection and moral hazard which affect how individuals act, and which may affect the ability of the health insurance market to function properly.

The existence of adverse selection, moral hazard, non-price competition and increasing costs and the inability to afford insurance premiums are likely to influence the effect that health insurance will have on the market for health care. Ultimately, these problems may mean that health insurance markets are flawed as a means of coping with the uncertainty in the incidence of ill health. Instead, the basic health insurance system may need to be modified and refined so that it might better cope with these problems, and so that it might better accommodate the incentives which health insurance has on the provision and consumption of health care.

Therefore, in the following chapter we shall explore a number of variations on the basic health insurance system outlined in this chapter. We shall see that the concepts discussed above allow us to explain the existence of the National Health Service in the UK where, in return for the payment of a sum of money, individuals are allowed free access to health care services as and when they are required, thus alleviating the problems associated with uncertainty in the health care market.

Appendix 5.1

Expected value

Suppose that the value of some variable X depends on the final state of the world that occurs. The expected value of X is the value of X that occurs *on average*. To find the expected value of X, weight the payoff from X in each state by the probability of that state of the world occurring. Suppose that there are two possible states of the world which may occur, that the payoff from X in state of the world 1 is X_1 and that the payoff from X in state of the world 2 is X_2. If the probability of state of the world 1 occurring is p, then the expected value of X ($EV[X]$) is given by:

$$EV(X) = [p \times X_1] + [(1 - p) \times X_2]$$

The expected value is therefore the sum of the payoff in each possible state of the world weighted by the probability that that state of the world will occur. Therefore, if there are n possible states of the world, and each state i has a payoff X_i and a probability of occurring p_i, then the expected value of X ($EV[X]$) is given by:

$$EV(X) = (p_1 \times X_1) + (p_2 \times X_2) + ... + (p_n \times X_n)$$

or, alternatively:

$$EV(X) = \sum_{i=1}^{n} (p_i \times X_i)$$

where 'Σ' means 'sum of'. Note that if all the possible n states of the world are correctly considered, it will be the case that:

$$p_1 + p_2 + ... + p_n = 1$$

or, alternatively:

$$\sum_{i=1}^{n} p_i = 1$$

This implies that it is certain that one of the states of the world will occur.

Appendix 5.2

Attitudes towards risk

Begg *et al.* (1994) argue that a risky situation has two characteristics: the likely outcome and the degree of variation in all the possible outcomes.

Suppose an individual is offered a 50 per cent chance of winning £10 and a 50 per cent chance of losing £10. On average the individual would expect to make no money, since the expected value of this gamble is zero (that is, $[+10 \times \frac{1}{2}] + [-10 \times \frac{1}{2}] = [+5] + [-5] = 0$). A gamble such as this, with an expected value of zero is called a *fair gamble*. A fair gamble is therefore one which, on average, will make exactly zero profit.

In contrast, suppose an alternative situation: the individual is offered a 25 per cent chance of winning £10 and a 75 per cent chance of losing £10. This is an *unfair gamble*. On average, an individual involved in such gambles will lose money. In this case, the expected value is negative and the individual will lose £5 on average (that is, $[+10 \times \frac{1}{4}] + [-10 \times \frac{3}{4}] = [+2\frac{1}{2}] + [-7\frac{1}{2}] = -5$).

Now suppose these chances of winning and losing are reversed so that the individual has a 75 per cent chance of winning £10 and a 25 per cent chance of losing £10. We can now say that this gamble is *favourable*, since on average the gamble is expected to be profitable. In this case, the expected value of the gamble is positive and the individual will gain £5 on average (that is, $[+10 \times \frac{3}{4}] + [-10 \times \frac{1}{4}] = [+7\frac{1}{2}] + [-2\frac{1}{2}] = +5$).

Now suppose an individual may choose between a gamble offering a 50 per cent chance of winning or losing £10, and a gamble with a 50 per cent chance of winning or losing £200. Both of these gambles are fair gambles, since the expected value is zero in each case (that is, $[+10 \times \frac{1}{2}] + [-10 \times \frac{1}{2}] = [+5] + [-5] = 0$, and $[+200 \times \frac{1}{2}] + [-200 \times \frac{1}{2}] = [+100] + [-100] = 0$). Therefore, on average, both these gambles will have the same result. However, the second gamble is *riskier* because, depending on the outcome, the individual will either do better or worse since the range of possible outcomes is greater.

These are the types of gambles, or risky situations, which are available. Now we can examine individuals' tastes towards these risks. Economists generally classify individuals into one of three groups: *risk averse*; *risk neutral*; and *risk loving*. This classification defines an individual's attitude to risk. The attitude towards risk of an individual will depend crucially on whether or not the individual will accept a fair gamble. We shall examine each group in turn.

1. Risk aversion

A risk-averse individual will *refuse* a fair gamble. This does not mean that they will never bet, only that the chance of winning needs to be sufficiently favourable so that the probable monetary gain from the gamble will overcome the dislike of risk. The more risk averse the individual, the more favourable the chances of winning must be.

2. Risk neutrality

A risk-neutral individual is *indifferent* between accepting and not accepting a fair gamble. A risk-neutral individual will only accept a gamble if it will yield a profit on average. Therefore, a risk-neutral individual will refuse a gamble where on average the expectation is to lose.

3. Risk loving

A risk-loving individual will *accept* a fair gamble, and will bet even when the chances of winning are unfavourable. The more risk loving an individual, the more unfavourable the chances of winning must be before the individual will not bet.

It is generally assumed that individuals are risk averse and, therefore, that they will not accept a fair gamble.

References

Begg D., Fischer S. and Dornbusch R. (1994) *Economics*. Fourth edition. London: McGraw-Hill, p. 236.
Parkin M. and King D. (1995) *Economics*. Ontario: Addison-Wesley, p. 460.

Suggested further reading

For an examination of insurance markets in general, and a discussion of the problems associated with insurance, see one of the following:

Begg D., Fischer S. and Dornbusch R. (1994) *Economics*. Fourth edition. London: McGraw-Hill, pp. 236–41.
Parkin M. and King D. (1995) *Economics*. Ontario: Addison-Wesley, pp. 460–70.

For a discussion of the relationship between health, health care and health insurance see:

Besley T. (1991) The demand for health care and health insurance. In: McGuire A., Fenn P. and Mayhew K. (eds.) *Providing health care: the economics of alternative systems of finance and delivery*. Oxford: Oxford University Press.

For methods for addressing the problem of adverse selection see:

Sloan F. (1992) Adverse selection: does it preclude a competitive health insurance market? *Journal of Health Economics* 11: 353–6.

For a discussion of health insurance and moral hazard see:

Friedman L.S. (1984) *Microeconomic policy analysis*. New York: McGraw-Hill, pp. 225–32.

6 Financing health care

In this chapter we examine different methods of financing, or paying for, health care. Alternative methods for structuring health care finance are examined, and the key features of each are presented. Potential problems associated with each method are also discussed, and an example is provided of a health care system where each option is used. The health care finance system in various countries is then examined and particular attention is paid to the economic incentives facing patients, GPs and hospitals.

Summary

1. There are a number of possible deviations from the basic health insurance model, and there are advantages and disadvantages associated with each. Six possible options are: direct out-of-pocket payment; private health insurance; Preferred Provider Organisations; Health Maintenance Organisations; public health insurance; and direct taxation.

2. It is the responsibility of the insurance company to pay for the health care required by insured individuals should they become ill. We therefore say that a third party payer is responsible for financing or paying for health care, rather than the patient. The introduction of health insurance therefore leads to a system of third party payment.

3. Third party payment may represent the introduction of two different types of third party payer responsible for paying for the health care of insured individuals: private insurance companies and governments.

4. Health care professionals may be paid by one of three basic methods: fee-for-service reimbursement; reimbursement by salary; and reimbursement by capitation.

5. Health care institutions may be paid either by retrospective reimbursement or by prospective payment. Prospective reimbursement to health care institutions may take one of two forms: global budgeting and prospectively set costs per case by diagnosis related groups (DRGs).

6. The effectiveness of methods for financing health care may be described in terms of their ability to cope with the following problems: catastrophic expenditure; no choice of providers by consumers of health care; adverse selection; consumer and producer moral hazard; non-price competition; and affordability of insurance premiums.

7. In reality the burden of paying health insurance premiums is often shared between individuals and their employers, where the employer pays a proportion of the insurance premium.

8. Direct out-of-pocket payment relates to a charge made to the individual who receives health care for the treatment received. Payment is made at the point of health care service use. This system of financing health care therefore captures exactly the features of the market framework where, for a price, health care providers supply health care to individuals who require treatment, and these individuals meet the full cost of treatment at their own expense.

9. Private health insurance involves an insurance contract between private insurance companies and individuals who consider themselves to be at risk of ill health. Individuals pay an insurance premium in exchange for the insurance company paying for treatment for the individual should they become ill. There is some degree of competition between private insurance companies for the custom of individuals.

10. Preferred Provider Organisations are a derivative of private health insurance, where individuals pay an insurance premium in exchange for the insurance company paying for treatment for individuals should they become ill. Private insurance companies contract selectively with certain health care providers (the Preferred Provider Organisations), and agree to channel individuals which they insure to these providers in return for lower fees charged for health care provided.

11. The main feature of a Health Maintenance Organisation is that the insurance company and the health care provider merge so that they become, in effect, the same organisation. There is, therefore, integration between the insurance company and the health care provider, and the Health Maintenance Organisation provides health care for the individual in return for an insurance premium, rather than just paying for it.

12. With the introduction of public health insurance, an individual has the opportunity to purchase health insurance from only one insurance company, which is the government. There is therefore no competition between insurance companies, because only one exists. Since the government is the only insurance company, it has considerable power over health care providers regarding rates of pay for health care performed on behalf of insured individuals.

13. Direct taxation systems are a derivative of public health insurance where the role of the insurance company is again played solely by the government. Health

insurance is compulsory and all individuals are required to pay insurance premiums to the government. Insurance premiums are collected through taxation and therefore the contribution by individuals to the government for their compulsory health insurance is part of their total tax payment.

Modifying the basic health insurance model

In the previous chapter we have seen how problems arising from the existence of uncertainty in the market for health care may be addressed with the introduction of health insurance.

Because of the potentially devastating effects of uncertainty surrounding the timing and size of expenditure on health care, most countries in the developed world provide health care through the operation of some form of health insurance market covering the provision of some if not all health care. Unfortunately, as we have seen in the previous chapter, whilst health insurance may be successful in reducing uncertainty it also introduces a number of other problems which may affect the efficient allocation of health care resources. In light of these problems, a number of different forms of health insurance system have developed, though each of these is a modification of the basic health insurance model presented in Chapter 5. It is the objective of this chapter to examine the possible deviations from the basic health insurance model and to ascertain the advantages and disadvantages associated with each.

Six options will be discussed in turn:

1. direct out-of-pocket payment;
2. private health insurance;
3. Preferred Provider Organisations;
4. Health Maintenance Organisations;
5. public health insurance;
6. direct taxation.

Whilst many derivations of the basic health insurance model exist, these six options will be examined because all health care systems conform to one or more of these basic structures. Initially, each option will be reduced to its simplest form in order that its key features might be determined.

Before proceeding to analyse each of these options in turn it is useful to first clarify a number of related concepts, namely:

1. third party payment;
2. reimbursing health care providers;
3. the effectiveness of methods of financing health care;
4. paying insurance premiums.

Third party payment

A market is said to exist in any situation where buyers and sellers meet. Therefore, in the basic market for health care, only two parties are involved: consumers of health care, or buyers, and providers of health care, or sellers. However, with the development of an insurance market a *third party* is introduced into the health care market, namely, an insurance company.

Once an individual has paid an insurance premium to the insurance company, that individual is insured. It is then the responsibility of the insurance company to pay for the health care required by the individual should they become ill. Therefore, with the introduction of health insurance, a *third party payer* is responsible for financing or paying for health care, rather than the patient. In this way, the introduction of health insurance results in a system of *third party payment*.

In Chapter 5, the third party payer of health care was simply called an insurance company. However, in reality, a system of third party payment may represent the introduction of two different types of third party payer responsible for paying for the health care of insured individuals:

1. private insurance companies;
2. governments.

As we shall see later in this chapter, there are advantages and disadvantages associated with both types of third party payer.

Reimbursing health care providers

The method of reimbursement refers to the way in which health care providers are paid. It is important to distinguish between reimbursement methods since these are likely to have different effects on the manner in which health care is provided. Specifically, the method of reimbursement is likely to affect both the quantity and the quality of health care provided to patients. It is helpful to distinguish between two types of health care provider and discuss methods for their reimbursement separately:

1. reimbursing health care professionals;
2. reimbursing health care institutions.

Reimbursing health care professionals

Theoretically, health care professionals may be paid by any one of three basic methods: fee-for-service; salary; and capitation. In reality, however, health care professionals may be paid by any combination of these for the different types of service that they provide.

1. Fee-for-service reimbursement

In the UK, fee-for-service reimbursement commonly applies to general practitioners (GPs) and doctors working in private practice. If health care professionals are paid on a fee-for-service basis then they receive payment for each individual item of health care provided. Therefore, fee-for-service reimbursement would imply that GPs, for example, are paid according to the volume of services that they provide. Remuneration on this basis provides both an opportunity and a financial incentive to induce demand and to increase income. If GPs were paid in such a way that they would obtain more income if they increased the services they provide, then they would have a financial incentive to overprovide those services so that their income might be increased.

2. Reimbursement by salary

In the UK, payment by salary commonly applies to nurses and to hospital doctors working in the National Health Service (NHS). If health care professionals are paid on a salaried basis this implies they will receive the same income regardless of the quantity of health care they provide. In this case, there is no incentive to increase the services which are provided and induce demand, since no financial rewards will be received for doing so. Instead, there is a financial incentive to *underprovide* services and to provide *low-quality* care. For example, if nurses receive the same income regardless of the amount of work they do and regardless of the effort which they put into that work, then they have a financial incentive to provide only the bare minimum of services and to provide health care which is of low quality and thus requires less effort. Therefore, with salary payment systems, the potential problems are not of overprovision and demand inducement, but rather of underprovision and poor quality.

3. Reimbursement by capitation

In the UK, GPs receive part of their funding through capitation payments. With reimbursement on a capitation basis, payment is made according to the number of patients registered with each GP. The income of GPs paid in this way therefore depends on the number of patients which they make themselves available to see: the more patients which are registered with an individual GP, the greater that GP's income will be. This method of payment provides an incentive for GPs to increase the number of patients who are registered with them. Whilst this may lead to utilisation levels with which the GPs are unable to cope, it also has a positive effect because GPs are likely to attract patients only if they provide high-quality health care.

Reimbursing health care institutions

Institutions that provide health care may be paid either retrospectively or pro-spectively. To analyse in greater detail the distinction between these two reimburse-ment methods, and to examine the financial incentives associated with each, we shall concentrate specifically on the payment of hospitals.

1. Retrospective reimbursement

Retrospective reimbursement implies not only that hospitals are paid *after* they have provided treatment, but also that the *size* of the payment is determined after treatment is provided. Retrospective reimbursement for hospitals is similar to fee-for-service payment for individual health care professionals in that this method of payment requires those paying for health care to pay the hospital for all expenditures incurred when treating the patient. Therefore, hospitals are paid according to the costs incurred when treating patients and on the volume of services that they provide. Payment on this basis gives exactly the same incentive that fee-for-service payment provides to health care professionals: a financial incentive to overprovide health care so that the income of the hospital might be increased.

2. Prospective payment

Prospective payment implies that the amount of money that a hospital is paid is decided in advance *before* the patient receives treatment. Prospective reimbursement does not necessarily imply that the hospital *receives* the payment in advance, only that the *size* of the payment is determined in advance. With this reimbursement method, payment is not directly related to the actual costs incurred by the hospital when treating patients. Prospective reimbursement to hospitals may take one of two forms: *global budgeting* and *prospectively set costs per case*.

With global budgeting in its simplest form, the overall budget which the hospital spends on treating patients is determined in advance, though the manner in which that budget is dispersed throughout the hospital on individual treatment cases is not.

With prospectively set costs per case, the amount to be paid for treatment is determined in advance by *diagnostic related groups (DRGs)*, where each individual treatment case is allocated a cost before the treatment is provided. Therefore, payment is determined in advance on the basis of individual cases.

With both forms of prospective payment, problems exist with regard to the financial incentives to underprovide health care and to provide health care of low quality. The hospital receives the same income regardless of whether the treatment be high quality or low quality, and it therefore has a financial incentive to provide low-quality care using the minimum amount of effort and incurring the minimum costs.

The effectiveness of methods of financing health care

The different methods of financing health care discussed in this chapter will be described in terms of their ability to cope with various problems which may impede the success of each method in allocating health care resources efficiently. These potential problems are as follows:

1. catastrophic expenditure;
2. no choice of providers by consumers of health care;
3. adverse selection;
4. moral hazard;
5. non-price competition;
6. affordability of insurance premiums.

Catastrophic expenditure

Health care expenditure may be catastrophic if it is necessary for individuals to spend large amounts of income on health care as a result of unexpected illness. Either individuals may be unable to afford this expenditure and so go without the health care which they need, or they may be able to afford the required health care but only at the expense of the consumption of other important goods and services, such as food and clothing. Therefore, the ability of individuals to cope with catastrophic health care expenditure may help to provide some evidence as to whether health care is financed in a way which is acceptable to society.

No choice of providers by consumers of health care

A further way of distinguishing between different methods of financing health care is by the amount of freedom that patients have in choosing the provider of their health care. For example, a financing system which allowed no choice as to where patients received treatment might be unacceptable to those patients who are dissatisfied with their health care provider yet who are unable to change.

Adverse selection

Adverse selection is defined as the phenomenon under which exactly the wrong individuals from the point of view of the insurance company choose to buy health insurance. This occurs because of the asymmetry of information between individuals who wish to buy insurance, who often know whether they are at high risk of becoming ill, and the insurance company, which does not know the risk a specific individual has of becoming ill.

Because of this informational asymmetry, insurance companies generally charge a community rate insurance premium, whereby the same insurance premium is charged to all individuals for health insurance regardless of their risk. However, only individuals with a high risk of illness have a financial incentive to buy health insurance charged at a community rate. Adverse selection arises because only those individuals who expect to benefit from health insurance (that is, those at high risk of illness) will choose to buy insurance. If individuals have a low risk of illness and believe they will not become ill then they may refrain from buying health insurance charged at the community rate insurance premium since they are unlikely to need health care and so are also unlikely to need money from an insurance company to pay for their treatment. Therefore, because of adverse selection, low-risk individuals may not buy the amount of health insurance which otherwise they would like. This will compromise the ability of these individuals to cope with catastrophic health care expenditure.

Moral hazard

Consumer moral hazard

Having paid an insurance premium, individuals receive all services covered by the insurance contract at zero cost, at the expense of the insurance company. Therefore, the effect of health insurance is to reduce the price of health care to patients from the market price to zero. This may introduce a problem of excess use where each individual has an incentive to obtain as much health care as possible, or at least not to limit their consumption in any way. Therefore, more health care expenditure will be incurred by an insurance company on behalf of an individual with health insurance than would be incurred by that same individual without insurance. This is the problem of consumer moral hazard.

Producer moral hazard

Under certain circumstances, providers of health care may seek to bring about a level of demand for their services which is greater than the level that would be demanded if consumers of health care were fully informed. This situation, known as supplier-induced demand, may arise because an insurance company is financing the provision of health care rather than the patient, and so providers have little incentive to moderate the amount of health care that they supply. Therefore, in the knowledge that its patients are insured, a health care provider may buy expensive medical equipment, and use medical and nursing staff inefficiently, and get reimbursed for this frivolous expenditure by the insurance company. This is the problem of producer moral hazard.

Non-price competition

With the introduction of health insurance it is unlikely that providers will supply health care at least cost, nor is there any incentive for them to do so, since price is no longer important to patients.

The effect of health insurance is to reduce the price of health care to the individual from the market price to zero. Therefore, having paid the insurance premium, the individual receives all services covered by the insurance contract at zero cost, at the expense of the insurance company. Since health care is therefore in effect free, patients will choose a health care provider not on the basis of price but, instead, on the basis of other non-price factors. In this case, non-price competition will emerge, where health care providers compete for the custom of patients on the basis of factors such as comfort, the pleasantness of surroundings and the quality of the food. This may result in a situation where costs will increase in the health care market and scarce resources will not be allocated efficiently.

Affordability of insurance premiums

Whilst the introduction of health insurance protects individuals from catastrophic expenditure, it still relies on individuals being able to afford health insurance premiums in the first place. Certain groups in the population, such as those earning low incomes, those at very high risk of illness, and the elderly, may find it difficult to afford health insurance. If these individuals are unable to buy health insurance then their ability to cope with unexpected illness will be impeded.

Paying insurance premiums

In Chapter 5 it was assumed that individuals pay premiums to the insurance company out of their own pocket. As we have seen, this may impose a significant burden on certain individuals in society who may be unable to afford insurance premiums, even if they are charged at the fair premium with no loading factor.

In reality, the burden of paying health insurance premiums is often shared between individuals and their employers, where the employer pays a proportion of the insurance premium. Clearly, this will make it easier for individuals to afford health insurance. Nevertheless, some individuals may still have difficulty in paying large health insurance premiums even with such a contribution. More importantly, unemployed individuals will not receive these benefits.

Direct out-of-pocket payment

Key features

Direct out-of-pocket payment relates to a charge made to the individual who receives health care for the treatment received. Payment is made at the point of health care service use. This system of financing health care therefore captures exactly the features of the market framework discussed in Chapter 3 where, for a price, health care providers supply health care to individuals who require treatment, and these individuals meet the full cost of treatment at their own expense. In other words, the fee charged to an individual for health care is the market price.

Catastrophic expenditure

With direct out-of-pocket payments, health care is purchased by those individuals who are willing and able to pay the market price. A system such as this has obvious problems for the consumer with regard to their ability to cope with catastrophic expenditure. Because of the uncertainty surrounding the incidence of ill health, a payment system which relies on patients having to pay for the health care they receive at the point of use therefore relies on patients' ability to pay as the criterion for deciding whether they receive health care. This will mean that a vast number of individuals will not be able to afford treatment for unexpected illness.

Consumer choice of health care provider

With a system of direct out-of-pocket payments for health care, the individual's choice of health care provider is limited only by the number of providers available and the amount of money which the individual is willing and able to spend on treatment. Potentially, patients therefore have a virtually unlimited choice of provider. With this system of payment, patients would be free to choose an alternative health care provider should they be dissatisfied with their current one, provided they were able to afford the prices charged.

Adverse selection

Adverse selection is a feature of insurance markets and is therefore unlikely to exist in a health care market with no health insurance where payment is made on a direct out-of-pocket basis.

Moral hazard

Both forms of moral hazard are unlikely to exist with direct out-of-pocket payments for health care because patients meet the full cost of treatment themselves. In this case, patients will not wish to obtain more health care than they otherwise need, and they are more likely to be aware of supplier-induced demand.

Non-price competition

With a system of direct out-of-pocket payments for health care, health care providers will generally compete for patients on the basis of price. Where patients meet the full cost of health care out of their own pocket, price will be important in deciding from which health care provider an individual will choose to receive treatment. Non-price competition is therefore unlikely to arise. Instead, there is more likely to be *price competition*.

Affordability of health insurance

The problem of affordable health insurance premiums is redundant with a system of direct out-of-pocket payment. However, affordable direct out-of-pocket payments *are* likely to be a problem.

Empirical example of direct out-of-pocket payment

Because of the effects of uncertainty surrounding the timing and size of expenditure on health care, most countries in the developed world provide health care through the operation of some form of health insurance market covering the provision of some if not all health care. For this reason, direct payment for health care is uncommon in developed countries. However, there are exceptions to this, such as direct out-of-pocket payments for the treatment of minor ailments and illnesses which are generally simple and cheap to treat. For example, in the UK it is possible to buy relatively weak pain-relieving pharmaceuticals over the counter from chemists and pharmacists in return for a small direct out-of-pocket payment. In 1995 in the NHS, direct out-of-pocket payments by patients totalled £1,296 million (OHE, 1995), comprising hospital charges, prescription charges, and dental charges (see Table 6.1).

Table 6.1 Direct out-of-pocket payments made by patients to the NHS in 1995.

Charge	£ million (%)
Hospital[1]	455 (35.1)
Prescriptions	303 (23.4)
Dental	480 (37.0)
Other[2]	58 (4.5)
Total	1,296 (100)

Notes:
[1] Including income received from patients for the supply and repair of appliances, drugs, medicines, amenity beds and private accommodation and treatment.
[2] Including receipts from sales of pre-payment certificates for prescription medicines, prescription charges collected by dispensing doctors and charges paid for dental services provided in health centres.
Source: OHE (1995).

Private health insurance

Key features

Private health insurance involves the development of an insurance contract between private insurance companies and individuals who consider themselves to be at risk of ill health. When individuals buy private health insurance, they enter into an agreement with an insurance company to pay an insurance premium in exchange for a payout by the insurance company should they become ill. Therefore, individuals pays a sum of money on the understanding that if they become ill, the insurance company will pay for the treatment that they require.

With the introduction of private health insurance, an individual has the opportunity to purchase health insurance from a number of private insurance companies, who compete with each other for the custom of the individual on the basis of price (that is, the size of the insurance premium). Therefore, there is competition between private insurance companies, to a greater or lesser extent. Insured individuals are able to choose the health care providers from whom they wish to receive treatment, and they receive payment from the private insurance company.

Catastrophic expenditure

Private health insurance protects individuals from potentially catastrophic expenditure on health care because it is the private insurance company that pays for any treatment that the individuals require. Insured individuals are therefore able to cope financially with unexpected illness.

Consumer choice of health care provider

In its simplest form, private health insurance allows individuals freedom to receive health care from the provider of their choice. Therefore, patients who are dissatisfied with the health care they receive are able to change provider. Choice may, in fact, be greater with private health insurance than with direct out-of-pocket payments since individuals are no longer limited in the choice of provider by their ability to afford the prices charged.

Adverse selection

Adverse selection is likely to be a problem with private health insurance. This is because only individuals with a high risk of illness have a financial incentive to buy health insurance. Adverse selection therefore arises because only those individuals who expect to benefit from health insurance will choose to buy it. Individuals with a low risk of illness may refrain from buying health insurance since they are unlikely to need health care and so are also unlikely to need money from an insurance company to pay for their treatment.

Moral hazard

For some illnesses, individuals may choose to obtain health care which they otherwise would not have done if they had not been insured. Therefore, the use of some health care services may be frivolous or unnecessary, and, in this way, consumer moral hazard may exist.

Producer moral hazard may also exist, because, if a private insurance company is financing the provision of health care rather than the patient, then health care providers have little incentive to moderate the amount of health care that they supply to patients.

Non-price competition

With the introduction of private health insurance, price is no longer important to patients because the price of health care to the individual is effectively reduced to zero. Therefore, patients will choose a health care provider on the basis of non-price factors, and non-price competition will emerge.

Affordability of health insurance

Certain population groups such as individuals earning low incomes, individuals at very high risk of illness, and the elderly, may not be able to buy private health insurance because the insurance premiums are unaffordable.

Empirical example of private health insurance

Private health insurance exists in some form or other in most countries in the developed world, though the size of the private health insurance sector and the extent to which individuals choose to buy private health insurance differ from country to country. In the UK, the private health insurance market is dominated by two private health insurance companies, British United Provident Association (BUPA) and Private Patients Plan (PPP) who account for approximately 80 per cent of total market subscription income (Booer, 1994). In 1995, 3.8 million individuals subscribed to private health insurance and 7.5 million individuals had private health insurance cover (OHE, 1995). Relative to the NHS, the market for private health care is small. In 1995, health care expenditure on the NHS was £41,517 million, or 87.8 per cent of total UK health care expenditure. Expenditure on private health care was £2,536 million, or only 5.4 per cent of total UK health care expenditure (OHE, 1995).

Preferred Provider Organisations

Key features

Preferred Provider Organisations (PPOs) are a derivative of private health insurance, and the insurance market operates in a similar manner. Individuals pay an insurance premium to a private insurance company in exchange for a payout by the insurance company for health care should they become ill. Health care is therefore still, in effect, free to the individual at the point of receipt.

Individuals still have the opportunity to purchase health insurance from different private insurance companies, who compete for the custom of the individual on the basis of the size of the insurance premium. However, whilst with private health insurance, insured individuals are able to choose the health care provider from which they wish to receive treatment, with a system of PPOs, the individual has much less of a choice of health provider. Private insurance companies contract selectively with certain health care providers (the *Preferred Provider Organisations*), and agree to channel individuals whom they insure to these providers in return for lower fees charged for health care provided. Therefore, the private insurance company benefits because the amount of money which they spend on the health care of insured individuals who become ill is lowered, and PPOs benefit since they are guaranteed patients from whom they may earn income.

With health care provided by PPOs, whilst there is a link between private insurance companies and health care providers, they are still separate entities in the health care market, and have different aims and objectives.

Catastrophic expenditure

A health care market with PPOs operates in much the same way as the pure private health insurance market. Insured individuals are therefore able to cope financially with potentially catastrophic health care expenditure since private insurance companies are responsible for paying for the health care of the insured individual.

Consumer choice of health care provider

With PPOs, the individual has very little choice as to the health care provider from which they receive treatment. In extreme circumstances, insured individuals have *no* choice of health care provider, but will be required to obtain health care from the PPO linked to the private health insurance company.

Adverse selection

Adverse selection is likely to be a problem with PPOs, for the same reason it is likely to be a problem with private health insurance: only individuals with a high risk of illness have a financial incentive to buy health insurance from private insurance companies, and individuals with a low risk of illness may refrain from buying health insurance.

Moral hazard

Consumer moral hazard may exist with PPOs because, in some situations, individuals may choose to obtain health care which they otherwise would not have done if they had not been insured.

Producer moral hazard may also be a problem. Producer moral hazard is essentially a problem of excess use caused by health care providers and is shown by an increase in the volume of services provided over that volume that would be provided if patients were fully informed. Whilst PPOs are guaranteed custom from private insurance companies in return for lower *unit costs*, the actual volume of services provided may still increase. Therefore, supplier-induced demand may still occur with PPOs, since although the unit cost of health care is likely to decrease, the *volume* of services provided may increase.

Non-price competition

Non-price competition is unlikely to be an issue with PPOs since consumers have much less freedom as to their choice of health care provider and will therefore remain unswayed by providers who compete for patients on the basis of non-price factors. Instead, health care providers will be forced to compete with each other on the basis of price in order to obtain PPO status from private insurance companies. Therefore, price competition is more likely to exist between health care providers, and prices will consequently decrease as health care providers compete with one another to make themselves more attractive to private insurance companies.

Affordability of health insurance

Just as with private health insurance, affordable insurance premiums may also be a problem with PPOs because the insurance premiums charged by private insurance companies may be too high for certain groups in the population to afford. However, insurance premiums are likely to be smaller than with private health insurance, because the lower treatment costs that health care providers charge third party payers in return for preferred provider status may be reflected in smaller insurance premiums.

Empirical example of PPOs

PPOs have developed mainly in the health care market in the US as a means of increasing the competitiveness of private health insurance companies. The number of

PPOs and individuals with health insurance receiving health care from PPOs is growing rapidly: in 1990 there were between 38 million and 48 million individuals in the US who had access to approximately 820 PPOs (McCarthy and Minnis, 1994).

Health Maintenance Organisations

Key features

Health Maintenance Organisations (HMOs) are another derivative of private health insurance, where individuals pay an insurance premium in exchange for receiving treatment should they become ill. As with private health insurance, health care is therefore, in effect, free to the individual at the point of receipt.

In its simplest form, the main feature of an HMO is that the insurance company and the health care provider *merge* so that they become different parts of the same organisation. There is therefore an *integration* between the insurance company and the health care provider, and the HMO *provides* health care for the individual in return for an insurance premium, rather than just pays for it.

Individuals still have the opportunity to purchase health insurance from different HMOs, who compete for the custom of individuals. However, the individual has no choice of health care provider since the insurance company and the health care provider are effectively one and the same: the choice of insurance company therefore also directly determines the choice of provider of health care.

Whilst with PPOs, private insurance companies and health care providers are still separate entities in the health care market, each with different aims and objectives, with HMOs, insurance companies and health care providers effectively become the *same* entity with the same goals and the same objectives.

Catastrophic expenditure

HMOs provide a way for individuals to cope financially with potentially catastrophic health care expenditure by agreeing to provide health care for the individual in return for an insurance premium. In this way, HMOs have the same effect as private health insurance companies.

Consumer choice of health care provider

Individuals have effectively no choice as to the health care provider from which they receive treatment should they become ill. Instead, individuals are required to obtain health care from the health care provider with which the insurance company is merged. Of course, individuals do have a choice as to the HMO from which they obtain health insurance.

Adverse selection

As with any other private-insurance-based system, adverse selection is likely to be a problem with HMOs because only individuals with a high risk of illness have a financial incentive to obtain health insurance.

Moral hazard

Consumer moral hazard may exist with HMOs if individuals choose to obtain more health care than they would have done had they not been insured.

Producer moral hazard is unlikely to be a problem because the insurance company and health care provider have effectively merged to become the same organisation. Therefore, the component of the HMO responsible for providing health care will only cause the organisation as a whole to *lose* money if it chooses to induce demand for health care. In fact, there is more likely to be a problem arising from the *underuse* of health care services, where individuals are denied the treatment they need in an effort to minimise the payout which the HMO must make when providing health care to insured individuals.

Non-price competition

Non-price competition between health care providers is unlikely to be an issue with HMOs because consumers have no freedom as to their choice of health care provider. Providers therefore have no incentive to compete for insured individuals since the provider and the insurance company are integrated, and even if individuals might be attracted to seek health care from alternative providers, they are required to obtain health care from the provider to which their insurance company is merged.

Affordability of health insurance

Affordable insurance premiums may be a problem with HMOs if the insurance premium charged is too high for certain population groups.

Empirical example of HMOs

HMOs have developed mainly in the US health care market as a means of competing with private health insurance. In recent years, the provision of health care through HMOs in the US has increased dramatically: in 1976, approximately 6 million Americans were members of some 250 HMOs, whilst in 1991 these numbers had increased, with approximately 37 million Americans being members of 550 HMOs (McCarthy and Minnis, 1994).

Public health insurance

Key features

Public health insurance involves the development of an insurance contract between an insurance company and individuals who consider themselves to be at risk of ill health. Having paid an insurance premium, if they become ill, individuals receive health care which is paid for by the insurance company. Therefore, health care is still, in effect, free to insured individuals. In this way, public health insurance is no different from private health insurance.

However, with private health insurance, an individual may purchase health insurance from any one of a number of private insurance companies who compete for the custom of individuals. There is, therefore, some degree of competition between private insurance companies. With the introduction of public health insurance, an individual has the opportunity to purchase health insurance from only *one* insurance company, which is the *only* third party payer of health care. In this case, there is *no* competition between insurance companies because only one exists. Individuals therefore have no choice of insurance company, though insured individuals are able to choose the health care provider from which they wish to receive treatment.

With a system of public health insurance, the role of insurance company is played by the *government*. Because this is the only insurance company, the government has considerable power over health care providers regarding rates of pay for health care performed on behalf of insured individuals: because there is only one insurance company which they are compelled to deal with, health care providers are forced to accept the rates of pay that the government offers in return for health care provided.

Catastrophic expenditure

Public health insurance protects individuals from catastrophic health care expenditure in exactly the same way that private health insurance does, only now it is the government who pays for any treatment which an insured individual might require. Insured individuals are therefore able to cope financially with unexpected illness.

Consumer choice of health care provider

Public health insurance allows individuals freedom to receive health care from the provider of their choice. Patients who are dissatisfied with the treatment they receive are free to change health care provider.

Adverse selection

If individuals have a choice of whether to buy health insurance, adverse selection is likely to be a problem because only individuals with a high risk of illness will buy health insurance, and those with a low risk of illness will refrain from doing so.

Moral hazard

Consumer moral hazard may exist if individuals choose to obtain more health care than they would have done had they not been insured.

Producer moral hazard may well exist with public health insurance because whilst there being only one insurance company implies that health care providers are forced to accept low rates of pay for the services they provide, there is not necessarily any restriction on the actual volume of services they provide. Producer moral hazard is essentially a problem of excess use caused by health care providers and this may occur with public health insurance, since although the unit costs of health care are likely to decrease, the volume of services provided may increase.

Non-price competition

Non-price competition is unlikely to occur with public health insurance. It *is* the case that health care providers must compete with each other for patients who receive health care for free, and therefore theoretically non-price competition may exist if patients choose a health care provider on the basis of other non-price factors. However, non-price competition implies that the cost of health care will inevitably increase, and if health care providers are forced to accept low payments by the government for health care provided, they are unlikely to want this to happen.

Affordability of health insurance

Affordable insurance premiums are a realistic possibility with public health insurance. This is because the existence of a single insurance company gives considerable power to the government in the amount that health care providers are paid for treating patients. Since treatment costs will therefore be kept low, this will be reflected in the insurance premiums which individuals are required to pay for health insurance.

Empirical example of public health insurance

The health care system in Canada is often referred to as an example of a public health insurance system. Provincial governments are, in effect, the sole insurance companies in any one geographical area and are responsible for financing all basic health care needs. Individuals are unable to obtain insurance from private insurance companies for basic health care provision, and this gives the government considerable power over rates of pay to health care providers.

Direct taxation

Key features

Direct taxation systems are a derivative of public health insurance. The role of insurance company is played solely by the government which therefore has considerable power over health care providers regarding payment for the treatment of insured individuals. As with public health insurance, this arises because there is effectively only one insurance company and health care providers are therefore forced to accept the payment that the government offers for health care provided.

A key feature of direct taxation is that health insurance is compulsory and all individuals are required to pay insurance premiums to the government. These insurance premiums are collected through *taxation* and therefore the contribution by an individual to the government for their compulsory health insurance is part of their total tax payment.

As with public health insurance, individuals have no choice of insurance company because there is effectively only one, which is the government. With a direct taxation system, individuals also have no choice as to whether or not they buy health insurance in the first place, since participation is compulsory. However, individuals are able to choose the health care provider from which they wish to receive treatment.

Catastrophic expenditure

Direct taxation systems protect individuals from catastrophic health care expenditure in exactly the same way that public health insurance does because the government pays for any health care that an insured individual might require.

Consumer choice of health care provider

Direct taxation systems in their simplest form allow individuals the freedom to change health care provider should they wish to.

Adverse selection

Adverse selection is not a problem with direct taxation. This is because individuals have no choice as to whether they choose to buy health insurance and it is compulsory for everyone. It is therefore not possible for only high-risk individuals to buy health insurance and low-risk individuals to refrain from doing so because *all* individuals, both high and low risk, are required to obtain insurance cover.

Moral hazard

Consumer moral hazard may exist with direct taxation systems because in certain situations individuals may choose to obtain health care which they otherwise would not have done if they had not been insured.

Producer moral hazard may well exist with direct taxation for exactly the same reason that it might exist with public health insurance: health care providers, whilst restricted in the size of the payments they receive from the government for individual treatments, are not necessarily restricted in the *volume* of individual treatments they provide.

Non-price competition

Just as with public health insurance, non-price competition is unlikely to occur with direct taxation because this implies that the cost of health care will increase, and if health care providers are forced to accept low payments by the government for health care provided, they are unlikely to want this to happen.

Affordability of health insurance

Health insurance is affordable to everyone with a system of direct taxation because all individuals pay insurance premiums as part of their total tax payment. In this way, the size of the insurance premium is determined by an individual's ability to pay: rich individuals earn high incomes and so pay high taxes and therefore contribute *more* to financing health care than poor individuals. However, whilst the rich pay higher insurance premiums than the poor this does not mean that the poor are denied treatment: *all* individuals have the same right of access to health care. Therefore, the rich *subsidise* the poor.

Empirical example of direct taxation

The NHS is an example of a direct taxation system, where the tax payment covers all basic health care finance so that the consumer is able to use health care services at zero price. No maximum quantity of health care services which an individual is able to use is stipulated, and therefore individuals have unlimited access to health care. In 1995, total NHS expenditure was £41,517 million (OHE, 1995). Of this total, 84.2 per cent was raised from general taxation, 12.7 per cent was raised from NHS contributions, and 3.1 per cent was raised from patient payments such as prescription

Table 6.2 Effectiveness of alternatives for financing health care.

Problem with finance system	Systems in which problem exists	Systems in which problem does not exist
Coping with catastrophic expenditure	Direct out-of-pocket payment	Private health insurance; PPOs; HMOs; public health insurance; direct taxation
Consumer choice of health care provider	PPOs; HMOs	Direct out-of-pocket payment; private health insurance; public health insurance; direct taxation
Adverse selection	Private health insurance; HMOs; PPOs; public health insurance	Direct out-of-pocket payment; direct taxation
Consumer moral hazard[1]	Private health insurance; PPOs; HMOs; public health insurance; direct taxation	Direct out-of-pocket payment
Producer moral hazard	Private health insurance; PPOs; public health insurance; direct taxation	Direct out-of-pocket payment; HMOs
Non-price competition	Private health insurance	Direct out-of-pocket payment; PPOs; HMOs; public health insurance; direct taxation
Affordable health insurance	Private health insurance; PPOs; HMOs	Direct out-of-pocket payment;[2] direct taxation; public health insurance

Notes:
[1] It is uncertain whether consumer moral hazard will be observed in practice since it seems unlikely that an individual would wish to obtain more health care just because treatment will be paid for by an insurance company.
[2] The problem of affordable health insurance premiums is redundant with direct out-of-pocket payment. However, affordable direct out-of-pocket payments *are* likely to be a problem.

charges (OHE, 1995). Therefore, the main source of finance for the NHS is general taxation. The bulk of funds from general taxation is obtained from income tax. Therefore, income tax provides the main source of funds for the NHS. NHS contributions paid by employers and employees via the National Insurance scheme may also be regarded as a form of taxation on earned income. Therefore, taxation accounts for 96.9 per cent of total NHS finance, where the insurance premium paid by individuals to finance the NHS is part of their total tax payment.

The discussion so far has concentrated on the various ways in which health care may be financed. We have examined each of the possible deviations from the basic health insurance model in its simplest form, and assessed the advantages and disadvantages associated with each. The conclusions of this discussion are summarised in Table 6.2, which shows each of the six different structures and their effectiveness as options for financing health care.

Financing health care in specific countries

In the discussion above, each option has been reduced to its simplest form so that its key features might be determined more clearly. In reality, it is unlikely that health care will be financed according to these rather oversimplified structures. Also, most countries in the developed world are likely to finance health care through a *combination* of these different systems, rather than relying on any one single option. For these two reasons, there follows a description of health care financing in a number of countries. This provides an opportunity to explore which method of paying for health care is preferred by health policy decision-makers, and to explore the ways in which the six basic structures outlined above have been modified to cope with the pressures exerted by the reality of scarce health care resources.

The method of financing health care in four countries will be discussed in turn:

1. Canada;
2. Germany;
3. Sweden;
4. the US.

Clearly, any number of countries could be selected for discussion, and these four have been chosen because, in one form or another, and for some proportion of health care services provided, they are comprised of each of the different financing structures.

The key participants in any health care system are: the patients; the payers of health care; GPs (or primary care doctors); and the hospital sector. Each of the selected health care systems will be discussed with regard to the following:

1. key features of the system;
2. the role of patients;
3. the role of payers;
4. the role of GPs;
5. the role of the hospital sector;
6. economic incentives inherent in the system.

Financing health care in Canada

Key features of the system

The health care system in Canada is a universal access, single third party payer, public health insurance system for basic health care. The system is comprised of twelve individual health insurance plans administered by the ten provinces and two territories. Each province individually determines the level of services in that geographical area that will be provided free to the individual in return for the insurance premium payment. This level of services must conform at least to the basic level of health care services mandated by the federal government. That is, provincial governments are required by the federal government to provide a level of health insurance cover that allows individuals to receive basic health care. This ensures that, although there are twelve separate public insurance plans in Canada, they are largely similar because all provinces must provide public health insurance for certain key health care services.

Supplemental private health insurance is available for health care services not covered by the public system, but is not permitted for services covered by provincial health care insurance.

In 1995, total health care expenditure in Canada was £41 billion, and spending on health care per person was £1,447 (OHE, 1995). Funding of health care in Canada comes from a combination of federal government, provincial government, and private contributions. In 1991, contributions by the governments accounted for 72 per cent of total health care expenditures and were raised largely through tax revenues (of this 72 per cent, approximately 25 per cent was accounted for by the federal government, and approximately 47 per cent was accounted for by the provincial government). Private sources of health care finance accounted for 28 per cent of total expenditure (Rozek and Mulhern, 1994).

The role of patients

In Canada, patients are treated according to need and not according to ability to pay. There is therefore no two-tier system in Canada, in the sense that high-income individuals are not allowed to purchase private health insurance for health care services covered by the public health insurance scheme run by provincial govern- ments. Therefore, richer individuals are not allowed to queue-jump ahead of poorer individuals, and so everyone has access to the same level of health care. There is a role for private health insurance, but only for those services not covered by the public health insurance system.

Patients receive health care but are not required to pay for those services when they receive them. Instead, federal and provincial governments collect taxes, a proportion of which pay for the provision of basic health care services.

The role of payers

Provincial governments hold the main responsibility for the finance and delivery of health care in Canada. Within each province, the Ministry of Health carries out these responsibilities. The specific methods of organising, financing and administering health care vary from province to province and the Ministry of Health has a significant control over the quality and quantity of health care consumed. For example, provincial health ministries negotiate fee schedules with provincial medical associations, and negotiate the size of annual global budgets for hospitals.

Private health insurance covers supplemental hospital, medical, vision and dental services not covered by the public health insurance system administered by each province. Private health insurance may be purchased either by individuals or by their employers.

The role of GPs

In 1991, spending on GPs' services accounted for approximately 15 per cent of total health care expenditure in Canada (Rozek and Mulhern, 1994). Patients may be registered with the GP of their choice, and, in general, patients first contact GPs when they are ill. The GP may then make a referral to see a specialist where necessary.

The majority of GPs are paid on a fee-for-service basis according to schedules negotiated between the Ministry of Health in each province and provincial medical associations.

The role of the hospital sector

In 1991, hospitals accounted for 39 per cent of total health care expenditure in Canada (Rozek and Mulhern, 1994). Hospitals are classified as public, federal or private. Neither public nor federal hospitals are operated to make a profit and both accept all patients regardless of their ability to pay. Private hospitals admit patients who pay for the services provided either through private health insurance or through direct out-of-pocket payments. There are 1,227 hospitals in Canada which provide a total of 182,222 beds. 95 per cent of hospital beds are available in the public hospitals.

Provincial governments fund expenditure by public hospitals through global budgets negotiated annually by each hospital and the Ministry of Health in that province.

Economic incentives inherent in the system

Patients

Patients may be treated by the health care provider of their choice, and they receive all basic health care services mandated by the federal government at zero cost when they receive them. Copayments exist for certain additional services. A general lack of knowledge regarding health care and a zero price at the point of receipt may give patients an incentive to consume more health care than they would otherwise.

GPs

Most GPs are paid on a fee-for-service basis with fee schedules determined through negotiation between the provincial medical association (representing GPs' interests) and the provincial Ministry of Health (representing the third party payer's interests). Fee-for-service payments for GPs provide a financial incentive for the excess provision of health care services.

Hospital sector

Hospitals operate under a system of annually determined global budgets, which provides an incentive for containing the costs incurred when treating patients. However, prospective payment systems of this kind may also have an adverse effect on the provision of health care. For example, in Canada there is an incentive for hospitals to keep beds occupied by patients requiring low-intensity care which prevents the use of these scarce beds for the treatment of patients who may be in greater need of high-intensity, high-cost health care.

Financing health care in Germany

Key features of the system

The health care system in Germany is based on a compulsory public health insurance scheme. This is a comprehensive system which covers all health care except for long-term or permanent care. The system is highly decentralised and is comprised of more than 1,000 health insurance funds (often called sickness funds). Approximately 90 per cent of the population are covered by these funds. Of the remaining 10 per cent of the population, 8 per cent are covered by private health insurance, and 2 per cent are civil servants for whom the government administers health care (Hoffmeyer, 1994a).

Health insurance funds are required to accept all individuals who qualify for membership. Insurance premiums are paid into the funds by means of a tax which is levied on income earned. Both the employer and the employee contribute equal insurance premiums into the health insurance funds.

Individuals who earn more than a certain predefined income may choose to opt out of this system and seek private health insurance instead.

In 1995, total health care expenditure in Germany was £108 billion, and spending on health care per person was £1,677 (OHE, 1995). Health insurance funds account for approximately 46 per cent of total health care expenditure (Hoffmeyer, 1994a), with the remainder coming from employers (17 per cent), pension funds (7 per cent), accident insurance (3 per cent), direct out-of-pocket payments by patients (7 per cent), government expenditure (14 per cent) and private health insurance (6 per cent).

The role of patients

In Germany, patients are treated according to need and not according to ability to pay. The system of payment for health care means that the richer members of German society support the poorer members to ensure equality in the provision of health care.

Patients have a right to seek treatment from any health insurance fund-accredited GP. GPs act as gatekeepers to the hospital sector and, within limits, GPs and patients have a free choice regarding the hospital to which patients are referred.

The role of payers

The majority of the German population belong to a health insurance fund. These are established as private corporations but are also under government control. The system is highly decentralised, and consists of different types of funds, which are either specific to a particular geographical region (called primary funds), or specific to a particular occupation or industry (called substitute funds).

Health insurance funds are obliged to accept as a member anyone who is eligible to join. They are therefore not allowed to engage in risk selection, where there is an incentive to recruit only those individuals with a low probability of illness. The health insurance fund guarantees a comprehensive health care package which is available to all insured individuals, and it is not possible for health insurance funds to deny payment to health care providers for the treatment of insured individuals.

Health insurance funds are not-for-profit organisations and receive no additional funding from the government. The financial contribution which members pay to their health insurance fund depends solely on ability to pay and is calculated as a proportion of income, up to an upper limit. Most health care is free when individuals receive it, though copayments exist for certain health care services, such as inpatient care in hospitals.

The role of GPs

All individuals have a free choice of GP who is normally the first contact that patients have with the health care sector. Patients may subsequently be referred elsewhere for further treatment. GPs in Germany are therefore of central importance in determining the amount of health care that is provided to insured individuals.

GPs are usually paid on a fee-for-service basis, with both GPs and health insurance funds collectively negotiating the fee schedule. In an effort to contain the costs incurred when treating patients, an overall health care budget is often also negotiated with health insurance funds.

The role of the hospital sector

In Germany, there are hospitals which care for the acutely ill, special (for example, military) hospitals, and hospitals which care for patients with long-term illnesses. Also, three different types of hospital ownership exist: public hospitals are owned by cities, counties and other public authorities; private voluntary hospitals are often owned by religious organisations; and private proprietary hospitals are often owned by doctors. Each group owns approximately one third of all hospitals (Hoffmeyer, 1994a).

Insured individuals often have a say as to which hospital they are referred to by a GP, though it is usual for patients to be referred to the nearest hospital geographically.

Health insurance funds contract with hospitals. Recent changes to the health care system have meant that health care is paid for by prospective payments on a cost-per-case basis by health insurance funds. It is possible for health insurance funds to withdraw funding from hospitals which are inefficient.

Economic incentives inherent in the system

Patients

Whilst copayments exist for certain additional services, a zero price at the point of receipt may give patients an incentive to consume more health care than they would otherwise.

GPs

GPs are paid on a fee-for-service basis which provides a financial incentive to treat as many patients as possible and to induce demand for their services.

Hospital sector

With prospective payments for health care services provided, there exists a financial incentive to underprovide health care or to provide health care of low quality, since hospitals will in effect receive the same fee regardless of the quality of the treatment provided. However, it is possible for health insurance funds to withdraw funding from hospitals which are inefficient.

Financing health care in Sweden

Key features of the system

The provision of health care in Sweden is primarily the responsibility of 26 public authorities divided by geographical region. These authorities, called county councils, are responsible for paying for and providing health care for their resident population. Within each region there are municipalities which also contribute to the finance of health care.

Health care is therefore predominantly the responsibility of county councils. Expenditure on health care is financed through taxation, which is levied on the resident population. County councils are also supported by state grants and receive a budget from the national insurance system.

The national insurance system, apart from funding health care provided by county councils, is also responsible for providing cash benefits such as sickness benefits and maternity benefits. This national insurance system is also funded through compulsory income taxation, paid to the national government on a regional basis.

A very small private health insurance sector exists, the main role of which is to provide insurance against patient copayments for health care.

In 1995, total health care expenditure in Sweden was £12 billion, and spending on health care per person was £1,317 (OHE, 1995). Fifty-nine per cent of health care expenditure is funded out of county council taxation, and 7 per cent is funded by municipality taxation. Contributions from the national insurance scheme and the national government account for 23 per cent of health care expenditure, and the remaining 11 per cent comes from copayments by patients (Hoffmeyer, 1994b).

The role of patients

Within their specific county council, patients have a free choice of both GP and hospital. Furthermore, they may refer themselves directly to hospitals, rather than being referred there by a GP.

Copayments exist for most health care services, though there is an annual upper copayment limit. Individuals may privately insure against these payments.

The role of payers

It is the responsibility of county councils to pay for and provide health care in Sweden. Municipalities have responsibility regarding the provision of long-term health care for the elderly. Specifically, the provision of health care is the responsibility of the county council of the individual's county of residence. Therefore, patients have no choice of insurer, which implies that county councils need not compete for customers.

Swedes are required to pay municipality-based taxes, county council-based taxes and national taxes. A portion of each of these moneys is used to pay for health care. The national insurance scheme is financed on a regional basis through payroll taxes.

County councils have a total budget for financing health care which they are unable to exceed because they are not allowed to raise taxation beyond levels agreed with the national government.

The role of GPs

Within each county council there are public GPs and private GPs. Public GPs are salaried employees of the county council. Also, a small number of private GPs exist who are reimbursed on a fee-for-service basis by the national insurance system. GPs tend to group themselves in large group practices or health centres.

Public GPs are not in competition with each other, nor is there any incentive to compete since income is fixed regardless of work undertaken. Private GPs on the other hand do compete for patients.

The role of the hospital sector

There are three main types of hospital in Sweden: regional hospitals; county hospitals; and district hospitals. Sweden is divided into medical regions, each of which has a large regional hospital providing specialist facilities administered by the county council in which it is located, though funding also comes from all county councils which refer patients there. Each county also has at least one county hospital which is less specialised than regional hospitals, and within each county there are a number of district hospitals.

Patients have free choice as to which hospital they refer themselves to or, in consultation with a GP, are referred to, as long as the hospital is within the boundary of the county of residence.

Hospitals are reimbursed through annual budgets paid by county councils. The general method for allocating funds is by global budgeting.

Economic incentives inherent in the system

Patients

Patients may obtain health care from the GP and hospital of their choice, provided they fall within the boundaries of their county council. Non-price competition is unlikely because GPs are generally paid on a salaried basis and hospitals are reimbursed prospectively.

The use of copayments is extensive in Sweden, curtailing any incentive for patients to consume more health care than they would if health care were completely free.

GPs

Public GPs are generally paid on a salaried basis, and do not compete with each other. They also have little incentive to provide a high-quality service. On the other hand, private GPs are paid on a fee-for-service basis and therefore have a financial incentive to induce demand for their own services.

Hospital sector

Hospitals have an incentive to contain costs incurred through the provision of health care because they are financed on a global budget basis. However, since revenue is effectively fixed in advance, they, like public GPs, also have a financial incentive to minimise actual expenditure on treatment.

Financing health care in the US

Key features of the system

The health care system in the US is characterised by a mixture of health care financing systems. Health care is financed by direct out-of-pocket payments, private health insurance, PPOs, HMOs and public health insurance.

The public health insurance system includes both the *Medicare* and *Medicaid* schemes. Medicare is a federal government health insurance programme which covers all individuals aged 65 years or more. Medicaid is a joint state and federal health insurance programme which covers the very poorest individuals.

Private health insurance and its derivatives provide insurance cover for the majority of Americans. Competing in the same market as traditional private health insurance are PPOs and HMOs. In 1990, approximately 14 per cent of the population of the US (some 33 million individuals) were uninsured (McCarthy and Minnis, 1994). These individuals must rely on charity care, pay for services directly out of their own pocket or go without health care.

The health care delivery system in the US is also diverse and competitive. Health care providers are generally independent suppliers responsible for their own costs and revenues.

In 1995, total health care expenditure in the US was £741 billion, and spending on health care per person was £2,816 (OHE, 1995). The health care system in the US is financed as follows (see McCarthy and Minnis, 1994):

1. Government expenditure

Approximately 42 per cent of health care expenditure is financed by the government, comprising Medicare and Medicaid expenditure and other programmes.

    (a) Medicare public health insurance accounts for approximately 17 per cent of total health care expenditure in the US. This scheme is funded through a combination of taxes on income, insurance premiums and direct payments by patients, with both coinsurance and deductibles required.

    (b) Federal and state expenditure on the Medicaid health insurance programme accounts for approximately 11 per cent of total US health care expenditure. The scheme is financed mainly from federal and state general tax revenues.

    (c) Health care expenditures by the federal government outside of the Medicare and Medicaid programmes account for 14 per cent of total US health care expenditure. These programmes include the Civilian Health and Medical Program of the Uniformed Services (CHAMPUS), Veterans' Administration (VA) and Federal Employees' Health Benefits Program (FEHBP).

2. Private health insurance

Including traditional private health insurance, PPOs and HMOs, 33 per cent of health care expenditure in the US is financed by private health insurance.

3. Direct out-of-pocket payment

Out-of-pocket payments by consumers form a large share of total health care expenditure in the US (20 per cent).

4. Other private funds

Funds from a variety of private sources such as hospital non-patient revenues and charities account for 5 per cent of total health care expenditure.

The role of patients

In 1990, 86 per cent of Americans were protected from catastrophic health expenditure by some form of health insurance, public or private. However, 14 per cent of the population of the US (some 33 million individuals) were without any form of health insurance. Most uninsured individuals are poor, but not poor enough to qualify for Medicaid public health insurance, and too young to qualify for Medicare public health insurance. For these uninsured individuals, access to adequate health care is often not possible.

For those individuals who are able to afford insurance premiums, the growing cost of health care has increased the size of insurance premiums for private health insurance which are paid primarily by employers (generally, employers pay between 75 per cent and 90 per cent of the private health insurance premium).

The role of payers

Health care in the US is financed from both private insurance companies and state and federal governments.

Private insurance companies

Traditional private health insurance is often complex and can vary greatly in the benefits offered. Individuals with private health insurance often face zero price for health care in return for paying insurance premiums. There is increasing use of coinsurance and deductibles to discourage excess use of health care services.

There are a number of different types of traditional insurance company from which an individual can choose to buy health insurance, including commercial insurance companies, Blue Cross and Blue Shield and employers' self-insurance. Commercial insurance companies are organised as profit-maximising firms, and must compete with each other for custom. Blue Cross hospital and Blue Shield GP health insurance plans are national health insurance schemes that are private not-for-profit organisations governed locally. Self-insurance is a form of health insurance used by employers where the employers bear the financial risk of health insurance coverage for their employees.

Health insurance is also obtainable from HMOs, which provide a predefined comprehensive set of services to a voluntarily enrolled population within a specific geographical area. Health care may also be financed through PPOs.

Governments

Local, state and national governments participate in health care finance in the US for those individuals generally not covered by private health insurance, including the elderly, the poor, the military and government employees. The majority of government health expenditure is provided via a few major health care programmes including: Medicare; Medicaid; CHAMPUS; VA; and FEHBP.

The role of GPs

GPs in the US directly or indirectly control over 70 per cent of all health expenditure through their contacts with patients, and their decisions regarding testing, treatment and hospitalisation (McCarthy and Minnis, 1994).

GPs in the US are paid through a variety of methods, each of which produces different financial incentives to the way in which health care is provided. With private health insurance, GPs are invariably paid on a fee-for-service basis, which provides a financial incentive to induce demand. HMOs and PPOs often pay GPs on either a capitation basis or a salary basis, both of which may provide incentives to underprovide services and to minimise the inputs to providing health care. Under the Medicare scheme, GPs are paid according to the *Resource-Based Relative Value Scale* (*RBRVS*) which is a uniform national fee schedule that bases payment of GPs on the resources used in providing health care to patients, adjusted geographically only for cost differences. This scale rewards GPs on the basis of their input into the treatment process and results in a bias towards time-intensive diagnostic and primary care procedures rather than speciality care and high-technology diagnostic and therapeutic health care services.

The role of the hospital sector

There are various types of hospital in the US: government hospitals (either federal, state or local, which account for approximately 41 per cent of the 6,700 total number of hospitals); not-for-profit hospitals (which account for approximately 48 per cent of the total); and for-profit hospitals (which account for approximately 11 per cent of the total) (McCarthy and Minnis, 1994).

The US health care system provides a great deal of choice to patients in the selection of a hospital. There is less choice for patients whose health care is financed by HMOs and PPOs, where the third party payer negotiates a contract with a hospital. However, individuals may enter into an insurance contract with HMOs and PPOs on the basis of the hospital with which the third party payer deals.

All hospitals are, therefore, to some degree or other, in competition with each other, and cost containment pressures imposed by third party payers provide an incentive for all hospitals to behave as profit maximising firms regardless of their status. Hospitals are able to set their own prices, but are increasingly forced to negotiate discounted prices with individual third party payers. These pressures have also caused hospitals to shift from inpatient treatment to outpatient treatment, which is generally less expensive.

Most hospitals are now paid on a prospective basis for the health care they provide, often involving prospectively set costs per case where the amount to be paid for treatment is determined in advance by *Diagnostic-Related Groups* (*DRGs*). By this reimbursement method, individual treatment cases are allocated a cost before the treatment is provided, and payment is therefore determined in advance. With this form of payment, problems may exist with regard to the financial incentives to underprovide health care and to provide health care of low quality.

Economic incentives inherent in the system

Patients

Patients in the US have substantial freedom to choose among numerous health insurance providers and health care providers. For those patients with health insurance there is an incentive to seek the very best health care regardless of its cost. However, over 33 million Americans have no health insurance and must pay for health care out of their own pockets, or go without treatment.

GPs

GPs are paid by a variety of methods including fee-for-service, salary and capitation, each of which provides its own financial incentives regarding the provision of health care.

Hospital sector

Hospitals, like GPs, are paid in a variety of ways, though considerable emphasis is placed on prospective pricing, with prospectively set costs per case. The amount paid for treatment is often determined using *Diagnostic-Related Groups* (*DRGs*), where each individual treatment case is allocated a cost before the treatment is provided. With this method of payment, the hospital receives the same income regardless of whether the treatment be high quality or low quality and therefore has a financial incentive to provide low-quality care using the minimum amount of effort and incurring the minimum costs.

Conclusion

In this chapter we have explored different methods for financing, or paying for, health care. We have examined six methods for structuring health care finance and explored the key features and problems associated with each. None of these systems is perfect, though some are less prone to the problems that arise from health insurance and third party payment.

We have also looked in some detail at the way in which health care is financed in a number of countries in the developed world. Whilst the number of different health care systems covered in this review does not pretend to be fully comprehensive, the countries selected do provide a broad discussion of the way in which health care is financed and the way in which the problems associated with health insurance are addressed in reality.

In the following chapter the discussion of financing health care is extended and we concentrate in much more detail on the finance and delivery of health care in one specific health care system, namely, the UK National Health Service.

References

Booer T. (1994) The health care system in the United Kingdom. In: Hoffmeyer U.K. and McCarthy T.R. (eds.) *Financing health care*. Dordrecht: Kluwer.

Hoffmeyer U.K. (1994a) The health care system in Germany. In: Hoffmeyer U.K. and McCarthy T.R. (eds.) *Financing health care*. Dordrecht: Kluwer.

Hoffmeyer U.K. (1994b) The health care system in Sweden. In: Hoffmeyer U.K. and McCarthy T.R. (eds.) *Financing health care*. Dordrecht: Kluwer.

McCarthy T.R. and Minnis J. (1994) The health care system in the United States. In: Hoffmeyer U.K. and McCarthy T.R. (eds.) *Financing health care*. Dordrecht: Kluwer.

Office of Health Economics (OHE) (1995) *Compendium of health statistics*. Ninth edition. London: OHE.

Rozek R. and Mulhern C. (1994) The health care system in Canada. In: Hoffmeyer U.K. and McCarthy T.R. (eds.) *Financing health care*. Dordrecht: Kluwer.

Suggested further reading

For an introduction to the different methods of financing health care see:

Donaldson C. and Gerard K. (1993) *Economics of health care financing: the visible hand*. Basingstoke: Macmillan, pp. 51–67.

For an analysis of the health care financing systems in various countries in the developed world see:

Hoffmeyer U.K. and McCarthy T.R. (eds.) (1994) *Financing health care*. Dordrecht: Kluwer.

For a presentation of total health care expenditures in various countries and an analysis of health care expenditure in the UK see:

Office of Health Economics (OHE) (1995) *Compendium of health statistics*. Ninth edition. London: OHE.

7   The UK National Health Service

In this chapter we extend our discussion of methods for financing health care and we concentrate on the finance and delivery of health care in the UK National Health Service. The organisational structure and the flow of funds through the system are both discussed in considerable detail, and we examine how health care resources are allocated via the NHS internal market.

Summary

1. The government's proposals for the future of the NHS were published in January 1989 in a white paper called 'Working for patients'.

2. The key changes announced in the white paper concerned the way in which health care would be provided in the NHS. These changes were primarily intended to increase competition between health care providers, and this was to be achieved by a variety of means: a separation of the roles of purchasers and providers in an NHS internal market; the creation of self-governing NHS Trusts to provide health care and earn revenue for the services they provided; the transformation of District Health Authorities into purchasers of health care for their resident populations; the opportunity for large general practitioner practices to become GP Fundholders, able to purchase limited hospital services for their patients; and the use of contracts as a means of providing links between purchasers and providers.

3. The organisational structure of the NHS is extremely complicated. The major components of the NHS are as follows: Secretary of State for Health; Department of Health; NHS Executive (HQ); NHS Executive (Regional Offices); Health Authorities; NHS Trusts; general practitioners; GP Fundholders; Total Purchasing Pilots; and Locality Commissions.

4. The flow of funds in the NHS is also extremely complicated. The system may be characterised by funding flows between the various components of the organisational structure.

5. In the NHS internal market, the buyers of health care are called purchasers and they buy health care for the population they serve. The sellers of health care are called providers, and they provide health care to this population.

6. Providers in the NHS internal market are NHS Trusts. They are responsible for delivering contracted health care services within the quality and quantity specifications delineated by contracts to one or more purchaser, in return for an agreed sum of money.

7. There are three types of purchaser in the NHS internal market: Health Authorities; GP Fundholders; and Total Purchasing Pilots. Each of these has a primary responsibility to ensure that, within available resources, health care services are secured to meet the health needs of the population it serves. Purchasers are therefore responsible for paying for, or purchasing, the health care required by the population they serve.

8. With regard to hospital services, the population served by each purchaser is determined by: the type of treatment that a patient requires (which may be either emergency or elective) and the type of doctor of the patient (who may be a general practitioner, a GP Fundholder or a Total Purchasing Pilot).

9. Purchasers receive a sum of money from Hospital and Community Health Services Revenue Funds with which to buy health care for the population they serve. The NHS internal market then works by purchasers deciding which providers they want to buy health care from for the population they serve, and then negotiating a contract with those providers. This contract essentially specifies the health care services to be provided by the provider and the sum of money to be paid for those services by the purchaser. The success of the NHS internal market as a means of allocating scarce health care resources in this way depends primarily on two factors: the ability of health care purchasers to choose from whom they wish to purchase health care for the population they serve, and competition between health care providers.

10. The main features of a contract are that it may stipulate a quantity of health care to be provided, the quality of health care to be provided and the price for that level of provision. However, the exact content will depend upon the type of contract. There are three types: block contracts ('simple' and 'complex'); cost-per-case contracts; and cost-and-volume contracts.

11. A proportion of patient referrals for health care are not covered by contracts between purchasers and providers. Such cases are known as extra-contractual referrals (ECRs), and occur when a patient seeks health care from a provider which is not covered by a contract negotiated with the patient's purchaser. There are two types of extra-contractual referral: emergency extra-contractual referrals and elective extra-contractual referrals.

12. The link between prices and costs in the NHS internal market is extremely important. The fundamental principles set out by the NHS Executive for the establishment of costs and prices are: prices should be based on average costs (in that prices should equal costs with no intent to make a profit); costs should generally be arrived at on a full cost basis (with all costs absorbed into the process so that the anticipated cost of the unit divided by the total anticipated activity will give a unit price); and there should be no planned cross-subsidisation between contracts (so that there will be no deliberate cost shifting to make one price lower at the expense of another).

13. Two features are likely to be extremely important if the NHS internal market is to be sustained as a tool for allocating scarce health care resources in the UK: competition between health care providers and pricing regulation to ensure average cost pricing by health care providers.

The UK National Health Service

The establishment of the UK National Health Service (NHS) in 1948 was an attempt to make health care available to the entire population of the UK via a system of direct taxation-based finance and universal provision. The NHS at that time was therefore available to everyone and it was comprehensive in the range of services that it provided.

A key principle underpinning the introduction of the NHS was that health care was to be provided on the basis of clinically defined need rather than on ability to pay or other considerations. Money to fund the NHS was raised through a combination of taxes and National Insurance contributions and there were, initially at least, no charges made for treatment. This ensured that health care was made universal to all. Later, NHS funds were supplemented by prescription charges and additional payments for dental treatment and eye tests.

Throughout the 1980s, expenditure on the NHS continually grew, but there developed a widening gap between the funds provided by the government for the NHS and the funding required to meet the increasing demands of an ageing population and advances in medical technology (Ham, 1995). The impact of the shortage of funding became particularly apparent in 1987 and was felt most acutely in the hospital services. That year, many health authorities had to take urgent action in order to keep expenditure within financing limits. This included cancelling non-emergency admissions, closing hospital beds on a temporary basis and not filling staff vacancies.

Behind these problems lay a funding system for health care services that failed to reward hospitals for treating extra patients (Ham, 1990). This so-called 'efficiency trap' was caused by the use of global budgeting for hospital services, which provided a fixed income regardless of the number of patients treated. This meant that hospitals were, in effect, penalised for productivity improvements because, whilst their expenditure on providing health care increased with the number of patients treated, the income received to cover that expenditure remained the same. In this situation, hospitals had little choice but to reduce workloads and to cut costs when their budgets ran out. The simplest way for hospitals to cut costs was to reduce the number of staff employed, so that, in addition to the financial pressures facing hospitals, problems were exacerbated by staff shortages.

The government responded to these problems in 1988 when the then Prime Minister, Margaret Thatcher, announced her decision to introduce a far-reaching ministerial review of the future of the NHS. The Prime Minister established and chaired a small committee of senior ministers to undertake the review, which was supported by a group of civil servants and political advisers.

In its early stages, this ministerial review focused on alternative methods for financing health care in the UK. This included examining the scope for increasing the role of private health insurance and moving from a direct taxation-based funding system to a public health insurance system, common in other European countries. However, this was soon overtaken by an analysis of how the provision of health care services could be reformed assuming the continuation of direct taxation-based health care finance.

It was on this basis that ideas originally put forward by an American economist called Alain Enthoven caught the attention of the ministerial review committee. In a report published in 1985, Enthoven argued that an internal market should be developed within the NHS and used as a basis for the provision of health care (Enthoven, 1985). This idea was acknowledged by the then Secretary of State for Health, Kenneth Clarke, who saw the merits of introducing choice and competition into the provision of health care in the UK in this way (Roberts, 1990).

The government's proposals for the future of the NHS, which were based on the outcomes of the ministerial review, were published in January 1989 in a White Paper called 'Working for patients' (Secretary of State for Health, 1989).

'Working for patients'

In 'Working for patients', the government announced that the basic principles on which the NHS was founded would be preserved (see Box 7.1). The NHS would continue to be available to all, regardless of income, and it would continue to be financed mainly out of general taxation.

The key changes announced in the white paper did not concern the way in which health care would be financed. Rather, they concerned the way in which health care would be provided. These changes were primarily intended to increase competition between health care providers, and this was to be achieved by a variety of means:

Box 7.1 *Extracts from 'Working for patients' (source: Secretary of State for Health, 1989)*

'Working for patients'

Foreword by the Prime Minister

'The National Health Service will continue to be available to all, regardless of income, and to be financed mainly out of general taxation.' [Foreword]

'We aim to extend patient choice, to delegate responsibility to where the services are provided and to secure the best value for money.' [Foreword]

Objectives

'. . . to give patients, wherever they live in the UK, better health care and greater choice of the services available'. [p. 3]

'. . . greater satisfaction and rewards for those working in the NHS who successfully respond to local needs and preferences'. [p. 4]

Key changes

'. . . hospitals will be able to apply for a new self-governing status as NHS Hospital Trusts . . . NHS Hospital Trusts will earn revenue from the services they provide . . . NHS Hospital Trusts will also be able to set the rates of pay of their own staff and, within annual financing limits, to borrow money to help them respond to patient demand.' [p. 4]

'. . . large GP practices will be able to apply for their own budgets to obtain a defined range of services direct from hospitals . . . GPs will be encouraged to compete for patients by offering better services . . . it will be easier for patients to choose (and change) their own GP as they wish.' [p. 5]

'. . . each DHA's duty will be to buy the best service it can from its own hospitals, from other authorities' hospitals, from self-governing hospitals or from the private sector. Hospitals . . . will have to satisfy Districts that they are delivering the best and most efficient services. They will be free to offer their services to different health authorities.' [p. 33]

'. . . as much power and responsibility as possible will be delegated to a local level'. [p. 4]

'. . . 100 new consultant posts will be created over the next three years'. [p. 5]

'. . . management bodies will be reduced in size and reformed on business lines'. [p. 5]

'. . . quality of service and value for money will be more rigorously audited'. [p. 5]

1. a separation of the roles of purchasers and providers in an NHS internal market;
2. the creation of self-governing NHS Trusts to provide health care and earn revenue for the services they provided;
3. the transformation of District Health Authorities into purchasers of health care for their resident populations;
4. the opportunity for large general practitioner practices to become GP Fund-holders, able to purchase limited hospital services for their patients;
5. the use of contracts as a means of providing links between purchasers and providers.

These and other key changes were outlined in 'Working for patients'. These NHS reforms were a response to acute funding problems in the NHS that developed during the 1980s. Although the reforms themselves did not tackle the problem of long-term underfunding, they did seek to provide a way of ensuring that existing health care resources were used as efficiently as possible and that hospitals were not penalised for productivity improvements.

Together with parallel changes in the provision of community care in the UK, the proposals outlined in 'Working for patients' were incorporated into the NHS and Community Care Bill, which was published in November 1989 and received Royal Assent in June 1990. This allowed the NHS internal market to come into being in April 1991.

With the introduction of the NHS internal market, the NHS underwent a series of reforms more fundamental than any experienced since its beginning in 1948 (Ham, 1990). Up to the present day, these reforms have had a major impact on the organisational structure of the NHS and on the flow of funds through the system. It is to this current organisational structure that we now turn.

Organisational structure of the NHS

The organisational structure of the NHS is extremely complicated. A simplified version of this, which shows the key relationships between all the major components, is presented in Figure 7.1. If we use this organisational structure as the basis for the following discussion, the major components of the NHS are as follows:

1. Secretary of State for Health;
2. Department of Health;
3. NHS Executive (HQ);
4. NHS Executive (Regional Offices);
5. Health Authorities;
6. NHS Trusts;
7. general practitioners;
8. GP Fundholders;
9. Total Purchasing Pilots;
10. Locality Commissions.

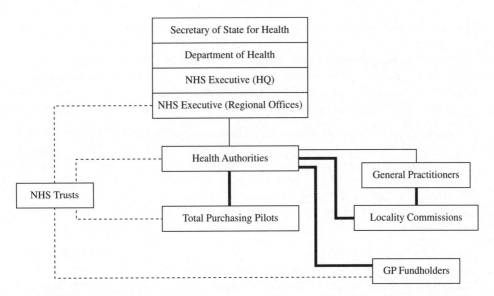

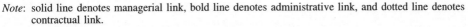

Note: solid line denotes managerial link, bold line denotes administrative link, and dotted line denotes contractual link.

Figure 7.1 Organisational structure of the NHS.

To understand the organisational structure more clearly, it is useful to discuss briefly the function of each of these components.

Secretary of State for Health

The Secretary of State for Health holds the ultimate responsibility for all health care provided by the NHS. He or she sits at the head of the Department of Health and is supported by a Minister of State for Health and a number of junior ministers. Additionally, some 5,000 civil servants work in the Department of Health under the Secretary of State for Health.

The Secretary of State for Health is accountable to Parliament for the provision of health services. The NHS is financed mainly out of public funds and it is the responsibility of the Secretary of State for Health to argue for these funds to be allocated to the NHS. Parliament votes on the size of expenditure devoted to the NHS and therefore has some say in how the money is spent. Members of Parliament are able to raise issues in correspondence and through parliamentary questions and debates, and the Secretary of State for Health is expected to be able to respond to these issues. In this way, the accountability of the Secretary of State for Health to Parliament has an important influence on the organisation and management of the NHS, and the provision of health care in the UK.

Department of Health

The Department of Health is responsible at a national level for the NHS and is also responsible for setting the policy and legislative framework for the provision of health care and related services. The Department of Health performs a number of functions, including the following:

1. making policy and issuing advice to Health Authorities (policy and advice are issued in various forms: major policy statements are set out in White Papers or Discussion Papers; more detailed advice and guidance is issued through Executive Letters [ELs], Finance Directorate Letters [FDLs] or Health Service Guidance Letters [HSGs]);
2. allocating resources to Health Authorities;
3. monitoring the performance of Health Authorities.

Management of the NHS is the responsibility of one division of the Department of Health, namely, the NHS Executive. The NHS Executive consists of centralised headquarters, NHS Executive (HQ), and regional outposts, NHS Executive (Regional Offices).

NHS Executive (HQ)

The NHS Executive (HQ) is chaired by the Chief Executive of the NHS and is concerned with operational matters within the strategy and objectives established by the Department of Health. A key role of the NHS Executive (HQ) is to allocate resources to Health Authorities. Also, the NHS Executive (HQ) monitors the performance of Health Authorities and NHS Trusts in order to assess the way in which they use resources. This involves discussion between the NHS Executive (HQ) and the NHS Executive (Regional Offices).

NHS Executive (Regional Offices)

Following the abolition of Regional Health Authorities (RHAs) in April 1996, the NHS Executive (Regional Offices) now plays a key role in the management of the NHS. The NHS Executive (Regional Offices) is the intermediate tier between the Department of Health and the Health Authorities, and it performs a number of functions, including the planning of the regional development of services within the context of national guidelines, and monitoring the performance of Health Authorities and NHS Trusts.

Health Authorities

In April 1996, the merger of District Health Authorities (DHAs) and Family Health Services Authorities (FHSAs) was made universal, and this led to the introduction of single agencies responsible for the management of health care services at a local level, namely, Health Authorities (HAs). Health Authorities play a key role in the organisation and management of the NHS, and they have a number of functions, including the following:

1. purchasing specified elective hospital services and community health services for the population served;
2. assessing the level of need for health care in the population;
3. planning services to meet those needs;
4. public health;
5. managing the contracts of family practitioners (that is, general practitioners, dentists, pharmacists and opticians);
6. allocating funds to family practitioners according to these contracts;
7. planning strategically with GP Fundholders regarding purchasing decisions;
8. providing information to the public;
9. interfacing with the population to ascertain public opinion;
10. dealing with complaints made by patients.

NHS Trusts

Hospitals and other units providing patient care, such as ambulance units and community care units, are now established as NHS Trusts. These are self-governing provider units within the NHS. They are run by a Board of Directors and are directly accountable to the NHS Executive, without any intervention from Health Authorities. NHS Trusts are free to:

1. determine their own management structure;
2. employ their own staff, and set their own terms and conditions of service;
3. acquire, own and sell their own assets;
4. retain surpluses achieved from the services they provide;
5. borrow money subject to annual limits.

Each NHS Trust is required to prepare an annual business plan outlining its plans for service development and capital investment which will be discussed with the NHS Executive. Each NHS Trust also prepares and publishes an annual report and statement of accounts.

NHS Trusts receive income from contracts with health care purchasers, and they are responsible to these purchasers for delivering the quantity and quality of health care specified in the contract.

General practitioners

General practitioners (GPs) are one component of the primary health care team, which may also include practice nurses, district nurses, health visitors, and other professions allied to medicine such as chiropodists, physiotherapists and dieticians. Primary health care teams are responsible for providing primary health care services in the NHS. GPs not in fundholding practices (hereafter simply called GPs) remain under the direct control of, and are managed by, Health Authorities.

GPs play an important role in the provision of health care in the NHS, since they are often a patient's first contact with the health care services. GPs have many important functions. Some of the more obvious include:

1. providing medical advice;
2. prescribing medications;
3. referring patients to hospital or other health care services.

GP Fundholders

GP Fundholders are large GP practices which hold their own budgets in order to buy a defined range of health care services on behalf of the patients on their list. In addition to providing medical advice, prescribing medications and referring patients to hospital or other health care services, all of which are possible without fundholding status, GP Fundholders are also able to purchase health care services from NHS Trusts. Specifically, GP Fundholders are able to purchase the following services:

1. specified elective hospital services (including elective surgical services, outpatient services, and diagnostic tests and investigations);
2. community health services (including health visiting; district nursing; dietetic services; chiropody services; mental health outpatient and community services; mental health counselling; health care services for people with learning difficulties; and referrals made by health visitors, district nurses, community psychiatric nurses and community mental handicap nurses).

Total Purchasing Pilots

Since 1994, a number of pilot projects have been initiated in which GPs have taken responsibility for purchasing the *full* range of health care services. These GPs are known as Total Purchasing Pilots. In addition to being able to purchase specified elective hospital services and community health services, Total Purchasing Pilots are therefore also able to purchase all other health care services, including emergency hospital services.

Locality Commissions

Alongside GP Fundholding and Total Purchasing Pilots, there have emerged additional methods for enhancing the involvement of GPs in purchasing decisions. Locality Commissions provide a method for increasing GP input into the purchasing decisions made by Health Authorities. They consist of local GPs who group together in an attempt to influence the range of services purchased by Health Authorities and, in this way, attempt to secure more practice-sensitive purchasing which reflects specific local needs and preferences. Health Authorities may, if they wish, disregard the preferences of Locality Commissions.

Flow of funds in the NHS

The flow of funds in the NHS is also extremely complicated. A simplified version of this flow, showing the key features of the system, is presented in Figure 7.2. The system may be characterised by funding flows between the various components of the organisational structure. These funding flows are numbered (1) to (10) in Figure 7.2. Each may be examined separately.

1. From: General Population (Taxation and National Insurance)
To: Treasury

From discussion of the various methods for structuring health care finance delineated in Chapter 6, we ascertained that the NHS is a direct taxation system. The key feature of this financing method is that all individuals are required to pay insurance

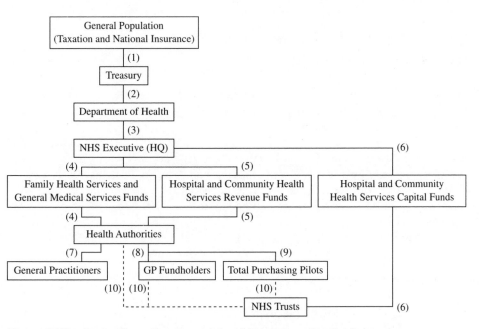

Note: solid line denotes direct allocation, and dotted line denotes allocation by contract.

Figure 7.2 Flow of funds in the NHS.

Table 7.1 NHS expenditure and sources of finance.

Year	NHS expenditure £ million	Taxation £ million	% of total	NHS contributions £ million	% of total	Patient payments[1] £ million	% of total
1974	3,970	3,610	90.9	235	5.9	105	2.6
1975	5,315	4,737	89.1	451	8.5	127	2.4
1976	6,303	5,554	88.1	597	9.5	152	2.4
1977	7,001	6,152	87.9	671	9.6	178	2.5
1978	8,032	7,072	88.0	761	9.5	199	2.5
1979	9,321	8,200	88.0	882	9.5	239	2.6
1980	11,954	10,591	88.6	1,042	8.7	321	2.7
1981	13,768	12,030	87.4	1,344	9.8	394	2.9
1982	14,543	12,487	85.9	1,594	11.0	462	3.2
1983	16,470	14,187	86.1	1,741	10.6	542	3.3
1984	17,417	14,935	85.8	1,846	10.6	636	3.7
1985	18,578	15,873	85.4	2,016	10.9	689	3.7
1986	19,901	16,936	85.1	2,228	11.2	737	3.7
1987	21,700	18,180	83.8	2,725	12.6	795	3.6
1988	23,829	19,517	81.9	3,419	14.3	893	3.8
1989	26,193	21,034	80.3	4,117	15.7	1,042	4.0
1990	28,900	23,505	81.3	4,261	14.7	1,134	4.0
1991	32,394	26,653	82.3	4,497	13.9	1,244	3.8
1992	36,361	30,292	83.5	4,646	12.8	1,323	3.7
1993	38,211	32,189	84.2	4,674	12.2	1,348	3.6
1994	39,968	33,648	84.2	4,962	12.4	1,358	3.4
1995	41,517	34,952	84.2	5,269	12.7	1,296	3.1

Note:
[1] Includes hospital charges, prescription charges, and charges for dental and ophthalmic services.
Source: OHE (1995).

premiums to the government. These insurance premiums are collected via taxation so that the contribution by individuals to the government to pay for their health care is part of their total tax payment.

As shown in Table 7.1, of total NHS expenditure in 1995 (£41,517 million), 84.2 per cent was financed out of general taxation and 12.7 per cent was financed by NHS contributions paid by employers and employees via the National Insurance scheme. Taxation in one form or another therefore accounts for 96.9 per cent of total NHS finance, where the contribution of individuals to the NHS is part of their total tax payment.

Therefore, the initial flow of funds in the system is from the general population via taxation and National Insurance payments to the Treasury.

2. From: Treasury
   To: Department of Health

Resources are allocated annually from the Treasury to the Department of Health following negotiations which take place in the government's annual Public Expendi-

Table 7.2 NHS expenditure as a proportion of total public expenditure; figures relate to central government and local authority expenditure, excluding charges.

Year	Total public expenditure £ million	NHS %	Defence %	Education %	Housing %	Social Security %	Others[1] %
1974	35,012	11.0	11.7	13.3	12.0	19.5	32.5
1975	46,550	11.1	11.1	14.2	9.5	19.1	34.8
1976	52,162	11.8	11.9	14.0	9.8	21.5	30.9
1977	54,694	12.5	12.5	15.3	10.0	27.7	22.0
1978	64,107	12.2	11.8	14.3	9.4	27.9	24.4
1979	75,624	12.0	11.9	13.6	9.6	27.8	25.1
1980	91,654	12.7	12.5	13.9	9.2	27.8	23.9
1981	102,434	13.1	12.3	14.0	7.0	30.3	23.3
1982	112,786	12.5	12.8	13.6	5.8	32.3	23.0
1983	122,232	13.0	13.0	13.4	6.1	32.1	22.4
1984	129,361	13.0	13.2	13.1	6.2	32.6	21.9
1985	137,806	13.0	13.2	12.5	5.1	33.6	22.6
1986	142,605	13.4	13.4	13.5	5.7	35.0	19.0
1987	148,501	14.1	12.8	14.0	5.5	35.1	18.5
1988	156,930	14.6	12.6	14.4	5.4	34.6	18.4
1989	174,711	14.4	12.0	14.2	4.6	32.8	22.0
1990	193,041	14.4	11.9	13.8	4.0	32.6	23.3
1991	207,652	15.0	11.2	14.1	4.2	35.5	20.0
1992	233,489	15.0	10.5	13.7	4.4	36.2	20.3
1993	251,095	14.7	9.7	13.5	4.4	37.1	20.6
1994	257,867	15.0	9.5	13.5	4.4	36.6	21.0
1995	269,873	14.9	8.8	13.4	4.3	36.9	21.7

Note:
[1] Including personal social services, transport, etc.
Source: OHE (1995).

ture Survey. It is through the Public Expenditure Survey that priorities for different areas of public expenditure are determined. The sum allocated to the Department of Health for all NHS expenditure is fixed for one year.

Ultimately, the sum of money devoted to the NHS each year is a political decision, and is decided in the broader context of expenditure across all public sectors. Total NHS expenditure as a proportion of total expenditure across all public sectors is presented in Table 7.2. In recent years, the NHS has been allocated approximately 15 per cent of total public expenditure, and therefore receives the second largest share of public funds after Social Security.

3. From: Department of Health
To: NHS Executive (HQ)

The Department of Health allocates funds to the NHS Executive (HQ) which then distributes the bulk of the NHS budget to Family Health Services and General Medical Services Funds, and Hospital and Community Health Services Revenue and

Capital Funds. Both the Department of Health and the NHS Executive (HQ) retain a small proportion of funds to resource their own operations.

4. From: NHS Executive (HQ)
   To: Family Health Services and General Medical Services
          Funds
   To: Health Authorities

Resources are allocated from the NHS Executive (HQ) to Health Authorities for family health services. This allocation is made from Family Health Services Funds. On receiving these funds, Health Authorities pass the majority on to family practitioners (GPs, dentists, pharmacists and opticians), retaining a small proportion to cover the costs they incur. Family Health Services Funds comprise the following:

1. General Medical Service Funds, ultimately allocated to GPs, GP Fundholders and Total Purchasing Pilots;
2. General Dental Service Funds, ultimately allocated to dentists;
3. General Pharmaceutical Service Funds, ultimately allocated to pharmacists;
4. General Optical Service Funds, ultimately allocated to opticians.

With the exception of certain payments to GPs from General Medical Services Funds (see below), allocations from the NHS Executive (HQ) to Health Authorities via Family Health Services Funds are generally not fixed in advance but determined by the demand for services.

5. From: NHS Executive (HQ)
   To: Hospital and Community Health Services Revenue
          Funds
   To: Health Authorities

Resources are allocated from the NHS Executive (HQ) to Health Authorities for hospital and community health services. This allocation is made from Hospital and Community Health Services Revenue Funds. The allocation to each Health Authority is determined with reference to a funding policy which is based on a weighted capitation formula. There are four stages in setting allocations to Health Authorities using the weighted capitation formula:

1. Estimate the resident population in each Health Authority

This is so that the greater the number of individuals living in a Health Authority, the greater the Hospital and Community Health Services Revenue Fund allocation received.

2. Apply age weights

This is to reflect the age distribution in each Health Authority and the fact that certain age groups require more health care than others. The greater the proportion of elderly or very young individuals in the population, the greater the Hospital and Community Health Services Revenue Fund allocation received.

3. Apply needs weights

This is to reflect the level of ill health in each Health Authority, so that the more unhealthy the population, the greater the Hospital and Community Health Services Revenue Fund allocation received.

4. Apply market forces weights

This is to reflect the fact that the cost of providing health care varies across the country, so that Health Authorities in London and the South East receive a greater share of Hospital and Community Health Services Revenue Funds.

As well as allocations received via the weighted capitation formula, Health Authorities also receive funds for various additional functions, including: management and administration of resources; surveillance of communicable diseases; nursing home registration; and provision of health promotion services.

6. From: NHS Executive (HQ)
   To: Hospital and Community Health Services Capital
          Funds
   To: NHS Trusts

Since 1993, land, buildings, equipment and motor vehicles with a cost or value of £5,000 or more are defined as capital. A capital allocation by the NHS Executive (HQ) to NHS Trusts from Hospital and Community Health Services Capital Funds is made on the basis of individual applications for funds submitted by NHS Trusts to the NHS Executive (HQ).

7. From: Health Authorities
   To: GPs

The allocation of funds from Health Authorities to GPs is made from General Medical Services Funds and comprises numerous components:

1. payments based on the population served (determined by the size and structure of the population served, these include capitation fees, basic practice allowances and deprivation payments);

2. item of service payments (including payments for child health surveillance, night visits, minor surgery services, health promotion clinics and maternity medical services);
3. target payments (based, for example, on the achievement of targets for screening for cervical cancer and childhood immunisation);
4. premises costs (including rent, rates and improvement grants);
5. staff costs (including reimbursement of the cost of employing suitable practice staff);
6. seniority payments;
7. post-graduate education allowances.

Rent payments, improvement grants and reimbursement of the cost of employing suitable practice staff are all paid on an annual basis and are fixed in advance. All other allocations from General Medical Services Funds are not. Instead, funds are allocated to GPs by Health Authorities under the terms of nationally agreed contracts. Payments to GPs via these contracts are not fixed in advance, but are determined by the demand for services and by how GPs choose to treat patients.

8. From: Health Authorities
To: GP Fundholders

The budget allocated to GP Fundholders by Health Authorities comprises three components:

1. Practice staff reimbursement

First, Health Authorities allocate funds to GP Fundholders from General Medical Services Funds for practice staff reimbursement. Health Authorities reimburse all GP Fundholders for an agreed proportion of practice staff, including practice nurses and receptionists. This proportion is originally set by the Health Authority which determines the staff that are appropriate for reimbursement.

2. Medications

Secondly, the allocation for expenditure on medications by GP Fundholders is set by the Health Authority, and is also allocated from General Medical Services Funds. This allocation is based upon existing prescribing patterns adjusted for any known or planned changes either to the practice's prescribing policies, or the structure or number of patients on the practice's list.

3. Hospital and community health services

Thirdly, GP Fundholders are able to purchase the following services:

- specified elective hospital services (including elective surgical services, out-patient services, and diagnostic tests and investigations);

- community health services (including health visiting; district nursing; dietetic services; chiropody services; mental health outpatient and community services; mental health counselling; health care services for people with learning difficulties; and referrals made by health visitors, district nurses, community psychiatric nurses and community mental handicap nurses).

The budget for the purchase of these services is allocated from Health Authorities to GP Fundholders from Hospital and Community Health Services Revenue Funds. The allocation is based on the practice's referral pattern and list size.

Whilst the budget allocated to GP Fundholders is calculated under three headings, it is offered as a single amount. As a consequence of this, GP Fundholders may transfer money allocated in the budget between the three components.

Underexpenditures achieved in any one year become savings once the practice accounts have been audited. Whilst regulations laid down by the Department of Health bar GP Fundholders from benefiting personally from these savings, they may be spent for the benefit of patients on the practice list, which, in the long term, may result in personal benefits to GP Fundholders.

9. From: Health Authorities
   To: Total Purchasing Pilots

The allocation of funds from Health Authorities to Total Purchasing Pilots is similar to the allocation from Health Authorities to GP Fundholders, above, except the ability of Total Purchasing Pilots to purchase the full range of health care services from NHS Trusts means that they receive a larger allocation for the purchase of hospital and community health services. Therefore, the budget allocated to Total Purchasing Pilots also comprises three components:

1. Practice staff reimbursement

This is allocated by Health Authorities from General Medical Services Funds. This reimbursement is made for an agreed proportion of practice staff, such as practice nurses and receptionists. The proportion is originally set by the Health Authority, which determines the staff who are appropriate for reimbursement.

2. Medications

This is allocated by the Health Authorities from General Medical Services Funds. This allocation is based upon existing prescribing patterns adjusted for any known or planned changes either to the practice's prescribing policies or the structure or number of patients on the practice's list.

3. Hospital and community health services

This is allocated by Health Authorities from Hospital and Community Health Services Revenue Funds. The allocation is based on the practice's referral pattern and list size, and rather than just covering specified elective hospital services and community health services, it covers the provision of all health care services.

10. From: Health Authorities, GP Fundholders, Total Purchasing Pilots
To: NHS Trusts

Funds are distributed from Health Authorities, GP Fundholders and Total Purchasing Pilots to NHS Trusts in return for the provision of hospital and community health services to the populations served. The relationship between Health Authorities, GP Fundholders, Total Purchasing Pilots and NHS Trusts is characterised by what has become known as the NHS internal market, and is determined by the contracts which exist between purchasers and providers of health care. The contracting process and the workings of the internal market are discussed in greater detail in the next section.

The internal market

One of the most important elements of the NHS reforms introduced in April 1991 was the separation of the roles of purchasers and providers of health care in a market called the *NHS internal market*.

As explained in Chapter 2, a market may be defined as any institution where parties can communicate with each other in order to buy and sell goods and services. A market is therefore, in effect, any institution where buyers and sellers meet. This principle has been applied to the NHS internal market, which is an arrangement between buyers and sellers who meet to buy and sell health care.

In the NHS internal market, the buyers of health care are called *purchasers* and they buy health care for the population they serve. The sellers of health care are called *providers*, and they provide health care to this population. The purchasers and providers in the NHS internal market are presented in Box 7.2.

Providers

Providers in the NHS internal market are NHS Trusts. They are responsible for delivering contracted health care services within the quality and quantity specifications delineated by contracts to one or more purchasers in return for an agreed sum of money.

Purchasers

There are three types of purchaser in the NHS internal market: Health Authorities; GP Fundholders; and Total Purchasing Pilots. Each of these has a primary responsibility to ensure that, within available resources, health care services are secured to

Box 7.2 *Purchasers and providers in the NHS internal market*

PROVIDERS	*PURCHASERS*
NHS Trusts	Health Authorities
	GP Fundholders
	Total Purchasing Pilots

The role of providers in the NHS internal market
NHS Trusts deliver contracted health care services within the quality and quantity specifications delineated by contracts to one or more purchasers in return for receipt of agreed charges.

The role of purchasers in the NHS internal market
Health Authorities, GP Fundholders and Total Purchasing Pilots have a primary responsibility to ensure that, within available resources, health care services are secured to meet the health needs of the populations they serve.

---

meet the health needs of the population it serves. Purchasers are therefore responsible for paying for, or purchasing, the health care required by the population they serve.

With regards to hospital services, the populations served by each purchaser are described in Table 7.3. These are determined by:

1. the type of treatment that a patient requires (which may be either emergency or elective);
2. the type of doctor of the patient (who may be a general practitioner, a GP Fundholder or a Total Purchasing Pilot).

Therefore, one of six scenarios may arise, numbered (1) to (6) in Table 7.3. These may be used to determine the purchaser of hospital treatment for a particular patient, as follows:

Table 7.3 Purchasing hospital services.

Type of treatment required by patient	Type of doctor which patient may have		
	GP	GP Fundholder	Total Purchasing Pilot
Elective	Scenario (1) HA	Scenario (2) GPFH	Scenario (3) TPP
Emergency	Scenario (4) HA	Scenario (5) HA	Scenario (6) TPP

GP = general practitioner
GPFH = GP Fundholder
TPP = Total Purchasing Pilot
HA = Health Authority

Scenario (1)

A patient requires *elective* treatment and the patient's doctor is a *GP*. In this case, the treatment is purchased by the *Health Authority* where the patient lives.

Scenario (2)

A patient requires *elective* treatment and the patient's doctor is a *GP Fundholder*. In this case, the treatment is purchased by the patient's doctor, that is, by the *GP Fundholder*.

Scenario (3)

A patient requires *elective* treatment and the patient's doctor is a *Total Purchasing Pilot*. In this case, the treatment is purchased by the patient's doctor, that is, by the *Total Purchasing Pilot*.

Scenario (4)

A patient requires *emergency* treatment and the patient's doctor is a *GP*. In this case, the treatment is purchased by the *Health Authority* where the patient lives.

Scenario (5)

A patient requires *emergency* treatment and the patient's doctor is a *GP Fundholder*. In this case, the treatment is purchased by the *Health Authority* where the patient lives.

Scenario (6)

A patient requires *emergency* treatment and the patient's doctor is a *Total Purchasing Pilot*. In this case, the treatment is purchased by the patient's doctor, that is, by the *Total Purchasing Pilot*.

In summary, if the patient's doctor is a GP, then the Health Authority pays for all hospital treatment (both elective and emergency). If the patient's doctor is a GP Fundholder, then that GP Fundholder pays for all elective hospital treatment and the Health Authority pays for all emergency hospital treatment. If the patient's doctor is a Total Purchasing Pilot, then that Total Purchasing Pilot pays for all hospital treatment (both emergency and elective).

The contracting process

Purchasers receive a sum of money from Hospital and Community Health Services Revenue Funds with which to buy health care for the population they serve. The NHS internal market then works by purchasers deciding which providers they want to buy health care from for the population they serve, and then negotiating a contract with those providers. This contract essentially specifies the health care services to be provided by the provider and the sum of money to be paid for those services by the purchaser.

The success of the NHS internal market as a means of allocating scarce health care resources in this way depends primarily on two factors:

1. the ability of health care purchasers to choose from whom they wish to purchase health care for the population they serve;
2. competition between health care providers.

A key feature of the introduction of an NHS internal market is that health care purchasers now have freedom of choice regarding the provider from whom they wish to purchase health care for the population they serve. Given this freedom, the intention is that purchasers will 'shop around' when deciding from whom to purchase health care in order to obtain a high standard of health care at a reasonable price.

Health care providers, realising that purchasers now have this choice, must ensure they are providing a high standard of health care at a reasonable price so that they attract the custom of purchasers. Providers who do not provide high-quality health care at reasonable prices will be unable to obtain contracts with purchasers, who will choose to obtain services elsewhere. Providers are therefore required to compete with each other in order to attract contracts from purchasers.

The relationship between a purchaser and provider is secured by a contract between both parties specifying the range and volume of services to be provided by the provider and the sum of money paid by the purchaser for the provision of those services. In this way, the system of competitive contracting in the NHS internal market is designed to introduce price competition and to enhance the achievement of efficiency.

The main features of a contract are that they may stipulate a quantity of health care to be provided, the quality of health care to be provided, and the price for that level of provision. However, the exact content will depend upon the type of contract.

Types of contract

There are three types of contract in the internal market:

1. block contracts ('simple' and 'complex');
2. cost-per-case contracts;
3. cost-and-volume contracts.

Block contracts

With *block contracts*, the provider is paid an annual sum of money by the purchaser, in monthly instalments, in return for granting access to the population served by the purchaser to a defined range of health care services.

There are two types of block contract: 'simple' block contracts and 'complex' (or 'sophisticated') block contracts. With simple block contracts, the actual volume of health care services to be provided is not specified in advance. With complex block contracts, whilst some variation is possible in the actual volume of services to be provided, floors and ceilings are stipulated, which indicate the minimum and maximum volume of services to be provided. Any cases which are required above the ceiling stipulated in the complex block contract are treated on a cost-per-case basis.

Cost-per-case contracts

With *cost-per-case contracts*, the provider receives a sum of money for providing a specific health care service to an individual patient. Purchasers agree to pay for each case treated at a pre-agreed price which depends on the diagnosis of the patient.

Cost-and-volume contracts

With *cost-and-volume contracts*, the provider receives an agreed sum of money in return for providing a specific range and volume of health care services. Any cases which are required above the volume stipulated in the cost-and-volume contract are treated on a cost-per-case basis. Therefore, purchasers buy access to facilities up to a maximum agreed workload, and then purchase additional cases beyond this maximum at a cost-per-case rate.

Initially, the majority of contracts in the NHS internal market negotiated between purchasers and providers were simple block contracts. Increasingly, however, purchasers and providers have tended towards the use of complex block contracts, cost-and-volume contracts and cost-per-case contracts.

Extra-contractual referrals

A proportion of patient referrals for health care are not covered by contracts between purchasers and providers. Such cases are known as *extra-contractual referrals* (*ECRs*), and occur when a patient seeks health care from a provider which is not covered by a contract negotiated with the patient's purchaser.

There are two types of extra-contractual referral:

1. emergency extra-contractual referrals;
2. elective extra-contractual referrals.

Emergency extra-contractual referrals occur when a patient requires emergency treatment from a provider and the patient's purchaser has not negotiated a contract with that provider. This may occur if, for example, the patient is taken ill on holiday. Purchasers are obliged to pay for all emergency extra-contractual referrals.

Elective extra-contractual referrals occur when a patient requires elective treatment from a provider and the patient's purchaser has not negotiated a contract with that provider. This may occur if, for example, a patient decides they would rather receive treatment from a provider different to the one with which the purchaser has negotiated a contract. They may also occur if a patient requires a rare elective treatment for which the purchaser has not negotiated a contract with any provider. In the case of elective extra-contractual referrals, the provider is required to obtain approval from the purchaser before the treatment is provided.

Both types of extra-contractual referral are purchased on a cost-per-case basis (that is, each case is paid for individually by the purchaser).

Invoicing purchasers

All health care services, whether provided under the terms of a negotiated contract or as extra-contractual referrals, have to be invoiced by the provider to the purchaser for payment.

For hospital services covered by contracts, patients are admitted into hospital and allocated to a contract using two pieces of information:

1. the patient's postcode;
2. the name of the patient's GP.

The patient's postcode is used to determine the Health Authority of residence. The name of the patient's GP is used to determine whether the purchaser is a Health Authority, a GP Fundholder or a Total Purchasing Pilot.

The patient then receives the required treatment. After discharge, clinical codes are attached to the patient's notes in order to identify the type of treatment which was provided. With information on the type of treatment provided to the patient and the type of doctor of the patient, and using the taxonomy presented in Table 7.3, the provider is able to ascertain who will pay for the patient's treatment. An invoice may then be issued to this purchaser.

In the case of block contracts and cost-and-volume contracts, an invoice is sent each month from the provider to the purchaser for payment. In the case of cost-per-case contracts, an invoice must be drawn up within one month of discharge and sent to the purchaser. For emergency and elective extra-contractual referrals, invoicing is the same as with cost-per-case contracts, except that the invoice should be issued a maximum of six weeks after the end of the month in which the episode of care is completed. Additionally, with elective extra-contractual referrals, the provider must obtain authorisation from the purchaser before providing treatment.

Payment to providers

It is important from the providers' perspective that the settlement of payments by purchasers occurs promptly, since failure to do so is likely to present cash flow problems to providers. A framework of rules has been developed for settlement of payments, which incorporate the following:

1. payments for block contracts and cost-and-volume contracts are to be made on a monthly basis;
2. for cost-per-case contracts, purchasers and providers should agree payment terms;
3. for extra-contractual referrals, payment should be made within one month of the date at which the invoice is sent;
4. where an episode of care is likely to extend over a long period, invoices should be submitted monthly;
5. mechanisms for preventing delayed payment are established, including time limits specified for solving uncertainty about payments, and arbitration where necessary.

Setting prices

The link between prices and costs in the NHS internal market is extremely important. The fundamental principles set out by the NHS Executive (originally called the NHS Management Executive) for the establishment of costs and prices are (NHSME, 1990):

1. prices should be based on average costs (in that prices should equal costs with no intent to make a profit);
2. costs should generally be arrived at on a full cost basis (with all costs absorbed into the process so that the anticipated cost of the unit divided by the total anticipated activity will give a unit price);
3. there should be no planned cross-subsidisation between contracts (so that there will be no deliberate cost shifting to make one price lower at the expense of another).

Unfortunately, in practice, prices may not reflect true average costs (MacKerrell, 1993). This may occur because of a lack of available cost data so that there is no information on average costs on which to base prices, or because health care providers have a financial incentive to inflate prices artificially above average cost level in order to make profits from the services they provide. Both these features mean that the NHS internal market may not function perfectly as a means of allocating health care resources.

Competition and pricing regulation

Two features are likely to be extremely important if the NHS internal market is to be sustained as a tool for allocating scarce health care resources in the UK:

1. competition between health care providers;
2. pricing regulation to ensure average cost pricing by health care providers.

We shall now discuss the significance of each of these in turn.

Competition between health care providers

A major aim of the NHS internal market is to increase competition between health care providers in order to achieve the benefits from improved efficiency in the provision of health care services. The relationship between different health care providers all competing for contracts from purchasers is a fundamental feature required for the internal market to succeed, since it gives a strong incentive for providers to provide high-quality health care at reasonable prices.

Unfortunately, in some situations, competition of this kind may not arise between health care providers, since there may be only one health care provider in a particular geographical area. In this situation, rather than a competitive market, the provision of health care is, in fact, the responsibility of a single *monopoly* provider.

As discussed in Chapter 3, a monopoly exists when there is only one producer or provider of a good or service. In the context of the NHS internal market, without any competition, a monopoly provider is able to influence the price of the services it provides so that it is able to exploit its position and to discriminate in such a way so as to make profits at the expense of the purchaser. In this situation, the NHS internal market will fail to allocate health care resources efficiently, since the costs of providing any given level of health care will not be minimised.

Clearly, geographical monopolies may exist in the provision of health care in the UK if it is usual for there to be only a single provider of health care in any one geographical area. In this situation, the NHS internal market price for health care services will be higher than it would if a number of health care providers are forced to compete with each other for the custom of purchasers.

Pricing regulation to ensure average cost pricing by health care providers

In view of the potential for the lack of competition between health care providers, it has been recognised that some form of regulation is required in order to ensure that the prices set by health care providers will be fair and acceptable to purchasers.

As explained above, the main element of the NHS Executive's regulatory strategy is the imposition of an average cost pricing rule designed to ensure that prices are set at average procedure cost. In other words, prices for health care services should be based on the average cost of providing that service. This means that the total revenue generated by health care providers from all contracts should be just sufficient to cover the costs of the services provided.

Unfortunately, this rule requires information on the average cost of every treatment provided via the NHS internal market. Only when the average cost of all

Table 7.4 Average costs by speciality.

Speciality	Patients using a bed (including inpatients and day cases)		Patients not using a bed (including outpatients)
	Cost per episode (£)	Cost per patient day (£)	Cost per attendance (£)
Medical specialities			
Paediatrics	659	197	66
Geriatrics	2,388	111	76
Cardiology	1,330	278	66
Dermatology	917	151	39
Infectious diseases	1,312	259	86
Medical oncology	898	289	79
Neurology	1,521	185	75
Rheumatology	1,567	161	55
Gastroenterology	329	196	57
Haematology	740	234	50
Clinical immunology and allergy	1,118	212	62
Thoracic medicine	928	155	60
Genito-urinary medicine	1,376	416	59
Nephrology	1,058	229	76
Rehabilitation medicine	4,107	136	314
Surgical specialities			
General surgery	875	220	50
Urology	603	207	54
Orthopaedics	1,299	201	50
Ear, nose and throat	608	307	50
Ophthalmology	635	358	40
Gynaecology	555	245	51
Dental specialities	491	376	40
Neurosurgery	2,560	321	75
Plastic surgery	849	294	39
Cardiothoracic surgery	2,362	414	75
Paediatric surgery	1,174	427	64
Maternity specialities			
Obstetrics	654	229	54
General practice	431	145	50
Psychiatric specialities			
Mental handicap	11,161	120	51
Mental illness	6,149	117	70
Child and adolescent psychiatry	10,083	229	57
Forensic psychiatry	33,418	196	152
Psychotherapy	50,236	327	129
Old age psychiatry	7,534	108	72
Other specialities			
General practice (other than maternity)	1,436	99	21
Radiotherapy	1,220	235	94
Pathology	1,673	571	64
Anaesthetics	629	449	52
Accident and Emergency	253	2,001	26

Source: HFMA/CIPFA (1995).

treatments has been fully estimated is it possible for providers to base prices accurately on average procedure costs.

However, considering the range of services provided by the NHS, this is clearly a massive undertaking which involves a great deal of time, effort and money. It is therefore unsurprising that some procedures have yet to be individually costed, and that prices which are used in the NHS internal market are often based only on average speciality costs. That is, the prices used in the NHS internal market, rather than being based on the average cost of individual treatments, are in fact based on average costs of all treatments in one clinical speciality. Clearly, average speciality costs may not accurately reflect the true cost of providing particular individual procedures. Examples of average procedure costs by speciality are provided in Table 7.4.

This problem is exacerbated further with the fact that health care providers have a financial incentive to renege on the average cost pricing rule and to artificially inflate prices in order to earn profits from the services they provide. With a paucity of data on average costs, there is clearly an opportunity for health care providers to act in this way.

Conclusion

It is apparent that, whilst there is much to be had from introducing markets as a means of providing health care in the UK, there are potential problems and pitfalls which may be encountered that may undermine the success of the NHS internal market as a means of allocating health care resources. Nevertheless, this is not to say that the market framework should be abandoned. Rather, it is necessary to examine more closely how the NHS reforms might be taken forward in order to benefit patients and the general public.

Clearly, there are benefits to be made from introducing markets into the health care sector. In the next chapter, we examine a further application of markets in this way, in the context of the market for nursing labour.

References

Enthoven A.C. (1985) *Reflections on the management of the NHS*. London: Nuffield Provincial Hospitals Trust.

Ham C. (1991) *The new National Health Service: organisation and management*. Radcliffe Medical Press: Oxford.

Ham C. (1995) *Management and competition in the new NHS*. Radcliffe Medical Press: Oxford.

HFMA/CIPFA (1995) *Introductory guide to NHS finance*. Third edition. London: HFMA.

MacKerrell D.K. (1993) Contract pricing: a management opportunity. In: Tilley I. (ed.) *Managing the internal market*. London: Paul Chapman.

NHSME (1990) *Costing and pricing contracts*. London: HMSO.

Office of Health Economics (OHE) (1995) *Compendium of health statistics*. London: OHE.

Roberts J. (1990) Kenneth Clarke: hatchet man or remoulder? *British Medical Journal* 301: 1383–6.

Secretary of State for Health (1989) *Working for patients*. London: HMSO.

Suggested further reading

For a discussion of the background to the NHS reforms see:

Ham C. (1995) *Management and competition in the new NHS*. Radcliffe Medical Press: Oxford, pp. 1–9.

A discussion of the key changes to the NHS introduced in April 1991 is provided in:

Ham C. (1995) *Management and competition in the new NHS*. Radcliffe Medical Press: Oxford, pp. 10–31.

For an analysis of the organisational structure of the NHS see:

Ham C. (1991) *The new National Health Service: organisation and management*. Radcliffe Medical Press: Oxford, pp. 13–28.

For a readable and easy-to-understand exposition of issues relating to the flow of funds through the NHS see:

HFMA/CIPFA (1995) *Introductory guide to NHS finance*. Third edition. London: HFMA.

8   The nursing labour market

In this chapter we focus our attention on another application of markets to the health care sector, namely, the labour market for nurses. First, a theoretical framework is provided which may be used to examine the way in which labour markets operate and the relationship between wage rates, employment, workers and employers. Secondly, this theoretical framework is applied to the labour market for nurses in the UK National Health Service. The mechanisms by which this market operates are explored in considerable detail and the peculiarities of the market are discussed.

Summary

1. The production function shows the maximum output that can be obtained from possible combinations of inputs. The resources used as inputs into the production of goods and services are called the factors of production.

2. Labour is a factor of production and refers to all human resources that can be used in the production of goods and services. How labour is used, and how it is combined with the other factors of production, helps to determine the amount of a particular good or service provided. Just as there may be a market for goods and services, so there may be a market for the factors of production such as labour.

3. The demand for labour is defined as the number of workers which an employer is willing and able to employ in a particular time period.

4. The most important variable that will have an effect on the quantity of labour demanded is its price, which is the wage rate paid to workers by employers. As the wage rate increases, the number of workers demanded will fall. Conversely, as the wage rate falls, then the number of workers demanded will rise. There is therefore an inverse relationship between the wage rate and the demand for workers.

5. The inverse relationship between the wage rate and the number of workers demanded is explained by the substitution effect of labour and the income effect of labour.

6. Marginal physical product is the change in production of a good or service resulting from the employment of an additional worker.

7. The Law of Diminishing Marginal Returns states that as increasing quantities of a variable factor of production are used in conjunction with a fixed factor of production, the marginal physical product of the variable factor will decrease.

8. Marginal revenue product is the change in revenue to the employer resulting from the employment of an additional worker. The marginal revenue product may be calculated as the marginal physical product multiplied by the price of the good which the worker is used to produce.

9. The decision regarding the optimal number of workers for an employer to employ depends upon the marginal revenue product of additional workers and the wage rate. If the employer wishes to maximises profits, it pays to continue employing more workers up until the point at which the marginal revenue product equals the wage rate. In this way, marginal revenue product may be used to determine the number of workers employed at each wage rate. The marginal revenue product curve is therefore the demand curve for labour because it shows the relationship between the number of workers employed and the wage rate.

10. There are many factors which affect the level of demand for labour, including: the wage rate; the productivity of labour; the price of output; and the substitutability of labour with other factors of production.

11. The supply of labour is defined as the number of workers who are willing and able to be employed in a particular occupation in a particular time period.

12. The variable which is likely to have most significance on the supply of labour is the wage rate. As the wage rate increases, the number of workers supplied will rise. Conversely, if the wage rate falls, then the number of workers supplied will fall. We can therefore say that there is a positive relationship between the wage rate and the number of workers supplied.

13. The effect of changes in the wage rate on the quantity of labour supplied will be affected most significantly by workers outside the labour market. As the wage rate increases, more workers will be attracted into the labour market, and as the wage rate falls, workers are likely to leave the labour market and move to other occupations.

14. The equilibrium wage rate is the wage rate at which the wishes of the employers and workers coincide. At the equilibrium wage rate, the quantity of labour demanded is exactly the same as the quantity of labour supplied. This quantity is called the equilibrium quantity of labour. Equilibrium occurs when the quantity of labour demanded and the quantity of labour supplied are equal, so that at the corresponding equilibrium wage rate there are no unsatisfied employers or workers.

Diagrammatically, the equilibrium wage rate and the equilibrium quantity of labour are defined by the intersection of the demand curve for labour and the supply curve for labour.

15. Wage rates in the labour market provide signals to both employers and workers regarding the quantities of labour to demand and supply. If there are unemployed workers in the labour market, then the market wage rate will fall. If there is a shortage of workers in the labour market, then the market wage rate will increase.

16. In the context of the NHS, the employers of nursing labour are health care providers such as NHS Trusts, who employ nursing staff in order to provide health care services for the patients which they are contracted to treat. It is therefore health care providers who demand nursing labour. The workers in the nursing labour market are nurses themselves, who work for health care providers in return for the receipt of wages. It is therefore nurses who supply nursing labour.

17. There are a number of reasons why the market for nursing labour may not function as conventional economic theory predicts, including: the importance of wage rates in the demand for nursing labour; the importance of wage rates in the supply of nursing labour; quantifying the role of nursing in the production of health care; the length of training period to become a nurse; the possibility of overshoot; and the existence of monopoly and monopsony.

18. In the context of labour markets, a monopoly exists when there is a single supplier of a particular form of labour. A monopsony exists when there is a single employer of a particular form of labour. With the existence of a monopoly supplier of labour, wage rates are likely to increase. With the existence of a monopsony employer, wage rates are likely to fall. In the labour market for nurses in the NHS, there exist both a monopoly and a monopsony. The monopoly is formed of all individuals who are qualified as nurses: nurses as a collective group effectively form a monopolistic supplier of their own labour. The monopsony in the nursing labour market is the NHS.

19. With the existence of both a monopolistic supplier of nurses and a monopsonistic employer of nurses the market wage rate will be determined by the relative bargaining power of each party in wage negotiations. The monopolistic supplier of nursing labour aims to increase the wage rate payable to nurses. The monopsonistic employer of nursing labour aims to reduce the wage rate payable to nurses. The actual wage rate paid to nurses will depend on the relative bargaining power of each group.

20. In theory, three methods may be used to determine the number of nurses employed by health care providers: top-down planning; bottom-up planning; and historical planning. In reality, whilst these theoretical models are likely to have some

influence, the number of nurses employed is more likely to be affected by the budget of health care providers. This in turn is influenced by government spending plans.

21. Since 1983, nurses' pay has largely been determined by the independent Pay Review Body for Nurses, Midwives and Health Visitors. This system was implemented mainly because of the apparent fairness it provided: the Pay Review Body is independent of nursing, NHS or government control, and the government is obliged to accept the recommendations on pay that it provides. In setting pay recommendations, the Pay Review Body must base its decisions on three types of evidence which form the basis for wage negotiations between nurses and their employers: evidence from nurses and their representatives; evidence from managers and employers and their representatives; and evidence from the wider economy.

22. Two features of the NHS are of particular importance to the labour market for nurses: the size of the budget allocated to the NHS and the relative bargaining power of nurses and employers in wage negotiations.

Markets and scarce resources

In previous chapters we have explored methods for allocating scarce health care resources via the use of markets, which have been defined as institutions where parties can communicate with each other in order to buy and sell goods and services.

Markets may be used to allocate resources as a result of decisions made by individual buyers and sellers acting in their own self-interest. It is assumed that buyers of goods and services do so in such a way so as to maximise their utility, and that sellers of goods and services do so in such a way so as to maximise their profits. The interaction of utility-maximising buyers and profit-maximising sellers ensures that the quantity of a good that consumers demand, or wish to buy, is the same as the quantity that producers supply, or wish to sell. Within this framework, the goods and services which will be produced are those which individuals are willing and able to spend their money on, and those that may be supplied profitably by producers.

The focus of much of this book so far has been on the way in which the markets for goods and services, and particularly the market for health care, function. In this chapter, we concentrate on the market for *labour*, which is a factor of production, and an input into the production of health care.

Production function

We use the notion of a *production function* in order to describe the relationship between the inputs into the production of goods and services and the output ultimately produced.

The production function shows the maximum output that can be obtained from possible combinations of the inputs. For convenience, we often express the relationship between inputs and outputs defined in the production function as follows:

$$Q = f(X_1, X_2, X_3, ..., X_n) \tag{8.1}$$

where Q represents the output and $X_1, X_2, X_3, ..., X_n$ represent the quantities of the various inputs used to produce that output. Therefore, the production function shows the effects of the inputs into the production of goods and services. Equation 8.1 states that output Q is related in a specific way, that is, is *a function of,* the inputs $X_1, X_2, X_3, ..., X_n$. These inputs are called the factors of production.

Factors of production

The answer to the basic economic question of 'what goods shall we produce?' depends essentially upon the resources which are available to produce goods and services and how efficiently those resources are used.

It is useful to divide resources into a number of categories, the most important of which are labour and capital. Collectively, these resources are used as inputs into the production of goods and services and are called the *factors of production.*

Labour

The term *labour* refers to all human resources that could be used in the production of goods and services. How labour is used and how it is combined with the other factors of production help to determine the amount of a particular good or service produced.

Just as there may be a market for goods and services such as chocolate bars and health care, so there may be a market for the factors of production such as labour. In this chapter we shall concentrate on issues concerning the market for labour. Having looked at the basic principles of labour markets, we shall then go on to look more closely at the market for nursing labour in the UK National Health Service.

We begin by describing the factors that determine the demand for labour.

Demand for labour

Derived demand

The demand for labour, as a factor of production, is a *derived demand*. This means that the demand for labour is derived from the demand for the good or service that it is used to produce. Therefore, the demand for labour clearly depends upon there being a demand for the good that it is used to produce, and factors of production are demanded not for their own sake but for the demand for these goods and services.

In the context of the demand for nursing labour, this too is a derived demand, since it is derived from the demand for health care, which, as discussed in Chapter 3, is in turn derived from the demand for health. Therefore, we do not demand nursing labour for its own sake but, rather, because we demand health care.

In a market situation, those parties that demand goods or services are often known as buyers or consumers. In the market for labour, parties that demand labour are generally employers, who demand labour in order to produce goods and services. In the following discussion we will therefore use the term *employers* to refer to parties or individuals who demand labour. It is generally the case that employers act in such a way so as to maximise their profits.

The demand for labour is defined as the number of workers which an employer is willing and able to employ in a particular time period. This will be influenced by many variables.

In Chapter 2 we saw that the most important variable to have an effect on the demand for goods and services is the price of that good or service. Analogous to this, and invariably the most important variable that will have an effect on the quantity of labour demanded, is its price. However, the price of labour is, in fact, the *wage rate* paid to workers by employers.

As the wage rate increases, the number of workers employed (that is, the quantity of labour demanded) will fall. Conversely, if the wage rate falls, then the number of workers employed will rise. We can therefore say that there is an inverse relationship between the wage rate and the number of workers demanded (analogous to the theory of demand of goods and services presented in Chapter 2, there is an inverse relationship between price and quantity demanded).

We can demonstrate this relationship between the wage rate and the number of workers employed graphically, by constructing a demand curve for labour (see Figure 8.1).

The demand curve for labour D is downward sloping from left to right. We say that it has a negative slope, reflecting the negative relationship between the wage rate and the number of workers employed. At a relatively high wage rate such as W_1, a relatively low number of workers will be employed, N_1. As the wage rate falls to a lower value, such as W_2, then number of workers employed will increase to N_2.

The simple explanation for this is that when the wage rate falls, labour becomes cheaper. Therefore, all other things being equal, employers will wish to employ more labour. This occurs for two reasons: the substitution effect of labour and the income effect of labour.

1. The substitution effect of labour: if the wage rate falls, employers will employ more labour because it is cheaper. This is the effect of a change in the wage rate on the number of workers employed due to the fact that the price of labour relative to other factors of production has changed.
2. The income effect of labour: if the wage rate falls, employers will employ more labour because it leaves more budget to spend. This is the effect of a change in

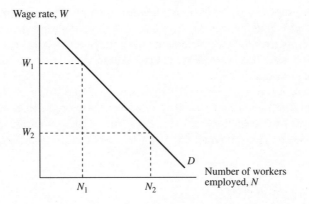

Figure 8.1 Demand curve for labour.

the wage rate on the number of workers employed due to the fact that the employers' real budget has changed. If the wage rate falls, employers are likely to employ more workers, and also more of the other factors of production as well. This is because since the wage rate has fallen, employers have more of their budget left available to buy all factors of production.

These two effects provide intuitive reasons why there is a negative relationship between the wage rate and the number of workers employed. A more involved explanation of why the demand curve for labour has a negative slope is provided by the theory of marginal productivity of labour.

Marginal productivity of labour

The demand for labour will depend, at least in part, upon its productivity. That is, it will depend upon the effect that labour has on the production of the good or service that it is used to produce. In order to examine the effect that the productivity of labour is likely to have on demand, we first need to explain the following concepts:

1. marginal physical product;
2. the Law of Diminishing Marginal Returns;
3. marginal revenue product.

Marginal physical product

Marginal physical product (*MPP*) is the change in production of a good or service (that is, the change in output) resulting from the employment of an additional worker.

For example, suppose an NHS Trust decides to employ an extra nurse to work in the Accident and Emergency department. If everything else stays constant, the number of patients treated in the Accident and Emergency department and the quality of care provided are likely to increase. This increase is the marginal physical product of the additional nurse.

Whilst adding more workers to the production of a good or service is likely to increase output, the increases from each additional worker are likely to fall. In other words, output will increase but at a decreasing rate as more workers are added to the production process. This illustrates the Law of Diminishing Marginal Returns.

Law of Diminishing Marginal Returns

In the short run, the amount of some factors of production which an employer can employ will be fixed, whilst others the employer may be able to vary.

For example, in the production of health care, an NHS Trust will have an Accident and Emergency department of a certain size with which to provide health care to patients. This is therefore a fixed factor of production. However, the NHS Trust may add to this fixed factor variable factors of production such as labour, in the form of more nurses.

Under these circumstances, the production of output will be affected by the *Law of Diminishing Marginal Returns*. This states that as increasing quantities of a variable factor of production (such as labour) are used in conjunction with a fixed factor of production, the marginal physical product of the variable factor will decrease (note that this law is analogous to the Law of Diminishing Marginal Utility described in Chapter 2).

In other words, the Law of Diminishing Marginal Returns basically states that while overall output increases if more workers are added to the production process, the marginal physical product of each additional worker will fall. Therefore, employing more and more workers leads to smaller and smaller increases in output. Therefore, marginal physical product decreases as the number of workers employed increases. This is shown in Figure 8.2(a).

For example, as more and more nurses are employed in the Accident and Emergency department, the total number of patients treated and quality of care are both likely to increase, but this improvement is likely to be less for each additional nurse employed. At the extreme, too many nurses might be employed, which might actually have a detrimental effect on the number of patients treated and the quality of care as staff overcrowding may occur.

Marginal revenue product

Marginal revenue product (*MRP*) is the change in revenue to the employer resulting from the employment of an additional worker.

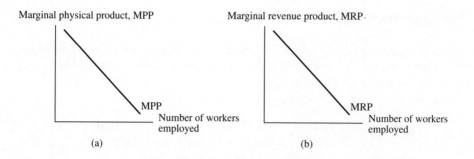

Figure 8.2 Marginal physical product and marginal revenue product of employing additional workers.

For example, in the NHS internal market, NHS Trusts earn revenue for the health care services they provide. The marginal revenue product of employing an additional nurse may be defined as the increase in revenue to the NHS Trust resulting from employment of the additional nurse.

Clearly, the marginal revenue product will depend upon the marginal physical product. However, it is also affected by the price of the good or service which the worker is used to produce. Specifically, marginal revenue product may be calculated as the marginal physical product multiplied by the price of the good which the worker is used to produce, or:

$$MRP = MPP \times p \tag{8.2}$$

where p denotes the price of the good which the worker is helping to make.

For example, the employment of an additional nurse by an NHS Trust may mean that it is possible to treat more patients. Since NHS Trusts earn revenue for the services they provide, this implies that the NHS Trust may earn additional revenue because of the nurse. Suppose the employment of the nurse means that an additional five patients per day may be treated in the Accident and Emergency department, this is therefore the marginal physical product of the additional nurse. Suppose the price which the NHS Trust charges for Accident and Emergency services is £26 (see Table 7.4). In this case, the marginal revenue product of the additional nurse is £130 per day (that is, five additional patients × £26 per patient).

Because of the Law of Diminishing Marginal Returns, which affects the marginal physical product of additional workers, and because marginal revenue product is closely related to marginal physical product, it is the case that marginal revenue product will also decrease as the number of workers employed increases, as shown in Figure 8.2(b). In other words, the additional revenue earned by the employer from employing additional workers falls as the number of workers employed increases.

Using this information on marginal revenue product, we may now construct the demand curve for labour.

Marginal revenue product and the demand curve for labour

With information on marginal revenue product, the employer may decide whether or not to employ an additional worker. The decision will depend upon a comparison of the marginal revenue product and the wage rate.

One of three situations may arise:

1. marginal revenue product is greater than the wage rate ($MRP > W$);
2. marginal revenue product is less than the wage rate ($MRP < W$);
3. marginal revenue product equals the wage rate ($MRP = W$).

We shall examine each situation in turn.

Marginal revenue product is greater than the wage rate ($MRP > W$)

If the marginal revenue product is greater than the wage rate, then the employer makes a profit from employing the additional worker since the additional revenue is greater than the additional wage bill. It therefore pays for an employer to employ a worker whose marginal revenue product is greater than the wage rate. The employer should employ more workers.

For example, if an additional nurse working in the Accident and Emergency department of an NHS Trust has a marginal revenue product of £130 and is paid £50 per day, then she results in the NHS Trust making a net gain of £80 (that is, £130 revenue − £50 wage bill). In this case, it pays for the NHS Trust to employ the nurse.

Marginal revenue product is less than the wage rate ($MRP < W$)

If the marginal revenue product is less than the wage rate, then the employer makes a loss from employing the additional worker since the additional revenue is less than the additional wage bill. It therefore pays for an employer not to employ a worker whose marginal revenue product is greater than the wage rate. The employer should employ fewer workers.

For example, if the additional nurse has a marginal revenue product of £130 and is paid £150 per day, then she results in the NHS Trust making a net loss of £20 (that is, £130 revenue − £150 wage bill). In this case, it pays for the NHS Trust not to employ the nurse.

Marginal revenue product equals the wage rate ($MRP = W$)

If the marginal revenue product equals the wage rate, then the employer is breaking even from employing the additional worker (that is, not making a profit or a loss) since the additional revenue is equal to the additional wages bill. The employer should employ neither more nor fewer workers. The employer should employ no more workers than the number now employed, or they will begin to make a loss, since the marginal revenue product of the next additional worker will be less than the wage rate due to the Law of Diminishing Marginal Returns. The employer should employ no fewer workers than the number now employed, or they will not maximise their profits, because they could earn more profits by employing additional workers.

For example, if an additional nurse working in the Accident and Emergency department of an NHS Trust has a marginal revenue product of £130 and is paid £130 per day, then she results in the NHS Trust breaking even, or making a net gain of £0 (that is, £130 revenue − £130 wage bill). In this case, it pays for the NHS Trust to employ the nurse, but not to employ any more or any fewer nurses.

We can therefore see that the decision regarding the optimal number of workers for an employer to employ depends upon the marginal revenue product of additional workers and the wage rate. If the employer wishes to maximise profits, it pays to continue employing more workers up until the point at which the marginal revenue product equals the wage rate (that is, up until $MRP = W$).

This information is presented diagrammatically in Figure 8.3. This shows the marginal revenue product curve, and it is downward sloping to indicate the effects of the Law of Diminishing Marginal Returns. The optimal number of workers to employ depends upon the wage rate.

At wage rate W_1, the optimal number of workers to employ is N_1. If fewer than N_1 workers are employed at this wage rate (such as N_2 workers) then the marginal

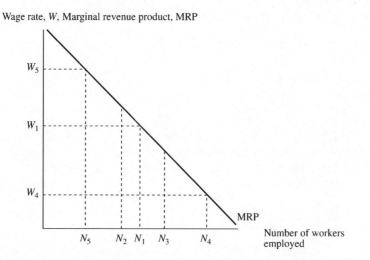

Figure 8.3 Using marginal revenue product and the wage rate to determine the number of workers employed.

revenue product is greater than the wage rate, so the employer can make gains from employing more workers. If more than N_1 workers are employed at this wage rate (such as N_3 workers) then the marginal revenue product is less than the wage rate, so the employer is making a loss from employing this number of workers and should employ fewer. At wage rate W_1, only when N_1 workers are employed is the employer maximising profits.

We can also see from Figure 8.3 that if the wage rate decreases from W_1 to W_4, then the employer should employ more workers (in this case, N_4 workers). If the wage rate increases from W_1 to W_5, the employer should employ fewer workers (in this case, N_5 workers) because only in these cases does marginal revenue product equal the wage rate.

We have therefore derived the demand curve for labour. What we have shown is how marginal revenue product may be used to determine the number of workers employed at each wage rate. This analysis therefore shows that the marginal revenue product curve is precisely the demand curve for labour because it shows the relationship between the number of workers employed (that is, the quantity of labour demanded) and the wage rate (that is, the price of labour).

Determinants of the demand for labour

Clearly, there are many factors which affect the level of demand for labour. These include the following:

1. wage rate;
2. productivity of labour;
3. price of output;
4. substitutability of labour with other factors of production.

We shall examine each of these briefly in turn.

Wage rate

As we have already seen, the number of workers employed is likely to be influenced by the wage rate. If the wage rate increases, the number of workers employed is likely to fall. Conversely, as the wage rate falls, the number of workers employed is likely to increase. The relationship between the wage rate and the number of workers employed is presented in Figure 8.1.

Productivity of labour

Since the demand for labour is determined at least in part by the marginal physical product of additional workers, then clearly the productivity of labour is an important factor in the number of workers employed.

If labour becomes more productive then the marginal physical product of additional workers will increase. Marginal revenue product will also increase (because $MRP = MPP \times p$, in Equation 8.2). Therefore, the number of workers employed will increase because the use of labour becomes more attractive to the employer relative to the other factors of production which are used as inputs in the production process.

Conversely, as productivity decreases, the number of workers employed will decrease.

Price of output

Since marginal revenue product is calculated using the price of output (that is, the price of the good or service which labour is used to produce), then the price of this output will also be an important factor in the number of workers employed.

If the price of the output increases, then the marginal revenue product of additional workers will increase because $MRP = MPP \times p$ (see Equation 8.2). Therefore, the number of workers employed will increase as the employer will wish to employ more workers to produce a greater output and thus increase profits.

Conversely, as the price of output decreases, the number of workers employed will decrease.

Substitutability of labour for other factors of production

The number of workers employed will also depend upon the substitution possibilities with other inputs into the production process.

If labour is easily substitutable with another factor of production, such as capital equipment in the form of, say, robots, then the number of workers employed will depend on the wage rate relative to the cost of capital to the employer.

If labour and capital equipment are easily substitutable and the wage rate increases relative to the cost of capital equipment, then the number of workers employed will fall as the employer switches to using capital equipment instead of labour in the production process.

If the wage rate decreases relative to the cost of capital equipment, then the number of workers employed will increase as the employer switches to using labour instead of capital equipment in the production process.

Clearly, the relative cost of each input becomes important only if the factors of production are easily substitutable for one another in the production process.

Supply of labour

Now that we have examined the demand for labour, we shall turn to the other side of the labour market, which focuses on the supply of labour. It is useful to distinguish between two forms of labour supply:

1. the total supply of labour;
2. the individual supply of labour.

The total supply of labour

The *total supply of labour* is the pool of workers who are willing and able to work in a particular geographical area in a particular time period.

The basic determinant of the total supply of labour is the size of the population. Of course, the entire population in a particular geographical area is not always available for work. In reality, the size of the total supply of labour is affected by many factors, including:

1. the number of births;
2. the number of deaths;
3. the number of people migrating in and out of the area;
4. the number of people who choose to stay at home and look after their families;
5. the number of people at school;
6. the number of people in further or higher education;
7. the number of people who are retired.

Each of these will affect the number of individuals available for work in any given geographical area.

The individual supply of labour

The *individual supply of labour* is the quantity of labour that individuals wish to offer for employment in a particular time period.

In Chapter 2 we saw how the decisions about how much of a good or service to supply were made by suppliers who were responsible for supplying the goods or services under consideration. This principle may be equally applied to the supply of labour because the provision of this too is, in effect, the responsibility of the supplier. However, the supply of labour does not act in quite the same way as the supply of goods and services because it is workers themselves who are responsible for supplying their own time and effort: workers themselves decide whether or not they want to work in a particular occupation for a particular employer and they decide how much of their time and effort they wish to supply to that employer. Therefore, it is the responsibility of individual workers to decide on their own input into the labour market. Individuals must decide whether they want to work in the first place, what they would like to do, where they would like to work, how much time they would like to devote to work and the effort they would like to put into working.

The supply of labour is therefore defined as the number of workers who are willing and able to be employed in a particular occupation in a particular time period.

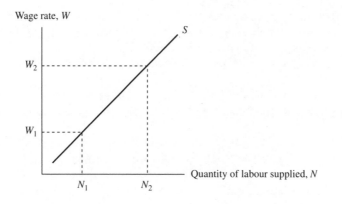

Figure 8.4 Supply curve for labour.

Just as in the case of the demand for labour, the factor which is likely to have most significance on the supply of labour is the wage rate.

The supply curve for labour

In Chapter 2 we saw that the most important variable to have an effect on the supply of goods and services was the price of that good or service. Analogous to this, invariably the most important variable that will have an effect on the quantity of labour supplied is the *wage rate* paid to workers.

As the wage rate increases, the number of workers supplied will generally rise. Conversely, if the wage rate falls, then the number of workers supplied will fall. We can therefore say that there is a positive relationship between the wage rate and the number of workers supplied (analogous to the theory of supply of goods and services presented in Chapter 2, where there is a positive relationship between price and quantity supplied).

We can demonstrate this relationship between the wage rate and the number of workers supplied graphically, by constructing a supply curve for labour (see Figure 8.4).

The supply curve for labour S is upward sloping from left to right. We say that it has a positive slope, reflecting the positive relationship between the wage rate and the number of workers supplied. At a relatively low wage rate such as W_1, a relatively low number of workers will be supplied, N_1. As the wage rate increases to a higher value, such as W_2, then the number of workers supplied increases to N_2.

Supply of labour and the wage rate

The simple explanation for the positive relationship between the supply of labour and the wage rate is that when the wage rate increases, so the returns from entering the labour market of a particular occupation increase. Therefore, all other things being equal, workers will supply more labour to that occupation. Conversely, as the wage rate falls, the quantity of labour supplied will fall.

This result has an intuitive appeal for two reasons, which apply to:

1. workers currently working in the labour market;
2. workers outside the labour market.

Workers currently working in the labour market

The relationship between supply of workers currently working in the labour market and the wage rate depends upon the alternatives open to individuals and their preferences towards those alternatives.

At any given wage rate, an individual working in the labour market fundamentally has two choices: to work, or not to work (that is, to be at leisure). Therefore, at any given wage rate, individuals must decide how much of their time to devote to work and how much to devote to leisure. In order to delineate the relationship between the wage rate and the supply of labour from workers currently in the labour market, we must ascertain what happens as the wage rate changes.

The effect of a change in the wage rate on workers currently in the labour market will depend upon the relative importance of two effects, namely:

1. The income effect of changes in the wage rate

The *income effect of changes in the wage rate* means that as the wage rate increases, so workers currently in the labour market will choose to work less, since at a higher wage rate they can devote less time to work for the same income. Conversely, as the wage rate falls, workers currently in the labour market will choose to work more in order to retain the same level of income.

2. The substitution effect of changes in the wage rate

The *substitution effect of changes in the wage rate* means that as the wage rate increases, workers currently in the labour market will choose to work more, since with a higher wage rate they can earn an even greater income by devoting only a little more time to work. Conversely, as the wage rate falls, workers currently in the labour market will choose to work less, since the rewards from working are less.

The *total effect of a change in the wage rate* is a result of both the income effect and the substitution effect of changes in the wage rate. Each effect has a different impact on the supply of labour following changes in the wage rate. For example, the income effect of changes in the wage rate means that as the wage rate increases individuals will work less, and the substitution effect of changes in the wage rate means that as the wage rate increases individuals will work more. Depending upon the relative magnitude of each effect, therefore, the supply of labour from workers currently working in the labour market may increase, decrease or stay the same following a change in the wage rate.

Workers outside the labour market

As the wage rate increases, so it becomes higher relative to wage rates in labour markets for other occupations. Workers outside the labour market may therefore find it attractive to enter this particular labour market in order to earn the higher wages. Therefore, as the wage rate increases, so more workers will enter the labour market and the quantity of labour supplied will increase. Conversely, as the wage rate falls, workers are likely to leave the labour market and move to other occupations where they may earn relatively higher wages.

Overall effect of changes in the wage rate on workers currently working in the labour market and workers outside the labour market

When the effects of changes in the wage rate on workers currently working in the labour market and on workers outside the labour market are added together, the overall effect of changes in the wage rate on the quantity of labour supplied may be ascertained.

It is generally the case that the ability of workers currently working in the labour market to work more or less following changes in the wage rate will be minimal, due to the nature of their contracts. Therefore, the effect of changes in the wage rate on the quantity of labour supplied will be affected most significantly by workers outside the labour market. Because, as the wage rate increases, more workers will be attracted into the labour market, and because, as the wage rate falls, workers are likely to leave the labour market and move to other occupations, it will be the case that there will be a positive relationship between the wage rate and the quantity of labour supplied.

Wage rate determination in the labour market

We have now examined the two components of a labour market, namely, the demand for labour and the supply of labour. Demand for labour is the number of workers demanded in a specific period of time and, all other things being equal, more workers will be employed at a lower wage rate, and vice versa. By the supply of labour we mean the quantity of labour that individuals wish to offer for employment in a specific period of time. All other things being equal, more labour will be supplied at a higher wage rate, and vice versa.

We can now put these two components together to see how they interact to form a labour market. We may combine our analyses of the demand for and supply of labour to show how a competitive wage rate is determined.

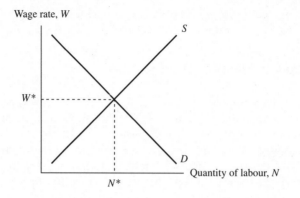

Figure 8.5 Labour market equilibrium.

The equilibrium wage rate

The *equilibrium wage rate* is the wage rate at which the wishes of the employers and workers coincide. At the equilibrium wage rate, the quantity of labour demanded is exactly the same as the quantity of labour supplied. This quantity is called the *equilibrium quantity of labour*.

Equilibrium therefore occurs when the quantity of labour demanded and the quantity of labour supplied are equal, so that at the corresponding equilibrium wage rate there are no unsatisfied employers or workers.

Diagrammatically, the equilibrium wage rate and the equilibrium quantity of labour are defined by the intersection of the demand curve for labour and the supply curve for labour. Superimposing Figures 8.1 and 8.4 on to each other, we can plot and overlap both curves on the same graph, using 'wage rate' and 'quantity of labour' as the axes, as presented in Figure 8.5. At the intersection of the demand curve for labour and the supply curve for labour, the quantity of labour demanded, which is read off the demand curve for labour, is exactly the same as the quantity of labour supplied, which is read off the supply curve for labour. The wage rate corresponding to this equilibrium quantity of labour is the equilibrium wage rate.

In Figure 8.5 the equilibrium wage rate is denoted by W^*, which is the prevailing wage rate at the intersection of the demand curve for labour D and the supply curve for labour S. The equilibrium quantity corresponding to the equilibrium wage rate is denoted by N^*. We can therefore say that in this labour market, the *equilibrium position* is defined by the point W^*N^*.

Disequilibrium wage rates

The equilibrium wage rate is the wage rate at which the quantity of labour demanded equals the quantity of labour supplied. However, the equilibrium wage rate may

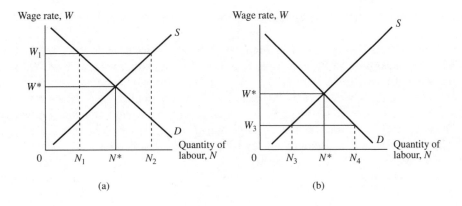

Figure 8.6 Excess supply of and excess demand for labour.

differ from the *market wage rate*. The market wage rate is the wage rate that actually exists in the market for labour at any one time. One of three situations may arise:

1. the market wage rate is greater than the equilibrium wage rate ($W > W^*$);
2. the market wage rate is less than the equilibrium wage rate ($W < W^*$);
3. the market wage rate is equal to the equilibrium wage rate ($W = W^*$).

We can examine the effects of these three situations in turn, with reference to Figure 8.6.

Market wage rate is greater than equilibrium wage rate, $W > W^*$

This situation is demonstrated in Figure 8.6(a). The market wage rate, denoted by W_1, is greater than the equilibrium wage rate, W^*. With a market wage rate of W_1, from the demand curve for labour D, N_1 is the quantity of labour demanded; from the supply curve for labour S, N_2 is the quantity of labour supplied. It is the case that N_2 is greater than N_1 and we therefore are in a position of *excess supply of labour*, where quantity of labour supplied is greater than quantity of labour demanded.

In a situation of excess supply of labour, workers will be *unemployed* because there is an excess number of workers.

In this situation, the market wage rate will *fall*. This will occur for two reasons:

1. workers, realising they are or may become unemployed, will accept lower wage rates, in an effort to make their services more attractive to employers;
2. employers, realising there are unemployed workers, will offer to employ workers at lower wage rates.

Both of these pressures will push the market wage rate *down*. Therefore, when there is an excess supply of labour and the market wage rate is greater than the equilibrium wage rate so that there are unemployed workers, the market wage rate will *fall*.

Market wage rate is less than equilibrium wage rate, $W < W^*$

This situation is demonstrated in Figure 8.6(b). The market wage rate, denoted by W_3, is less than the equilibrium wage rate, W^*. With a market wage rate of W_3, from the demand curve for labour D, N_4 is the quantity of labour demanded; from the supply curve for labour S, N_3 is the quantity of labour supplied. It is the case that N_4 is greater than N_3 and we therefore are in a position of *excess demand for labour*, where quantity of labour demanded is greater than quantity of labour supplied.

In a situation of excess demand for labour, workers will be highly sought after, because there is a *shortage* of workers.

In this situation, the market wage rate will *increase*. This will occur for two reasons:

1. employers, finding themselves unable to employ as many workers as they would like, will offer to employ workers at higher wage rates in an attempt to attract more workers;
2. workers, realising they are being sought after by employers, will begin to ask for higher wage rates for their services.

Both of these pressures will push the market wage rate *up*. Therefore, when there is excess demand for labour and the market wage rate is less than the equilibrium wage rate so that there is a shortage of workers, the market wage rate will *increase*.

Market wage rate is equal to equilibrium wage rate, $W = W^*$

Only when the market wage rate equals the equilibrium wage rate is there neither excess demand for labour nor excess supply of labour. In this situation, there are neither unemployed workers nor a shortage of workers.

The role of the labour market in the allocation of labour resources

In the labour market, employers and workers adjust the quantities of labour demanded and supplied in response to signals produced by changing labour market conditions. We have seen how changes in the wage rate signal the need for changes in the quantity of labour demanded and the quantity of labour supplied to which both employers and workers respond.

Wage rates in the labour market therefore provide signals to both employers and workers regarding the quantities of labour to demand and supply. The analysis so far has led us to two general conclusions:

1. if there are unemployed workers in the labour market, then the market wage rate will fall;

2. if there is a shortage of workers in the labour market, then the market wage rate will increase.

By this mechanism, labour markets will ensure that the equilibrium number of workers in the labour market is employed, and that the appropriate wage rate is paid to those workers. In the next section, we apply this theoretical framework to one particular labour market, namely, the labour market for nurses. Specifically, we discuss the demand and supply mechanisms which operate in the labour market for nurses in the UK National Health Service.

The nursing labour market in the UK

In the UK, approximately 80 per cent of qualified nurses work in the National Health Service (NHS) and approximately 20 per cent of qualified nurses work in the private sector (Project Steering Group On The Future Of The Healthcare Workforce, 1996). For the remainder of this chapter we shall therefore concentrate on the nursing labour market in the NHS, and we shall apply the general analysis of labour markets above specifically to this market. In the nursing labour market, the two key players are:

1. the employers of nursing labour;
2. the workers.

Employers of nursing labour

In the context of the NHS, the employers of nursing labour are health care providers such as NHS Trusts who employ nursing staff in order to provide health care services for the patients which they are contracted to treat. It is therefore *health care providers* who demand nursing labour.

Workers

The workers in the nursing labour market are nurses themselves, who work for health care providers in return for the receipt of wages. It is therefore *nurses* who supply nursing labour.

The demand for and supply of nursing labour

The demand for nursing labour in the NHS may therefore be defined as the number of nurses that health care providers are willing and able to employ in a particular time period. The supply of nursing labour in the NHS may be defined as the number of individuals who are willing and able to be employed as nurses by health care providers in a particular time period.

Applying directly the theoretical concept of labour markets to the nursing labour market in the NHS would imply that health care providers will continue to employ more nurses until the point at which the marginal revenue product from employing an additional nurse equals the wage rate. Also, individuals will seek and remain in employment with health care providers as nurses if the wage rate is sufficiently high relative to the value that individuals place on their leisure time, and to the wage rates in other labour markets.

Unfortunately, whilst the theoretical principles of labour markets described above do have intuitive appeal and do appear initially at least to be partially relevant to the nursing labour market in the NHS, there are a number of reasons why the market for nursing labour may not function as conventional economic theory predicts. These reasons include:

1. the importance of wage rates in the demand for nursing labour;
2. the importance of wage rates in the supply of nursing labour;
3. quantifying the role of nursing in the production of health care;
4. the length of training period to become a nurse;
5. the possibility of overshoot;
6. the existence of monopoly and monopsony.

We shall now examine the impact of each of these on the labour market for nurses in the NHS.

Importance of wage rates in the demand for nursing labour

As discussed in Chapter 7, the NHS is responsible for providing health care to the population of the UK, and nursing labour is an important input into the production process. Approximately 80 per cent of qualified nurses in the UK are employed by the NHS (Project Steering Group On The Future Of The Healthcare Workforce, 1996). In 1995, the size of the nursing pay bill for the NHS in Great Britain was £7,783 million (see Table 8.1). Total expenditure on the NHS in 1995 was £41,517 million (OHE, 1995). Therefore, the nursing pay bill accounts for approximately 20 per cent of total NHS expenditure, clearly a significant proportion of the total quantity of resources devoted to the NHS.

We would generally expect there to be an inverse relationship between the wage rate and the number of nurses employed by the NHS, so that as the wage rate increases fewer nurses will be employed, and vice versa. Furthermore, we would expect that health care providers will continue to employ more nurses up until the point at which the marginal revenue product of employing an additional nurse equals the wage rate.

In reality, the demand for nursing labour in the NHS is likely to be determined not by the marginal revenue product of employing additional nurses and the wage rate, but instead by the amount of resources allocated to health care providers for the provision of health care services.

Table 8.1 Nursing pay bill for Great Britain, 1995–6.

Component	£ million (% of total)
Basic pay	5,864.5 (75.3)
Special duty payments	606.5 (7.8)
Overtime	61.7 (0.8)
London allowance	123.2 (1.6)
Other allowances[1]	200.6 (2.6)
Other non-pay-related allowances[2]	11.5 (0.1)
Employers' costs[3]	793.8 (10.2)
Agency staff costs	120.7 (1.6)
TOTAL	7,782.5 (100)

Notes:
[1] Including geriatric lead, psychiatric lead, Regional Secure Unit allowance, on-call allowance, stand-by allowance, redundancy and maternity pay, protection and notice payments, flexible pay pilot scheme.
[2] Including uniform and initial expenses allowances.
[3] Employers' National Insurance contributions and superannuation.
Source: Review Body for Nursing Staff, Midwives, Health Visitors and Professions Allied to Medicine (1996).

As explained in Chapter 7, resources are allocated annually from the Treasury to the Department of Health for the provision of health care in the NHS. The size of the budget allocated to the NHS is decided following negotiations which take place in the government's annual Public Expenditure Survey, through which the priorities for different areas of public expenditure are determined. Ultimately, therefore, the sum of money devoted to the NHS is the result of a political decision made by the government, and is decided in the broader context of expenditure across all public sectors.

Funds originally allocated by the Treasury to the Department of Health for the NHS are passed through the system via the NHS internal market and eventually to health care providers. Through the allocation of funds by the NHS internal market, each health care provider is effectively allocated an annual budget with which it is required to provide all contracted health care services. The costs incurred in providing contracted health care services, including the costs of employing nurses, must be met from this budget. As presented in Table 8.1, the costs of employing nurses are considerable and, therefore, in determining the sum of money devoted to the NHS, the government is effectively determining the number of nurses employed by health care providers within the NHS each year.

In this situation, the wage rate for nurses will clearly be an important factor in determining the number of nurses which a health care provider is able to employ. The lower the wage rate for nurses then the greater the number of nurses that health care providers will be able to employ with their limited budgets, and vice versa. In this sense, therefore, the wage rate is important in determining the demand for nursing labour. However, because of the size of budgets allocated to health care providers, the number of nurses employed generally cannot be explained by health care providers choosing to employ that number of nurses which results in the marginal revenue product of an additional nurse equalling the wage rate, as predicted by economic theory. It is more likely that health care providers will employ as many nurses as they are able given the size of their budget.

In summary, therefore, whilst the wage rate is important in determining the number of nurses employed by health care providers in the NHS, and even though there will be an inverse relationship between the wage rate for nurses and the number of nurses employed, it is unlikely that the wage rate will be used by health care providers in the way that conventional economic theory predicts.

Importance of wage rates in the supply of nursing labour

A career in nursing has many characteristics which could be considered as unpleasant. Tasks can be dirty, tedious and repetitive, and nurses face a substantial risk of illness from their constant exposure to it. Also, nurses are often required to work varying shifts and professional freedom is limited as nurses are subject to supervision from various sources, including ward sisters, managers and doctors.

On the other hand, there are many positive features associated with nursing, one of the most often cited being the satisfaction derived from helping others. Also, nursing frequently offers stable employment and jobs in the profession are often readily available.

There are therefore many reasons why an individual might choose to become a nurse, and the wage rate may or may not feature as an important consideration, depending upon the individual concerned. If the wage rate is not important to an individual when deciding whether to become a nurse, or if an individual chooses to become a nurse and does not care what the wage rate is, then obviously the positive relationship between the quantity of nursing labour supplied and the wage rate predicted by conventional economic theory may not be realised.

It would probably be incorrect to argue that individuals choose to become nurses in order to maximise their income, and that this is the main reason why individuals choose to become nurses. It might be more appropriate to argue that the reasons for choosing to become a nurse are centred much more on improving the health of patients. However, whilst the wage rate may not be the most important factor in choosing to become a nurse, clearly it will have some impact and there is no reason to suppose that wage rates are any less important to nurses than they are to individuals in other occupations.

Quantifying the role of nursing in the production of health care

When deciding how many nurses to employ, one factor which is likely be taken into consideration by health care providers is the impact of nursing staff on the level of provision of health care.

The importance of productivity on the demand for labour has been analysed in detail above, where the relationship between the number of workers employed and the wage rate is explained by the theory of the marginal productivity of labour. On this basis, the number of workers employed will be affected by the marginal physical product of employing additional workers, the Law of Diminishing Marginal Returns and the marginal revenue product of employing additional workers.

Clearly, the number of nurses employed by health care providers may similarly be affected by the productivity of additional nurses. Unfortunately, it is difficult to measure the contribution of nurses (and any other input in the production process, for that matter) to the provision of health care, and it is therefore also difficult to measure marginal physical productivity. This difficulty arises for two reasons:

1. No satisfactory method exists for measuring the output of the NHS (for example, should output be measured in terms of the number of patients treated? the number of patients successfully treated? the number of patients seen by a doctor? or some other alternative measure? Clearly none of these is ideal as a means of accurately measuring the output of the NHS).
2. It is extremely difficult to separate out the specific contribution of various inputs, including types and grades of staff, to patient care and the provision of health care (for example, suppose we decided to measure the output of the NHS in terms of the number of patients successfully treated. Since there are many different inputs into the treatment process, including doctor and nurse time, medical supplies and major capital equipment, it is extremely difficult to measure the impact of individual nurses on this output).

Because of these two factors, it is often not possible to quantify the role of nursing in the production of health care. In this situation, it is difficult for health care providers to calculate the number of nurses that, under ideal conditions, they might wish to employ. Therefore, even if health care budgets were sufficiently large to allow freedom for health care providers to decide the number of nurses to employ, lack of data on the productivity of nurses will mean they are unable to do this in a meaningful way.

Since health care providers are unlikely to be able to estimate the marginal physical product of employing additional nurses, then they will be unable to calculate the number of nurses at which marginal revenue product equals the wage rate.

Length of training period to become a nurse

From the analysis of labour markets above we ascertained that, if there is a shortage of workers in the labour market, the market wage rate will increase in order to attract more workers. This is a general conclusion of the analysis and it ensures first that the optimal number of workers in the labour market is achieved, and secondly that the appropriate wage rate is paid to those workers.

This conclusion is applicable to the nursing labour market in that, should there be a shortage of nursing labour, one solution to this problem would be to increase the wage rate payable to nurses in order to attract more individuals into the profession.

This is a plausible and obvious response to a shortage of nursing labour. Unfortunately, in the nursing labour market, responding to a shortage of nurses in this way is likely to encounter problems because of the length of time it takes to train to become a nurse.

The time it takes to train to become a qualified nurse is generally three years, though it may often take longer. Suppose, then, that there is a shortage of nurses. In response to this shortage, health care providers increase the wage rate payable to nurses in an attempt to attract individuals into the profession. With the increase in wage rates, let us suppose enough individuals do decide to become nurses in order to eliminate the shortage completely. Unfortunately, the shortage problem will not be solved immediately, because once these individuals decide to become nurses they must train for at least another three years until they become qualified. It is only after a minimum time period of three years, when students become qualified nurses, that the shortage problem will be solved.

Therefore, whilst increasing the wage rate may have the desired effect of increasing the number of individuals choosing to become nurses, as an immediate response to a nurse shortage it is flawed because of the length of the training period.

Possibility of overshoot

Given the length of time it takes to train to become a nurse, a further problem may arise from training too many individuals to become nurses, and therefore overshooting the number of nurses required to eliminate the shortage.

Suppose there is a shortage of nurses and in response to this health care providers increase the wage rate payable to nurses. Individuals are therefore attracted to the profession and train to become nurses. In the time it takes for these individuals to train, the nurse shortage will remain, and therefore the wage rate payable to nurses will remain high. This will have the effect of attracting more and more individuals to the nursing profession. Unfortunately, once all these individuals have eventually trained to become nurses some years later, there may well be an excess number of nurses. As explained above, two consequences of having an excess number of workers are, first, that some individuals will become unemployed, and secondly, that the wage rate will fall.

This problem highlights the difficulties in setting the wage rate payable to nurses and the importance of closely monitoring the number of individuals who train to become nurses.

Existence of monopoly and monopsony

Two concepts relevant to the nursing labour market in the NHS are monopoly and monopsony, which are defined as follows:

1. in the context of labour markets, a *monopoly* exists when there is a single *supplier* of a particular form of labour;
2. in the context of labour markets, a *monopsony* exists when there is a single *employer* of a particular form of labour.

Monopolies exist in labour markets when workers join together and act collectively, as is the case with trade unions. Because monopoly suppliers of labour are, by definition, the only suppliers of labour in the labour market they have considerable power over wage rates and, with the existence of a monopoly, wage rates are likely to *rise* because workers wish to earn higher wage rates. This is possible because monopoly suppliers will exploit their position and will refuse to supply labour to employers who do not agree to pay high wage rates. Confronted with monopoly suppliers of labour, employers are therefore forced to *increase* the wage rate.

Monopsonies exist in labour markets when all workers are employed by a single employer. Because monopsony employers are, by definition, the only employers of labour in the labour market they too have considerable power over wage rates and, with the existence of a monopsony, wage rates are likely to *fall* because employers wish to pay lower wage rates. This is possible because monopsony employers will also exploit their position and will not employ workers who refuse to work for a low wage rate. Confronted with monopsony employers, workers are therefore forced to accept a *lower* wage rate.

Therefore, with the existence of monopolies and monopsonies in the labour market, the following general results are likely to arise:

1. with the existence of a monopoly supplier of labour, wage rates are likely to increase;
2. with the existence of a monopsony employer, wage rates are likely to fall.

In the labour market for nurses in the NHS, there exist both a monopoly and a monopsony. The monopoly is formed of all individuals who are nurses. Nurses as a collective group effectively form a monopolistic supplier of their own labour. A large number of individuals acting together have a much greater influence than a single individual acting alone. Similarly, a large group of nurses acting together will have more influence than a single nurse acting alone. This explains the existence of professional nursing bodies such as the Royal College of Nursing of the United Kingdom (the RCN) which aim to improve employment conditions for nurses, and to increase wage rates.

The monopsony in the nursing labour market is the NHS. This is because, having qualified, most nurses (approximately 80 per cent [Project Steering Group On The Future Of The Healthcare Workforce, 1996]) then go on to work for health care providers in the NHS. The NHS is therefore effectively the single employer of nursing labour in the UK. Given the budget constraints imposed on the NHS by the government in terms of the funds allocated by the Treasury to the Department of Health for the NHS, NHS employers aim to *reduce* the wage rates payable to nurses.

Applying directly the theoretical concept of labour markets to the nursing labour market in the NHS would imply that health care providers will continue to employ more nurses up until the point at which the marginal revenue product from employing an additional nurse equals the wage rate. This determines the quantity of nursing labour demanded. Also, individuals will seek and remain in employment with health care providers as nurses if the wage rate is sufficiently high relative to the value that individuals place on their leisure time and to the wage rates in other labour markets. This determines the quantity of nursing labour supplied. On this basis, the prevailing wage rate is determined by the competitive interaction of the demand and supply for nursing labour.

With the existence of both a monopolistic supplier of nurses and a monopsonistic employer of nurses the determination of the market wage rate is not so straightforward and the wage rate in the nursing labour market will in fact be determined by the *relative bargaining power* of each party in wage negotiations. The monopolistic supplier of nursing labour aims to increase the wage rate payable to nurses. The monopsonistic employer of nursing labour aims to reduce the wage rate payable to nurses. The actual wage rate paid to nurses will depend on the relative strength of each group. If the bargaining power of nurses as a collective group is greater, then the wage rate payable to nurses will be high. If the bargaining power of the NHS is greater, then the wage rate payable to nurses will be low.

In reality, there are many factors which may influence the bargaining power of each party in wage negotiations. For example, the bargaining strength of the monopolistic supplier of nursing labour would tend to be greater in the following circumstances (note that the reverse is required for the bargaining strength of the monopsonistic employer of nursing labour to be greater):

1. when there is little scope for substituting other factors of production for nursing labour, so that nurses are irreplaceable;
2. when the provision of health care is unaffected by the wage rate payable to nurses, so that increasing the wage rate will have little impact on the provision of health care;
3. when the labour costs are a small proportion of the total costs of providing health care, so that increasing the wage rate will have little impact on the total costs of providing health care;
4. when the collective body of nurses is strong, so that it is unified and has significant resources at its disposal;
5. when health care providers earn substantial profits which may be devoted to higher wage rates;
6. when nurses are prepared to offer productivity deals in compensation, for example, by working longer hours in return for increased wages.

Because of the various peculiarities of the nursing labour market in the UK, there are numerous reasons why the market for nursing labour may not function as conventional economic theory predicts. However, demand and supply are still important factors in determining the number of nurses employed and the wage rate payable to nurses in the NHS, as we shall see in the following sections.

Number of nurses employed

In theory, three methods may be used to determine the number of nurses employed by health care providers:

1. top-down planning;
2. bottom-up planning;
3. historical planning.

Top-down planning

With *top-down planning*, the number of nurses employed is determined in relation to the number of beds made available by health care providers. Nursing requirements are decided with a formula that is constructed using a specific nurse/bed ratio stating the number of nurses that should be employed per available bed. Thus, the greater the number of beds, the greater the number of nurses employed.

The main problem with top-down planning is that it may be considered crude and inflexible because it does not allow for the individual nursing requirements of particular groups of patients.

Bottom-up planning

With *bottom-up planning*, the number of nurses employed is determined with reference to patient dependency rates for particular treatments. Nursing requirements are therefore decided by ascertaining the number of nurses needed for different patient groups and the treatment they typically receive. Average patient flows within the health care provider are then used to determine the number of nurses employed.

The main problem with bottom-up planning is that it requires a great deal of information for it to be implemented properly. Difficulties are likely to be encountered in determining the relationship between patient dependency and the required nursing care because it may be difficult to ascertain the ideal number of nurses required to treat a patient receiving a specific treatment.

Historical planning

With *historical planning*, the number of nurses currently employed is based on the number previously employed. Nursing requirements are set initially using some method based either on top-down planning or bottom-up planning. Over time, this formula becomes diluted so that ultimately the number of nurses employed is based simply on the number employed in the previous time period.

The main problems with historical planning are first that it suffers initially from the weaknesses of the system on which it is originally based and secondly that the number of nurses employed is not based on the specific requirements of patients.

In reality, whilst these theoretical models are likely to have some influence, the number of nurses employed is more likely to be affected by the budget of health care providers. This in turn is influenced by government spending plans.

As explained above, funds originally allocated by the Treasury to the Department of Health for the provision of health care in the NHS are passed through the system via the NHS internal market eventually to health care providers. By this mechanism, each health care provider is effectively allocated an annual budget with which it is required to provide all contracted health care services. The costs incurred in providing contracted health care services, including the costs of employing nurses, must be met from this budget. Therefore, in determining the sum of money devoted to the NHS, the government is effectively determining the number of nurses employed by health care providers within the NHS each year.

In summary, whilst the theoretical models described above may be used to some extent to determine the number of nurses employed, the freedom of health care providers to decide the number of nurses they wish to employ is likely to be restricted in reality by financial constraints imposed by limited health care budgets.

The total numbers of nursing and midwifery staff employed by the NHS in Great Britain between 1974 and 1995 are presented in Table 8.2.

Table 8.2 Number of nursing and midwifery staff employed by the NHS in Great Britain, 1974–95.

| | | Nursing and midwifery staff | | | |
	Qualified	Unqualified	Learners	Other[1]	Total
1974	189,567	90,219	93,285	4,563	377,633
1975	202,464	103,679	95,461	4,212	405,817
1976	213,225	99,822	98,961	2,953	414,961
1977	219,900	99,675	94,939	1,181	415,694
1978	226,904	104,154	92,433	813	424,304
1979	233,249	108,582	91,043	616	433,490
1980	240,462	115,808	91,983	571	448,824
1981	256,921	120,991	96,255	330	474,497
1982	265,109	119,504	97,044	216	481,873
1983	270,736	118,063	94,167	95	483,061
1984	276,602	114,200	91,369	44	482,215
1985	284,116	116,006	86,485	0	486,607
1986	287,715	116,410	83,148	0	487,273
1987	291,388	118,566	79,085	0	489,044
1988	294,828	117,454	77,284	0	489,574
1989	299,527	116,088	74,929	0	490,545
1990	297,320	114,273	71,645	3,774	487,012
1991	298,299	114,474	59,615	11,115	483,507
1992	300,698	115,431	44,879	6,714	467,723
1993	295,245	116,360	27,560	6,981	446,056
1994	291,070	116,138	13,945	8,061	429,214
1995	292,248	116,053	7,580	5,768	421,648

Note:
[1] Comprising nursing cadets and 'unknown' nursing and midwifery staff.
Source: Central Statistical Office (1986, 1997).

Nurses' pay

Since 1983, nurses' pay has largely been determined by the independent Pay Review Body for Nurses, Midwives and Health Visitors (hereafter, the Pay Review Body). The remit of the Pay Review Body is to make annual recommendations concerning pay based on evidence from staff, management and relevant economic data.

This system was implemented mainly because of the apparent fairness it provided: the Pay Review Body is independent of nursing, NHS or government control, and the government is obliged to accept the recommendations on pay that it provides.

In setting pay recommendations, the Pay Review Body must base its decisions on three types of evidence which form the basis for wage negotiations between nurses and their employers:

1. evidence from nurses and their representatives;
2. evidence from managers and employers and their representatives;
3. evidence from the wider economy.

Evidence from nurses and their representatives

Nurses and their representatives provide the first source of information to the Pay Review Body on which to base its recommendations. Nurses and their representatives are monopolistic suppliers of nursing labour and will therefore have considerable power in wage negotiations. They are likely to negotiate for increases in nurses' pay and to emphasise the need for fair pay for nurses which recognises their training and qualifications and their responsibilities.

Evidence from managers and employers and their representatives

Managers and employers and their representatives provide a second source of information to the Pay Review Body. Managers and employers and their representatives are monopsonistic employers of nursing labour and will therefore also have considerable power in wage negotiations. They are likely to negotiate for decreases or only very small increases in nurses' pay and to emphasise the need for pay levels which allow them to employ an adequate number of nursing staff within their limited budgets for the health care services they are contracted to provide.

Evidence from the wider economy

The wider economy provides the third source of information for the Pay Review Body on which to base its recommendations. This will include primarily two types of evidence: average pay increases across other occupations and predictions on the

Table 8.3 Average gross annual earnings for selected occupations in Great Britain by sex, 1991–6.

Occupation	Gross annual earnings (£)					
	1991	1992	1993	1994	1995	1996
Males						
Doctors	34,060	39,083	39,983	40,550	41,137	44,382
Nurses	15,506	16,510	16,546	17,701	17,794	19,141
Assistant nurses/nursing auxiliaries	10,540	10,889	10,899	10,847	11,560	11,190
Care assistants	9,636	9,636	10,041	10,795	9,927	10,634
Ambulance staff	13,556	14,404	15,319	16,026	16,510	16,962
Secondary school teachers	19,739	22,568	22,989	23,473	24,055	24,679
Police officers (sergeant and below)	19,926	21,772	22,396	22,552	23,239	25,246
All occupations	16,271	17,347	18,060	18,491	19,188	20,067
Females						
Doctors	26,697	31,652	32,245	32,703	34,845	36,306
Nurses	13,894	15,038	15,241	16,006	16,640	17,524
Midwives	16,401	17,586	18,091	18,918	19,417	20,764
Assistant nurses/nursing auxiliaries	8,850	9,396	9,636	9,911	10,884	10,832
Care assistants	8,029	8,445	8,616	8,892	8,762	8,939
Secondary school teachers	17,446	19,588	20,176	20,836	20,935	21,570
Police officers (sergeant and below)	16,879	18,678	19,656	19,854	20,836	22,225
All occupations	11,294	12,262	12,839	13,302	13,738	14,451

Source: Central Statistical Office (1992–7).

future costs of living. First, large increases in pay across other occupations are likely to provide a greater justification for substantial increases in nurses' pay, and vice versa. Secondly, if the future cost of living is likely to rise significantly, this also provides a greater justification for substantial increases in nurses' pay, and vice versa.

Whilst each of these three sources of information is likely to have some influence over the Pay Review Body in setting its recommendations, the actual wage rate paid to nurses is likely to depend primarily on the relative strength of each of the sources of evidence. Of particular importance is the relative bargaining power of nurses and their representatives, and managers and employers and their representatives, and the ability of each to present a strong case to the Pay Review Body.

The average gross annual earnings for selected occupations including nurses between 1991 and 1996 in Great Britain, by sex, are presented in Table 8.3.

Conclusion

This chapter has considered how the conventional economic theories of the demand for and supply of labour may be applied to the labour market for nurses. We have also considered the extent to which these theories require modification in light of peculiarities of the nursing labour market in the NHS.

Two features of the NHS are of particular importance to the labour market for nurses:

1. the size of the budget allocated to the NHS;
2. the relative bargaining power of nurses and employers in wage negotiations.

Size of the budget allocated to the NHS

The sum of money allocated annually by the Treasury to the Department of Health for the provision of health care in the NHS is the result of a political decision made by the government. Having passed through the NHS internal market, these funds eventually reach health care providers. Since the overall allocation of funds to the NHS is fixed, so too is the annual budget of individual health care providers. This has important implications for the employment conditions of nurses because with this limited budget health care providers are required to provide all contracted health care services. The costs incurred in providing these services, which include the costs of employing nurses, must be met from this budget. Therefore, the political decision made by the government concerning the size of the budget allocated to the NHS has important consequences both for the number of nurses employed and for the wage rate received by nurses.

Relative bargaining power of nurses and employers in wage negotiations

With the existence of both a monopolistic supplier of nurses (that is, nurses as a collective group) and a monopsonistic employer of nurses (that is, the NHS), the determination of the market wage rate is effectively determined by the relative bargaining power of each party in wage negotiations. If the bargaining power of nurses as a collective group is greater, then the wage rate payable to nurses will be high. If the bargaining power of the NHS is greater, then the wage rate payable to nurses will be low. Therefore, the relative bargaining power of nurses and employers in wage negotiations has important consequences for the wage rate received by nurses.

This chapter ends our discussion of markets and their application to the health care sector. In the following chapters we concentrate on an alternative method for addressing the problem of scarce health care resources, namely, economic evaluation.

References

Central Statistical Office (1986, 1997) *Annual abstract of statistics*. London: HMSO.
Central Statistical Office (1992–7) *New earnings survey; part D, analyses by occupation*. London: HMSO.

Office of Health Economics (OHE) (1995) *Compendium of health statistics*. London: OHE.
Project Steering Group On The Future Of The Healthcare Workforce (1996) *The future healthcare workforce*. Manchester: University of Manchester.
Review Body for Nursing Staff, Midwives, Health Visitors and Professions Allied to Medicine (1996). *Thirteenth report on nursing staff, midwives and health visitors 1996*. London: HMSO.

Suggested further reading

There are a great many economics textbooks available which might be used to obtain further reading on labour markets. However, a possible starting point might be any one of the following:

Begg D., Fischer S. and Dornbusch R. (1994) *Economics*. Fourth edition. London: McGraw-Hill, pp. 173–97.
Lipsey R.G. and Chrystal K.A. (1995) *An introduction to positive economics*. Eighth edition. Oxford: Oxford University Press, pp. 327–65.
Parkin M. and King D. (1992) *Economics*. Wokingham: Addison-Wesley, pp. 376–427.

9   Introduction to economic evaluation

Since the use of markets as a means of allocating health care resources may be inappropriate, an alternative method for resource allocation is required. In this chapter we examine an alternative possibility, namely, economic evaluation. A justification for economic evaluation is provided, that lays the foundation for the analysis of the following chapters. The discussion concentrates on explanation of the types of economic evaluation and the various tools employed. Methods for conducting an economic evaluation are also discussed.

Summary

1. The basic problem which economics attempts to address is that of scarce resources.

2. Because of scarcity, all economic decisions necessarily involve a choice in terms of what goods to produce, how to produce them and who shall receive them.

3. Since the application of markets to the health care sector may well be inappropriate, what is required is an alternative means of addressing the problem of scarcity and of determining how health care resources should be allocated. One possibility is to use economic evaluation.

4. Economic evaluation is a technique that has been developed by economists to assist in decision-making when choices need to be made between several courses of action. In essence, it entails estimating the costs and consequences associated with alternative options so that an appropriate choice can be made between them. The aim is to select those interventions that maximise the surplus benefits over costs.

5. The central criterion for appraisal in economic evaluation is opportunity cost. This reflects the sacrifice involved in a decision, measured in terms of the benefits forgone from choosing one alternative over another.

6. There are a number of specific forms of economic evaluation, distinguished by the way in which the benefits of alternatives are measured: cost-minimisation analysis; cost-effectiveness analysis; cost-utility analysis; and cost-benefit analysis.

7. There are several interrelated components of an economic evaluation: establishing the hypothesis to be tested; measuring effectiveness; measuring costs; and measuring cost-effectiveness.

8. Establishing the hypothesis to be tested involves: defining the study problem; specifying the objectives of the evaluation; defining the setting of the economic evaluation; defining the target group; determining the viewpoint of the analysis; determining the alternatives to be compared; and determining the form of economic evaluation.

9. There are two components to measuring the effectiveness or outcomes of alternatives included in an economic evaluation: choosing an outcome measure and obtaining effectiveness data.

10. There are four interrelated steps to measuring costs in an economic evaluation: identifying the range of resource inputs to include; valuing the unit cost of the resource inputs; measuring the volume of resource use; and multiplying the unit cost by the volume of resource use.

11. The final stage of an economic evaluation is to combine the collected evidence on costs and effectiveness in order to interpret which intervention represents the most cost-effective option. There are a number of steps to measuring cost-effectiveness: adjusting costs and outcomes for differential timing; constructing cost-effectiveness ratios; allowing for uncertainty; and constructing cost-effectiveness league tables.

The basic economic problem

In Chapters 2 and 3 we examined the problem of scarce resources and a response to this problem, namely, the market solution. Our discussion concentrated on both the demand for and supply of all goods in general, and on the demand for and supply of one specific good, health care. In subsequent chapters we examined further the application of economics to the health care sector and its empirical relevance and validity.

The problem of scarcity is thought to be exceptionally acute in health care because the need and demand for health care far exceed the resources available. It has been argued that, in light of this problem, some decision is needed regarding the appropriate allocation of resources. Ultimately, this allocative procedure will require some form of prioritisation.

The need for prioritisation in health care

Because health care resources are scarce, it is often not possible to provide individuals with the full amount of health care which they would ideally like. Because, for example, there are not enough doctors, nurses, hospitals and beds, it is necessary to make choices between different methods of treating an individual, or whether to treat one individual as opposed to another. Obviously these choices are not pleasant ones to have to make, and inevitably they will mean that people may suffer by not receiving benefits from the health care which they need. These choices imply an allocation of health care to one individual rather than to another, and patients may be denied the treatment they require. Perhaps an individual denied treatment may even die because of the choice made. However, such choices *are* necessary because of the existence of scarcity, and they do occur in clinical practice all the time, though often only implicitly (for example, through the use of waiting lists).

The existence of scarcity in the health care sector therefore implies that some sort of choice is required in order that limited resources are used in the best possible way. In light of the problem of scarcity, then, various questions arise which should be addressed:

1. What health care interventions or treatments should be made available?
2. How should these treatments be provided?
3. Who should receive these treatments?

In previous chapters we have examined the use of markets as a potential means of allocating health care resources, where purchasers and providers adjust their demand and supply of health care in response to signals produced by changing market conditions. Prices in the market provide signals to both purchasers and providers, and the prices change to ensure that scarce resources are used to produce the health care services that society demands. Under ideal conditions, resources will thus be allocated efficiently.

In this way, health care markets provide a framework for obtaining a solution to these three questions:

1. What health care interventions or treatments should be made available?

Via the price system, the health care market will decide which treatments should be made available and the quantity of those treatments which should be made available by finding the price for health care at which the quantity demanded equals the quantity supplied. The equilibrium quantity corresponding to this price defines how much of each treatment should be demanded and how much of each treatment should be supplied by health care purchasers and providers.

2. How should these treatments be provided?

A health care market also tells us who should provide different treatments, and the form of that provision: health care interventions will be supplied by those providers willing and able to supply health care at the market price.

3. Who should receive these treatments?

A health care market also tells us for whom the treatments will be provided: treatment is obtained for individuals by those purchasers who are willing and able to pay the market price.

Therefore, within the framework of a health care market, the treatments which will be produced are those which purchasers are willing and able to finance, and those that may be supplied by health care providers.

However, as discussed in Chapter 3 and subsequent chapters, the existence of market failure in the health care sector means that the introduction of a health care market may not result in an efficient allocation of resources. Specifically, market failure may arise in the health care sector through the existence of a number of circumstances, such as the following:

1. uncertain demand for health care;
2. the existence of externalities arising from the use or non-use of health care services;
3. imperfect knowledge on the part of patients;
4. patients unable to act free of self-interested advice from health care providers;
5. the existence of health care providers who act as monopolies.

We have also discussed how prices may have less significance in the health care market than in markets for other goods, and it is unlikely that the demand and supply of health care will behave in the way that economic theory requires for the formation of a perfect market. Furthermore, the market will provide health care only for those patients with purchasers who are willing and able to pay the equilibrium price. These features of a health care market may well be undesirable, and consequently, the introduction of a market for health care may well be considered unacceptable.

Therefore, the application of markets in the pure economic sense to the health care sector may well be inappropriate. In light of this, what is required is an alternative means of addressing the problem of scarcity and of determining how health care resources should be allocated. One possibility is to use *economic evaluation*.

Economic evaluation

Economic evaluation is a technique that has been developed by economists to assist in decision-making when choices need to be made between several courses of action. In essence, it entails estimating the costs and consequences associated with altern- ative options so that an appropriate choice can be made between them. With economic evaluation, questions are being asked such as 'is this treatment worth providing compared with other treatments that could be provided with the same resources?' and, more generally, 'are we satisfied that the health care resources should be used in this way rather than in some other?'

The guiding economic principle behind economic evaluation is efficiency, and the aim is to select those interventions that maximise the surplus benefits arising from a choice over the accompanying costs. This is useful for health care decision-makers who are responsible for allocating resources because it enables prioritisation between competing uses of scarce health care resources. In this way, the maximum benefit or health gain may be obtained from a given budget.

Note, then, that economic evaluation does not simply imply cutting costs. Rather, it involves considering both costs *and* benefits so that an appropriate allocation decision may be made.

The evaluation process itself relies on properly informed individuals comparing different ways of allocating resources on the basis of full knowledge of the costs associated with each option and of the consequences or outcomes associated with each option. Having attached the appropriate cost to each consequence, the highest valued outcome within the resource-constrained set of all possible outcomes would then be produced.

For the purposes of the following discussion, the terms 'intervention', 'treatment' and 'programme' will be used interchangeably to describe health care options which are the subject of the economic evaluation. The terms 'benefits', 'outcomes', 'consequences' and 'effectiveness' will be used interchangeably to reflect the output of a particular health care programme.

Economic evaluation and nursing

Wells (1995) states that: '[t]he implementation of a . . . market within the UK National Health Service has added impetus to the debate on how to distribute effectively, and equitably, the finite resources of state-funded health care. This discourse . . . has increasingly come to dominate the interface between managers, doctors and politicians . . . [N]ursing has yet to fully engage in, and attempt to influence, the course and outcome of this debate.'

Issues surrounding the allocation of health care resources via economic evaluation techniques have not yet been fully explored and exploited in the context of the nursing profession. This is surprising, since because of the size of the nursing workforce in the NHS, the resources devoted to nursing from health care budgets are considerable. However, the importance of applying the techniques of economic evaluation to nurses is slowly emerging.

In anticipation of this growing interest in economic evaluation, Lessner *et al.* (1994) delineate a number of methods by which efficient use of nursing resources may be achieved:

1. efficient self-organisation (relating to organisation of workload and priority setting by individual nurses across patients);

2. efficient use of equipment and supplies (in order to prevent wastage and duplication);
3. efficient delegation of work (relating to effective communication amongst all health care providers);
4. efficient planning and organisation of patient care (relating directly to health care given to patients);
5. efficient organisation of the health care environment (relating to use of space, placement of patients and location of equipment and supplies).

According to Wells (1995), the dilemma for nurses when confronted with scarcity in the clinical setting is how best to distribute nursing care. Problems addressing this issue are incurred primarily because difficulties arise in defining what is meant by the term 'best' in this sense, since this is often subjective. It has therefore been argued (see, for example, Reigle, 1989) that nurses need explicit guidelines in order to balance patient care requirements with available health care resources. The development of such guidelines, which may be used for the allocation and utilisation of nursing resources, may be conducted using economic evaluation techniques.

Unfortunately, there have been few economic evaluations of nursing procedures and services. However, with the realisation that health care resources are scarce, the pressures for thorough economic evaluation of all (and especially new) health care programmes involving nursing services are likely only to increase. In the medical profession, the number of economic evaluations examining the costs and outcomes of health care programmes is large and ever-increasing. Nursing services also need to be evaluated in this way so that their economic impact might be assessed. This and subsequent chapters examine the application of economic evaluation to the health care sector, particularly in the context of nursing services. To do this, we first need to describe the concept that economists use as the central criterion for appraisal in economic evaluation, which is called *opportunity cost*.

Opportunity cost

Limited resources have alternative uses. In choosing to use resources one way we are forgoing the opportunity to use them in another and a sacrifice is therefore involved. This sacrifice is called the opportunity cost of a decision. The cost of using resources one way can be measured in terms of the *benefits forgone* from other competing alternatives. Hence, the opportunity cost of providing a particular nursing service (for example, a community psychiatric nurse) is measured in terms of the benefits forgone from the alternative use of those resources (such as, say, providing hysteroscopies). Alternatively, the opportunity cost of providing a community psychiatric nurse is the benefit forgone from other methods of providing the same care (such as via general practitioners [GPs]).

The decision to provide a particular nursing service may well have a financial cost. In addition, it will also have an opportunity cost arising from the potential benefits forgone. For example, suppose a community psychiatric nurse is hired to work in a primary health care setting at a cost of £20,000. The *financial* cost of the community psychiatric nurse is therefore £20,000. Suppose that if that money were not spent on providing this nursing service, it would instead be spent providing fifty outpatient hysteroscopies at a cost of £400 each. The *opportunity* cost of the community psychiatric nurse is the lost potential benefit to the fifty patients who would have received the hysteroscopies had the money been diverted instead to fund those services.

Types of economic evaluation

Economic evaluation is therefore the comparative analysis of alternative courses of action, in terms of both their (opportunity) costs and their outcomes, in order to achieve efficiency in the allocation of scarce resources. There are a number of specific forms of economic evaluation, and these are well documented (see, for example, Drummond *et al.*, 1987, and Robinson, 1993). Each of these approaches involves the systematic identification, measurement and, where appropriate, valuation of all the relevant costs and outcomes of the options under review. These methods may be distinguished by the way in which the outcomes or benefits of an intervention are measured or valued. The four main approaches to economic evaluation are as follows:

1. cost-minimisation analysis;
2. cost-effectiveness analysis;
3. cost-utility analysis;
4. cost-benefit analysis.

Cost-minimisation analysis

Cost-minimisation analysis considers only the costs of options, and is an appropriate form of analysis to use when the outcomes of the options under consideration are known to be the same. If outcomes are the same so that there are no differences in effectiveness, then the decision regarding the most appropriate option can concentrate on finding the lowest-cost option.

If there is no evidence available that the outcomes are the same then concentrating solely on cost minimisation will run into the dangers of ignoring differences in outcome and obtaining misleading results. Unfortunately, it is often the case that differences in outcomes are ignored, and the lowest-cost option is selected so that costs are minimised as so-called 'efficiency savings'. These are, in effect, budgetary control exercises, and whilst they may be acceptable as cost-cutting measures, they are not good economic practice.

An example of a cost-minimisation analysis is presented by Tomson *et al.* (1995). The objective of this economic evaluation was to compare the costs and effects of two different interventions for the non-pharmacological treatment of raised cholesterol levels in a primary health care practice in Sweden. One treatment option, labelled the 'medium-intensity' programme, involved following national guidelines where individuals were screened for raised cholesterol levels by a practice nurse and then invited for a consultation with their GP, who offered a twelve month treatment programme comprising visits to a dietician. The alternative, labelled the 'low-intensity' programme, involved individuals shown to have raised cholesterol levels subsequent to screening by a practice nurse being sent a letter from their GP which explained that their cholesterol level was too high and that the therapy for this was a modified diet. Enclosed in the letter was a booklet with simple diet information. Both interventions were shown to result in small decreases in the cholesterol levels of those examined, and, in fact, there was shown to be no significant difference between the two groups. However, the cost per patient was SKr 753 (approximately £47) in the low intensity group, and SKr 3,614 (approximately £229) in the medium intensity group. It was therefore argued that because the effect of the two programmes was the same, the low intensity programme was preferred owing to its lower cost. This is an example of cost-minimisation analysis.

Cost-effectiveness analysis

Whilst cost-minimisation analysis is useful as a tool for comparing health care programmes which have the same outcome, few interventions actually do yield the same outcome in practice. *Cost-effectiveness analysis* is an appropriate technique to use when the outcomes of the alternatives under consideration may be expected to vary, but these outcomes are expressed in common units.

Common and convenient measures of effects in cost-effectiveness analyses often relate to one of the following:

1. measures of *physiology*;
2. measures of *morbidity*;
3. measures of *mortality*.

If the treatments under consideration are designed to have physiological effects, such as reducing blood pressure, outcomes may be gauged by measures such as the per cent reduction in blood pressure. If each alternative influences the level of morbidity, then outcomes may be gauged by measures such as the number of symptom-free or disease-free days. If mortality is affected by treatments being evaluated, changes in life expectancy or life-years gained may be used as a measure of effectiveness.

With a common unit of effectiveness across the options being compared, the different procedures may be expressed in terms of their cost per unit of outcome. The procedure with the lowest cost per unit of outcome may be deemed the most cost-effective use of resources.

For example, Milne et al. (1979) assessed the cost-effectiveness of utilising nurses to provide long-term follow-up care at work to employees in the US with previously undetected and untreated hypertension. The alternatives compared were using nurses to control hypertension at work and the normal practice of using GPs. Patients were screened for hypertension at work before being followed either by a nurse or by their GP for a time period of one year. Reduction in blood pressure was chosen as the measure of outcome, and cost-effectiveness was expressed as the cost per unit reduction in blood pressure. The average treatment cost per individual for the nurse-treated group was $682 (approximately £430), and the average treatment cost for the GP-treated group was $543 (approximately £342). The reduction in diastolic blood pressure averaged 12.2 mm Hg per individual in the nurse-treated group, compared to 6.5 mm Hg in the GP-treated group. Therefore, the cost-effectiveness of utilising nurses to control hypertension at work was £35 per mm Hg reduction in the nurse-treated group (that is, £430/12.2 mm Hg), compared to £53 per mm Hg reduction in the GP-treated group (that is, £342/6.5 mm Hg). On this basis, it was argued that whilst using nurses to control hypertension at work might be more expensive than relying on GPs, it is so much more effective that it is a cost-effective use of resources. This is an example of cost-effectiveness analysis.

Cost-utility analysis

Information from cost-effective analyses can be extremely useful in clarifying choices between different treatments for the same disease, where outcomes may be measured in common units. It is, however, limited in its ability to assist in decision-making between different treatments for different illnesses where the unit of outcome will vary across the options being compared. Because of this limitation, there has developed *cost-utility analysis*, which uses a utility-based measure of outcome which is usable across all treatments for all conditions. As we have seen in Chapter 2, in the context of health care, utility is usually referred to as the subjective level of well-being that people experience in different states of health. Therefore, with cost-utility analysis, the outcomes of the options to be compared are measured in terms of their utility.

Measures of utility usually attempt to incorporate some component of *quality of life* as well as *quantity* (or length) *of life* because it is generally assumed that quality of life is important, particularly for valuing health care programmes which have an impact on quality rather than length of life. *Quality adjusted life years (QALYs)* provide one method of combining information on the quality and quantity of life which is viable for cost-utility analyses. QALYs combine a measure of quality of life with a quantitative measure of life years to obtain a single measure of lifetime utility. Results may then be presented in terms of cost per QALY gained from the alternative treatments to be compared. The formulation and use of QALYs are discussed in greater detail in Chapter 10.

Since outcomes can be measured in commensurate units of utility, there is scope for comparison across different interventions for different illnesses. Options may be expressed in terms of their cost per QALY gained, and the procedure with the lowest cost per QALY gained may be deemed the most cost-effective use of resources.

Gournay and Brooking (1995) conducted a cost-utility analysis of utilising community psychiatric nurses for the treatment of non-psychotic patients in the primary health care setting. The alternatives compared were use of community psychiatric nurses and normal treatment by GP services. Costs and outcomes were assessed over a time period of 24 weeks. Outcomes were measured in terms of QALYs, and cost-effectiveness was assessed in terms of the cost per QALY gained. The additional cost of the community psychiatric nurse over and above the cost of standard GP care was calculated to be £48 per patient, and the gain in health outcomes per patient from the service was estimated to be 0.0017 QALYs. Therefore, the cost per QALY gained from the introduction of a community psychiatric nurse was estimated to be approximately £28,000 (that is, £48/0.0017 QALYs). This figure was compared with other cost-effectiveness data relating to treatment of patients with schizophrenia, with affective disorders and with neurotic disorders. Previous studies had estimated a cost per QALY gained of £6,000 for treatment of schizophrenia, of £10,000 for treatment of affective disorder and of £25,000 for treatment of neurotic disorder. This led the authors to conclude that there appears to be little justification for community psychiatric nurses continuing to provide treatment for non-psychotic patients in the primary health care setting, and that resources would be better allocated elsewhere. This is an example of cost-utility analysis.

Cost-benefit analysis

Among health economists, *cost-benefit analysis* is restricted to those forms of evaluation where both costs and benefits are measured in monetary terms (such as pounds sterling, £). This has a number of advantages. First, it allows for direct comparison across interventions because the effects of alternatives being compared are measured in commensurate units. In this regard, cost-benefit analysis is similar to cost-utility analysis, except in this case outcomes are measured in monetary terms rather than in terms of utility.

Cost-benefit analysis has an additional advantage in that, unlike the other forms of economic evaluation, it permits an estimation of the net benefit of a treatment (that is, the extent to which the benefits exceed the costs). Since costs and benefits are measured in the same units, it is possible to conclude directly whether a particular treatment option is worth providing. This occurs when the benefits are greater than the costs. This is not possible with other forms of economic evaluation, where costs and outcomes are measured in separate units (such as with cost-utility analysis, where costs are measured in monetary terms and outcomes are measured in terms of utility). When comparing one programme to another via cost-benefit analysis, programmes with the greatest net benefit (that is, benefit minus cost) are the most preferred.

Unfortunately, most health care services do not have explicit monetary benefits. Indeed, it is often extremely difficult to estimate the benefits of treatment in monetary terms. This has led economists to use various methods for estimating the monetary value of benefits, which include assessment of the *willingness-to-pay* for a given health benefit. Methods for estimating the outcomes of treatment alternatives in monetary terms are discussed in greater detail in Chapter 10.

Table 9.1 Forms of economic evaluation.

Form of economic evaluation	Measuring costs	Measuring outcomes
Cost-minimisation analysis	Opportunity costs in monetary terms	Same across alternatives
Cost-effectiveness analysis	Opportunity costs in monetary terms	Common units relating to physiology, morbidity or mortality
Cost-utility analysis	Opportunity costs in monetary terms	Utility-based measure of outcome with qualitative and quantitative components (e.g. QALYs)
Cost-benefit analysis	Opportunity costs in monetary terms	Monetary terms

O'Brien *et al.* (1995) conducted an economic evaluation in Canada which sought to assess the cost-effectiveness of a new antidepressant drug, moclobemide, relative to that of a traditional tricyclic antidepressant medication, amitriptyline. Side effects of antidepressant medications were identified, and seven of the ten most frequently reported side effects were observed less frequently with moclobemide. Ninety-five patients with depression were interviewed face-to-face by trained interviewers and presented with the probability of each of these seven adverse effects. In light of this information, respondents were asked what would be the maximum they would be willing to pay to have the new drug in preference to amitriptyline. Responses indicated that patients would be willing to pay Can$118 per month (approximately £61) for the new drug. Moclobemide costs Can$52 (approximately £26) more than amitriptyline per month. The net benefit of treating depression with moclobemide rather than with amitriptyline is therefore positive, with a value of Can$66 (approximately £35). In other words, the willingness to pay for the drug (that is, £61) minus the additional cost of the drug (that is, £26) is positive (that is, £61 − £26 = +£35). It may therefore be concluded that there is an overall net benefit from using moclobemide over amitriptyline in the treatment of depression. This is an example of cost-benefit analysis.

Note that whilst cost-effectiveness analysis is one specific form of economic evaluation, the aim of economic evaluation is generally to find the most 'cost-effective' alternative. This does not necessarily imply that cost-effectiveness analysis is the form of economic evaluation used. The most cost-effective alternative refers to that option which maximises the surplus benefits over costs, and this information may have been obtained via any form of economic evaluation.

A summary of the main features of each form of economic evaluation is presented in Table 9.1.

Choosing a form of economic evaluation

Whilst there are different types of economic evaluation, there is no one correct form which should always necessarily be used. Instead, the appropriate form of analysis

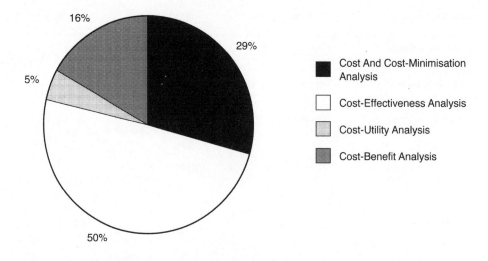

Figure 9.1 Form of economic evaluation (*source*: Backhouse *et al.*, 1992).

will depend on the treatment options being compared, and on the ability to obtain meaningful data. For example, cost-minimisation analysis is an appropriate form of economic evaluation to use when there is evidence that the outcomes of the options being compared are the same. Cost-minimisation is therefore inappropriate if there is no evidence of this similarity. Cost-effectiveness analysis may be used when outcomes differ across the options to be compared, but it is only an appropriate form of economic evaluation to use when comparison is required of different treatments for the same condition, where outcomes may be expressed in common units. Cost-utility analysis and cost-benefit analysis are both useful forms of economic evaluation for comparing different treatments for different conditions where outcomes may not be the same across the options being compared. However, cost-effectiveness analysis is often preferred to both cost-utility and cost-benefit analyses owing to the difficulties of obtaining meaningful data on quality of life and in measuring health outcomes in monetary units.

In a bibliography of the world literature on health economics, Backhouse *et al.* (1992) identified 1,171 economic evaluations conducted between 1964 and 1992. Of this total, 342 were cost-minimisation analyses (or calculated costs only), 580 were cost-effectiveness analyses, 58 were cost-utility analyses, and 191 were cost-benefit analyses (see Figure 9.1). The most frequently used form of economic evaluation is therefore cost-effectiveness analysis, comprising approximately 50 per cent of all economic evaluations.

Components of economic evaluation

We shall now outline in more detail a framework for conducting economic evaluations. This framework may be used both to interpret existing studies of the cost-effectiveness of nursing services, and to facilitate the design of future economic evaluations.

There are several interrelated components of an economic evaluation:

1. establishing the hypothesis to be tested;
2. measuring effectiveness;
3. measuring costs;
4. measuring cost-effectiveness.

We shall now address each of these issues in turn.

To illustrate more clearly the methods and uses of economic evaluation and the various techniques involved for assessment of the cost-effectiveness of nursing services, a *hypothetical* economic evaluation will be conducted of community psychiatric nurses in the primary health care setting. Examples will be provided where they are an appropriate and useful addition to the text.

1. Establishing the hypothesis to be tested

The first step in conducting an economic evaluation is to establish the hypothesis to be tested. This involves: defining the study problem; specifying the objectives of the evaluation; defining the setting of the economic evaluation; defining the target group; determining the viewpoint of the analysis; determining the options to be compared; and determining the form of economic evaluation.

(a) Defining the study problem

This involves identification of the issue for evaluation and consideration of the justification for implementing the particular intervention.

EXAMPLE _____

There are currently approximately 4,500 community psychiatric nurses (CPNs) working in the UK. These nurses are now increasingly based in general practice and community health centres rather than psychiatric hospitals and psychiatric care units. Referrals to CPNs are increasingly coming directly from GPs, while referrals from consultant psychiatrists are decreasing. Evidence suggests that CPNs favour more and more working with patients with non-psychotic disorders such as general anxiety, stress and relationship difficulties, where their main role is so-called 'primary prevention' via counselling.

The shift of CPNs towards working in the primary care setting with non-psychotic patients will have an effect both in terms of the costs of providing health care to non-psychotic patients and the health outcomes of those patients. It is therefore feasible and worthwhile to conduct an economic evaluation of the use of CPNs in the primary health care setting.

(b) Specifying the objectives of the evaluation

This involves stating clearly the aims and objectives of the evaluation. Ideally this will consist of a statement which encapsulates the study question to be addressed. The ultimate goal of the analysis following is to achieve this objective.

EXAMPLE

The objective of this economic evaluation is to assess the effectiveness, costs and cost-effectiveness of CPNs in the management of non-psychotic patients in the primary health care setting.

(c) Defining the setting of the economic evaluation

This involves stating where the economic evaluation will take place, and any other relevant background details concerning the study setting, such as the approximate number of patients receiving the intervention to be assessed, and the number of medical and nursing staff involved.

EXAMPLE

The economic evaluation will be carried out across five general practices which have a total of 36 GPs. The total number of patients registered at these practices is 62,000. Ten CPNs are attached to these practices.

(d) Defining the target group

This involves stating the cohort of individuals for whom the intervention is relevant. When the effectiveness and costs of the interventions will be assessed, it will be done so in the context of services provided to this group of individuals.

EXAMPLE

The target group of patients for inclusion in this economic evaluation are those who obtain help from their GP for non-psychotic problems such as: relationship/family problems; depressive symptoms; anxiety symptoms; phobic anxiety; bereavement; obsessive/compulsive disorder; post-traumatic stress disorder; and morbid jealousy. Of the 62,000 patients in the study setting, an estimated 1,200 experience the problems stated. These therefore form the target group for the analysis.

(e) Determining the viewpoint of the analysis

The next stage in conducting an economic evaluation is to determine the viewpoint or perspective of the analysis. Economic evaluation involves analysis of the costs and benefits relating to different options. What is counted as a cost and what is counted as a benefit is therefore important, but also likely to differ across the parties involved. For example, a patient may have very different ideas about what should be considered as a cost of treatment to those of the health care provider.

In order to delineate costs and benefits, it is necessary to decide on the correct viewpoint of the evaluation. This is an important practical dimension in any economic evaluation because it directly concerns the measurement of costs and benefits. In effect it determines what is regarded as an appropriate cost and what is regarded as an appropriate outcome from the intervention.

There are a number of potential viewpoints that may be taken:

- the patient;
- the third-party payer of services;
- the health care provider (either local, regional or national);
- society.

At its simplest, an economic evaluation might consider the costs and benefits only to patients or to the local health care provider. However, if this viewpoint alone is considered, this may result in a number of important costs and outcomes being omitted from the analysis.

The viewpoint adopted will generally depend on the decision-making context of the economic evaluation. An economic evaluation designed by the Department of Health to analyse the cost-effectiveness of a national programme to train nurse practitioners on how to prescribe drugs is unlikely to be interested in an evaluation which concentrates solely on the costs and outcomes to patients. More likely, a much wider viewpoint will be preferred which considers wider cost and health outcome implications on the NHS and society.

The *societal* perspective is the most general and therefore the most preferred viewpoint for an economic evaluation because it ensures that *all* costs and outcomes are considered. However, whilst it is recommended that this viewpoint is taken, in reality, practical difficulties encountered in assessing costs and outcomes across the whole of society usually result in a much less broad viewpoint being adopted.

EXAMPLE _____

The following viewpoints were considered for the economic evaluation of CPNs in the management of non-psychotic patients in the primary health care setting: the patient; the GP practices; the local Health Authority; the NHS; and society.

It is expected that the introduction of this service will involve costs being incurred by various parties, including: patients (from time off work); GPs (from treating patients); Health Authorities (from hiring CPNs to treat patients); non-psychiatric hospitals (from treating patients); Social Services (from caring for patients); and families and friends of patients (from caring for patients).

The costs that might be considered with each viewpoint are as follows:

Possible viewpoint	Costs included with this viewpoint
Patient	Costs to patients
GP practices	Costs to GPs
Health Authority	Costs to GPs; costs to Health Authorities
NHS	Costs to GPs; costs to Health Authorities; costs to non-psychiatric hospitals
Society	Costs to patients; costs to GPs; costs to Health Authorities; costs to non-psychiatric hospitals; costs to Social Services; costs to families and friends of patients

On this basis, the viewpoint taken in this economic evaluation will be that of society because this allows consideration of the full range of costs and outcomes from the interventions considered, and no important values will be omitted.

(f) Determining the alternatives to be compared

The next stage in conducting an economic evaluation is to define and select the different options to be compared in the analysis. This is obviously an extremely important stage in any economic evaluation because it involves deciding what exactly is to be evaluated.

Generally, an economic evaluation is geared towards examining the costs and outcomes of one specific health care programme. Deciding the options to be compared may therefore appear to be clear-cut because this will almost certainly involve the intervention which is the focus of the evaluation. However, it is equally important to select the correct options to compare with this intervention so that it will be possible to say whether one option is more or less costly than another and whether one option has more or less favourable health outcomes than another.

The strength of an economic evaluation depends on comparisons being made amongst the most appropriate options. If the aim is to assess the most cost-effective method of treating a particular illness, then it is necessary to ensure that reasonable options are selected for comparison. It would be unsurprising if one option were shown to be more cost-effective than another if that other option were a wholly inappropriate and unrealistic comparator.

When selecting the alternatives to be compared, comparison might include the current 'best-practice' option, and a 'do-nothing' option. Using the current best-practice option means that the intervention which is the focus of the economic evaluation will be compared with the currently favoured option. Should the intervention be shown to be more cost-effective than the best-practice option, this will provide a strong argument for its implementation.

Another obvious alternative for comparison is a do-nothing option, where the intervention that is the focus of the evaluation is compared with what would happen if no intervention at all were implemented. Should the intervention be shown to be less cost-effective than the do-nothing option, then this will provide a strong argument for not implementing this intervention.

To select the best options for comparison, a list of all potential options may be compiled and ranked to determine final selection. A number of factors may be worthy of consideration when compiling this list, including: feasibility; ethical acceptability; political acceptability; relevance; and real-world acceptability.

Finally, each option included in the economic evaluation should be well described so that it is clear exactly what is being compared with what in the analysis. It is also useful to state reasons why particular alternatives were not chosen for inclusion in the economic evaluation.

EXAMPLE

In order to assess the effectiveness, costs and cost-effectiveness of CPNs in the management of non-psychotic patients in the primary health care setting, two interventions will be compared:

1. Treatment of non-psychotic patients by GPs. Patients continue to see their GP as normal. GPs manage their patients as if treatment by CPN is not available. This is the current best-practice option.
2. Treatment of non-psychotic patients by CPNs. Patients are allowed to attend their GP if they wish, but they may see a CPN instead should they wish to do so. GPs initially suggest to patients (if appropriate) that they should see the CPN, but treat patients as normal if they decline to do so. CPNs follow their normal procedures and treat patients as they see fit.

A do-nothing option was considered but deemed inappropriate because it is unrealistic and ethically unacceptable.

(g) Determining the form of economic evaluation

The final stage in establishing the hypothesis to be tested is to determine the form of economic evaluation to be used. As discussed above, an economic evaluation may take one of a number of forms: cost-minimisation analysis; cost-effectiveness analysis; cost-utility analysis; and cost-benefit analysis.

This decision is important because it indicates in what form outcomes are to be measured in the analysis: whether they are considered to be the same across the interventions to be assessed (in the case of cost-minimisation analysis); whether they will be measured in common units relating to physiology, morbidity or mortality (in the case of cost-effectiveness analysis); whether they will be measured in terms of a utility (in the case of cost-utility analysis); or whether they will be measured in monetary terms (in the case of cost-benefit analysis).

EXAMPLE _____

In the economic evaluation of CPNs in the management of non-psychotic patients in the primary health care setting, the form of economic evaluation to be used will be cost-utility analysis. This form of analysis has been chosen firstly because both quality and quantity of life are likely to be important to the patients treated by CPNs, but also because it enables comparison with treatments for other illnesses.

---

2. Measuring effectiveness

There are two components to measuring the effectiveness or outcomes of options included in an economic evaluation: choosing an outcome measure; and obtaining effectiveness data.

(h) Choosing an outcome measure

Corresponding to the different forms of economic evaluation, the three main categories of outcome measures in economic evaluations are: common units of outcome relating to measures of physiology, morbidity or mortality; utility-based units of outcome with qualitative and quantitative components; and units of outcome measured in monetary terms. The exact choice of outcome measure will thus depend on the form of economic evaluation employed.

The chosen measure will ultimately depend on the health care programme being evaluated. It may be possible to estimate the incidence of various outcome endpoints such as death, symptoms and functional restrictions. A time dimension may be incorporated so possible endpoints might also include life years gained and symptom-free days. Additionally, quality of life data may be incorporated so that effectiveness may be measured in both qualitative and quantitative terms, as is the case with quality-adjusted life years (QALYs) gained.

(i) Obtaining effectiveness data

The availability of data on the effectiveness of the programmes being assessed is crucial to the accuracy of any economic evaluation. Data on effectiveness may be obtained in a number of ways: via clinical trials; via existing research; and via expert professional opinion.

Ideally, economic evaluations should be built alongside clinical trials so that relevant data on costs and effectiveness can be collected at the same time. However, setting up and conducting appropriate clinical trials is often time-consuming and expensive. Because of this, many economic evaluations often rely on existing research, or on expert professional opinion.

The use of data from existing research raises issues of quality and relevance. Research needs to be of a high quality and needs to be relevant to the economic evaluation in hand. Unfortunately, there is often a lack of good epidemiological evidence relating health inputs to outputs, particularly in the case of new health care programmes which are commonly the focus of economic evaluation. Even when outcome data are available, it is important to ensure that they are relevant in the context of the current evaluation.

If no good clinical evidence of effectiveness exists, then the study may proceed by making assumptions regarding the various parameters involved. These baseline assumptions may be obtained from asking, for example, a Delphi panel of expert health professionals to value the appropriate outcomes.

See Chapter 10 for a detailed account of methods for measuring effectiveness in an economic evaluation.

3. Measuring costs

There are four interrelated steps to measuring costs in an economic evaluation: identifying the range of resource inputs to include; valuing the unit cost of the resource inputs; measuring the volume of resource use; and multiplying the unit cost by the volume of resource use.

Once the relevant costs to be included in the analysis have been identified, cost measurement then proceeds by estimating the unit cost of a particular resource and then estimating the total volume of that resource used. The unit cost may then be multiplied by the volume of resources used to give the total cost incurred from a particular resource input.

(j) Identifying the range of resource inputs to include

If an economic evaluation is to consider all the relevant costs from a particular treatment programme, then three main categories of cost should be considered: health service costs; costs borne by patients and their families; and costs borne by the rest of society.

Health service costs include labour costs, non-labour costs, capital costs and overheads. These items may be divided into variable costs, which may vary according to the level of activity, and fixed costs, which are incurred whatever the level of activity. In an economic evaluation, all health service costs, both fixed and variable, are referred to as *direct costs*.

Costs borne by patients and their families include out-of-pocket expenses such as travel costs, and any costs resulting from care activities provided by the family. These are both direct-cost items. In addition, there may also be *indirect costs* arising from income lost due to absence from work (which is a production loss to society), and any stress and anxiety experienced by patients or their families.

Costs borne by the rest of society may be incurred when individuals not directly involved in a health care programme experience increased costs because of it. In most cases these effects are very small and do not merit inclusion in the analysis, but there may be some occasions when they are large enough to require attention.

(k) Valuing the unit cost of the resource inputs

The valuation of opportunity cost requires a unit cost to be attached to each resource input identified. Therefore, once the relevant range of costs has been identified, the individual items must then be valued. This requires each item to be measured in monetary terms.

For most direct-cost items, *market prices* will be available. For example, the labour costs may be valued according to current wage rates, and non-labour costs may be valued according to manufacturers' retail prices. Strictly speaking, economic evaluation should seek to value all inputs in terms of their opportunity cost, and occasionally opportunity costs will diverge from market prices. For example, if an individual working as a nurse would otherwise be unemployed, then his or her opportunity cost would be zero and not the hourly wage rate. Unfortunately, in reality, opportunity costs are difficult to calculate, and so for most practical purposes it is usual to use market prices unless there is strong evidence that they diverge appreciably from opportunity costs. Information on unit costs is generally obtained from published sources.

Indirect costs are a controversial subject because they are difficult to measure since estimation of indirect costs entails examination of production losses or lost income. Often, they are omitted from economic evaluations.

(l) Measuring the volume of resource use

In a similar fashion to collecting data on effectiveness, information regarding the volume of resources used may be obtained from various sources: via clinical trials; via existing research; and via expert professional opinion. A fourth approach is to measure the volume of resource use using strictly defined options.

The most direct and comprehensive approach is to conduct an empirical data collection exercise in which information on resource use is collected alongside a clinical trial. However, such methods are costly in terms of research time, resources and effort. A number of short cuts may be taken to produce crude estimates of resource use. These might involve the use of current research, in the form of financial accounts and internal market prices, or best guesses and estimates and informed assumptions regarding resource use and cost by expert professional opinion.

(m) Multiplying the unit cost by the volume of resource use

Total costs are estimated by calculating the volume of resources used and multiplying these data by the unit cost of that resource.

See Chapter 11 for a detailed account of methods for measuring costs in an economic evaluation.

4. Measuring cost-effectiveness

The final component of an economic evaluation is to combine the collected evidence on costs and effectiveness in order to interpret which intervention represents the most cost-effective option. There are a number of steps to measuring cost-effectiveness: adjusting costs and outcomes for differential timing; constructing cost-effectiveness ratios; allowing for uncertainty; and constructing cost-effectiveness league tables.

(n) Adjusting costs and outcomes for differential timing

An important issue in any economic evaluation relates to the fact that costs and consequences of health care programmes may have different time profiles. On a conceptual level, it is argued that we are not indifferent to the timing of costs and benefits, and that we prefer to postpone costs and bring forward benefits. The most widely accepted means of incorporating this phenomenon into an economic evaluation is to use *discounting*, and to discount costs and outcomes occurring in the future to *present values*. The basis for discounting is *time preference*.

The discounting procedure therefore has the effect of giving less weight to future events. Economic evaluation may weight future costs and benefits with a *discount rate*, according to the year in which they accrue, before adding them up and expressing total costs and benefits in present value terms (that is, values in the current year).

(o) Constructing cost-effectiveness ratios

The ultimate aim of an economic evaluation is to bring together and interpret results on costs and consequences in order to determine which intervention represents the most cost-effective option.

The basic methodology for doing this is to construct cost-effectiveness ratios where an estimate is made of the *cost per unit of outcome*. These cost-effectiveness ratios may be compared across the options being evaluated so that the intervention which has the lowest cost per unit of outcome is the most cost-effective. In its simplest form, this ratio may be estimated by dividing the total costs of the programme by the number of units of effectiveness resulting from that programme. However, it is possible to make a number of errors in comparing cost-effectiveness ratios between interventions. It is especially important that the relevant *additional* costs and *additional* benefits are calculated.

(p) Allowing for uncertainty

Given the difficulties in measuring costs and outcomes, most economic evaluations address the issue of uncertainty surrounding estimates of cost-effectiveness. Uncertainty regarding the true value of an estimate may arise for numerous reasons and the traditional manner in which to control for uncertainty is through *sensitivity analysis.*

Sensitivity analysis is a useful means of exploring how sensitive the results of an evaluation are to varying parameter values. For example, an investigator may feel that particular costing data are not reliable, and may use sensitivity analysis to establish the importance of such data to the result of the evaluation. To do so, the investigator may alter the value of the cost by, for example, doubling, trebling or halving the value to assess the importance of this parameter in reaching a final result.

Therefore, sensitivity analysis permits the robustness of the results to be tested in light of variations in the values of the key variables. By using sensitivity analysis it is possible to show whether the results of a particular study are robust over a range of assumptions or whether the results hinge on the accuracy of particular assumptions.

(q) Constructing cost-effectiveness league tables

When the costs of different interventions are assessed using economic evaluation and their outcomes are calculated in common units, then it is possible to rank the interventions in terms of their cost per unit of outcome. By this method, cost-effectiveness league tables may be constructed where those interventions with the lowest cost per unit of outcome are ranked at the top of the league table, and those with the highest cost per unit of outcome are ranked at the bottom. Using this method, a decision-maker interested in providing only the most cost-effective health care programmes would choose to provide those interventions found higher up the league table.

The ultimate use of economic evaluation and cost-effectiveness league tables is to guide resource allocation decisions by shifting resources away from those interventions that are costly in terms of the health benefits they generate and towards health care interventions that are of relatively low cost. Utilising this method, health care decision-makers can ensure that benefits or health gains are being maximised from a given budget.

The construction of such league tables is therefore extremely useful for health care decision-makers since it provides an easy way to gauge the cost-effectiveness of different health care interventions relative to one another.

See Chapter 12 for a detailed account of methods for measuring cost-effectiveness in an economic evaluation.

Conducting an economic evaluation

In summary, there are a number of components to conducting an economic evaluation:

1. Establishing the hypothesis to be tested:

    (a) defining the study problem;
    (b) specifying the objectives of the evaluation;
    (c) defining the setting of the economic evaluation;
    (d) defining the target group;
    (e) determining the viewpoint of the analysis;
    (f) determining the alternatives to be compared;
    (g) determining the form of economic evaluation.

2. Measuring effectiveness:

    (h) choosing an outcome measure;
    (i) obtaining effectiveness data.

3. Measuring costs:

    (j) identifying the range of resource inputs to include;
    (k) valuing the unit cost of the resource inputs;
    (l) measuring the volume of resource use;
    (m) multiplying the unit cost by the volume of resource use.

4. Measuring cost-effectiveness:

    (n) adjusting costs and outcomes for differential timing;
    (o) constructing cost-effectiveness ratios;
    (p) allowing for uncertainty;
    (q) constructing cost-effectiveness league tables.

Addressing the problem of scarcity using economic evaluation

Economic evaluations conducted in the manner discussed above provide a useful tool for decision-makers in the allocation of scarce health care resources. Such analyses enable estimation of the most cost-effective health care programmes and in this way economic evaluation provides a framework for obtaining a solution to the three questions relating to the basic economic problem of scarcity:

1. What health care interventions or treatments should be made available?

The health care interventions which should be made available are those from which the maximum benefit or health gain may be obtained from a given budget, that is, the most cost-effective programmes, which incur the least cost per unit of outcome.

2. How should these treatments be provided?

Economic evaluation also tells us how these treatments should be provided: health care interventions should be provided by the most cost-effective means possible, that is, by the method that maximises benefits or health gains from a given budget, which incurs the least cost per unit of outcome.

3. Who should receive these treatments?

Economic evaluation also tells us for whom the treatments should be provided: treatment is provided to individuals such that the maximum benefit or health gain is obtained from a given health care budget.

Therefore, within the decision-making framework of economic evaluation, the provision of health care is determined by ascertaining which health care programmes are the most cost-effective.

In the following chapters we explore the techniques involved in conducting an economic evaluation in much more detail. In the next chapter we turn to issues relevant to measuring the effectiveness of health care programmes.

References

Backhouse M.E., Backhouse R.J. and Edey S.A. (1992) Economic evaluation bibliography. *Health Economics* supplement: 1–236.

Drummond M.F., Stoddart G.L. and Torrance G.W. (1987) *Methods for the economic evaluation of health care programs.* New York: Oxford Medical Publications.

Gournay K. and Brooking J. (1995) The community psychiatric nurse in primary care: an economic analysis. *Journal of Advanced Nursing* 22: 769–78.

Lessner M.W., Organek N.S., Shah H.S., Williams C.A. and Bruttomesso K.A. (1994) Orienting nursing students to cost-effective clinical practice. *Nursing and Health Care* 15: 458–62.

Milne B.J., Logan A.G., Campbell W.P., Achber C. and Haynes R.B. (1979) Cost-effectiveness of utilising nurses to control hypertension at work. *Preventive Medicine* 8: 197.

O'Brien B.J., Novosel S., Torrance G.W. and Streiner D. (1995) Assessing the economic value of a new antidepressant: a willingness-to-pay approach. *PharmacoEconomics* 8: 34–45.

Reigle J. (1989) Resource allocation decisions in critical care nursing. *Nursing Clinics of North America* 24: 1009–15.

Robinson R. (1993) Economic evaluation and health care. *British Medical Journal* 307: 670–3, 726–8, 793–5, 859–62, 924–6, 994–6.

Tomson Y., Johannesson M. and Aberg H. (1995) The costs and effects of two different lipid intervention programmes in primary health care. *Journal of Internal Medicine* 237: 13–17.

Wells J.S. (1995) Health care rationing: nursing perspectives. *Journal of Advanced Nursing* 22: 738–44.

Suggested further reading

For a brief introduction to economic evaluation, see the series of articles by Ray Robinson in the *British Medical Journal*:

Robinson R. (1993) Economic evaluation and health care. *British Medical Journal* 307: 670–3, 726–8, 793–5, 859–62, 924–6, 994–6.

For a complete introductory guide to conducting an economic evaluation, including examples, see:

Drummond M.F., Stoddart G.L. and Torrance G.W. (1987) *Methods for the economic evaluation of health care programs*. New York: Oxford Medical Publications.

For a guide to the principles and practice of economic evaluation placed in the context of a specific health care service see:

Tolley K. and Rowland N. (1995) *Evaluating the cost-effectiveness of counselling in health care*. London: Routledge.

For a review of the world literature on the economic evaluation of health care programmes see:

Backhouse M.E., Backhouse R.J. and Edey S.A. (1992) Economic evaluation bibliography. *Health Economics* supplement: 1–236.

10   Measuring effectiveness

In this chapter we explore the various ways in which the effectiveness of health care programmes may be measured. Numerous methodologies are examined, discussing both methods for choosing an outcome measure in an economic evaluation and for obtaining effectiveness data. Where appropriate and useful, examples are provided.

Summary

1. There are two components to measuring the effectiveness of alternatives included in an economic evaluation: choosing an outcome measure and obtaining effectiveness data.

2. Relating to the different forms of economic evaluation, there are three main types of outcome measure which may be used: common units of outcome relating to measures of physiology, morbidity and mortality; utility-based measures of outcome; and valuation of outcome measured in monetary terms.

3. The number of different common units of outcome relating to measures of physiology, morbidity and mortality is unlimited, since outcome measures may be specifically geared to the health care programme being assessed.

4. Many different outcome measures have been used by researchers conducting economic evaluations, though the actual choice of outcome measure to be used in cost-effectiveness analyses will depend upon the objectives of the health care programme being evaluated: if there is one unambiguous objective of this health care programme, this provides a clear dimension along which effectiveness may be assessed.

5. Utility is usually referred to as the subjective level of well-being that people experience in different states of health. Measures of utility usually attempt to incorporate some component of quality of life as well as quantity (or length) of life, since it is generally assumed that quality of life is an important feature of the utility that an individual experiences in a specific health state.

6. There are a number of steps to be taken when measuring quality of life: identifying the relevant health states to be valued; choosing individuals to obtain utility values from; choosing the technique to be used in eliciting the value of health states; and measuring utility values.

7. Quality-adjusted life years (or QALYs) combine a measure of the quality of life experienced in a particular health state with a quantitative measure of life years in order to obtain a single measure of lifetime utility. QALYs therefore represent years of life adjusted for the quality of those years of life.

8. There are a number of methods which may be used to place monetary values on the benefits which arise from health care programmes. These may be divided into three main categories: the human capital approach; the observed preferences approach; and the stated preferences approach.

9. The method which is used to measure the outcome of health care programmes in monetary terms via stated preferences is called the willingness-to-pay (or WTP) approach. This is based on the premise that the maximum amount of money that an individual is willing to pay for a health care programme is an indicator of the value of that programme to that individual.

10. Data on effectiveness may be obtained in a number of ways: via clinical trials; via existing research; and via expert professional opinion.

11. The basic approach to measuring effectiveness via clinical trials (also called intervention sudies) is by means of a comparison between the rates of the outcome of interest in the treatment group and the corresponding rates of outcome in a comparison group or groups. Key considerations are the ethics, feasibility and cost of clinical trials.

12. There are a number of issues to consider when designing and conducting clinical trials to ensure that high-quality results are obtained. These include: selecting a study population; allocating individuals to study groups; maintaining compliance; ensuring complete follow-up; blinding and use of placebos; and choosing the correct sample size.

13. When it is not possible to conduct a clinical trial in order to obtain information on the effectiveness of a particular health care intervention, then it may be appropriate to look to existing research for the information required. Obtaining effectiveness data via existing research in this way involves reviewing the literature in order to obtain evidence on the effectiveness of a particular health care programme.

14. There are a number of steps to carrying out a review of the literature: statement of objectives; literature search; comparison of studies found with inclusion

and exclusion criteria; data collection; assessment of study quality; pooling of results; and sensitivity analysis.

15. There are several different methods of obtaining expert opinion for the purposes of economic evaluation: Delphi panels; modified Delphi panels; nominal group processes; and expert panels.

16. There are a number of stages to measuring effectiveness via the Delphi panel approach: developing a questionnaire; selecting the experts; eliciting answers from the experts; and collecting and disseminating results.

Measuring effectiveness in an economic evaluation

In this chapter we concentrate specifically on methods for measuring effectiveness in economic evaluations. There are two components to measuring the effectiveness or outcomes of health care programmes, as follows:

1. choosing an outcome measure;
2. obtaining effectiveness data.

Choosing an outcome measure

As we have seen in Chapter 9, there are a number of specific forms of economic evaluation. Each of these approaches involves the systematic identification, measurement and, where appropriate, valuation of all the relevant costs and outcomes of the options under review. These methods may be distinguished by the way in which the outcomes or benefits of an intervention are measured. The four main approaches to economic evaluation are as follows:

1. cost-minimisation analysis;
2. cost-effectiveness analysis;
3. cost-utility analysis;
4. cost-benefit analysis.

Relating to these different forms of economic evaluation, there are three main types of outcome measure which may be used in an economic evaluation:

1. common units of outcome relating to measures of physiology, morbidity and mortality;
2. utility-based measures of outcome;
3. valuation of outcome measured in monetary terms.

These different measures relate to cost-effectiveness analysis, cost-utility analysis and cost-benefit analysis, respectively. (Note that cost-minimisation analysis considers only the costs of options. This is an appropriate form of analysis to use only when the outcomes of the options under consideration are known to be the same. If outcomes are the same, so that there are no differences in the effectiveness of options, then the decision regarding the most appropriate option can concentrate on finding the lowest-cost option.) We shall now examine each of the three different types of outcome measure in more detail.

Common units of outcome relating to measures of physiology, morbidity and mortality

Common units of outcome relating to measures of physiology, morbidity and mortality are used to measure effectiveness in cost-effectiveness analyses. The actual choice of outcome measure to be used in cost-effectiveness analyses will depend upon the objectives of the health care programme being evaluated and the ability to measure a single dimension of output. If there is one unambiguous objective of this health care programme, this provides a clear dimension along which effectiveness may be assessed.

In order to decide upon a common unit of outcome relating to measures of physiology, morbidity or mortality suitable for a cost-effectiveness analysis, the following steps are necessary:

1. Clarify the objectives of the health care programme which is the subject of the economic evaluation.

   EXAMPLE _____

   The objective of this economic evaluation is to assess the effectiveness, costs and cost-effectiveness of Community Psychiatric Nurses (CPNs) in the management of non-psychotic patients in the primary health care setting.

   The target group for inclusion into this economic evaluation consists of patients who obtain help from their GP for non-psychotic problems such as: relationship/family problems; depressive symptoms; anxiety symptoms; phobic anxiety; bereavement; obsessive/compulsive disorder; post-traumatic stress disorder; and morbid jealousy.

2. If a single major dimension for the measurement of the success of this health care programme is apparent, use this dimension.

   EXAMPLE _____

   The most common problems experienced by individuals in the target group are depressive symptoms. Thus, one possible dimension for the measurement of the success of CPNs in the management of non-psychotic patients in the primary health care setting involves improvements in these symptoms. One possible measure of effectiveness might therefore be the 'number of patients successfully treated for depressive symptoms'. A cost-effectiveness analysis conducted using this measure of effectiveness would therefore seek to measure the 'cost per patient successfully treated for depressive symptoms'.

3. Assess the possibility of alternative measures of success being used as measures of outcome.

EXAMPLE

Whilst depressive symptoms might be the most common problems experienced by the target group in this economic evaluation, these individuals also experience other problems which affect their psychological well-being. These include relationship and family problems, anxiety problems and obsessive/compulsive disorder. The existence of these other problems indicates that other measures of effectiveness may also be appropriate.

4. Examine the feasibility of employing more sophisticated forms of outcome measure if it turns out that there is more than one outcome measure which may be appropriate. For example, measuring outcomes in terms of utility or in monetary terms may be more appropriate since these measures may incorporate the effects of a number of dimensions relevant to the health care programme.

EXAMPLE

With the existence of other problems in addition to depressive symptoms, to measure effectiveness solely in terms of 'number of patients successfully treated for depressive symptoms' would be inappropriate. Indeed, because more than one outcome measure may be used, it would be more appropriate to measure effectiveness in terms of utility, since this will enable all dimensions of outcome relevant to the health care programme to be included.

The number of different common units of outcome relating to measures of physiology, morbidity and mortality is unlimited because outcome measures may be specifically geared to the health care programme being assessed. Many different outcome measures have been used by researchers conducting economic evaluations, and possibilities might include: lives saved; life years gained; pain-free days gained; symptom-free days; complications avoided; cases detected; cases prevented; and cases treated appropriately.

Final health outcomes versus intermediate outcomes

It is also necessary to distinguish between *final health outcomes* and *intermediate outcomes* when deciding on the choice of outcome measure for an economic evaluation. Final health outcomes (such as life expectancy) attempt to show the ultimate effect of the health care programme being assessed on the health of the patients to whom it is provided. Intermediate outcomes (such as patients appropriately treated or cases detected) do not show the ultimate effect of the health care programme on the patient, though they show some measure of outcome which may contribute to the final health outcome, or which will have an effect on the final health outcome as an intermediate step.

Intermediate outcomes are important in an economic evaluation since they may provide the link between the health care programme and its final impact on the health of the patient, though they may be of only limited use as a primary measure of outcome if the objective of the health care programme being evaluated is ultimately to improve health.

EXAMPLE _____

Intermediate outcomes which are relevant to the use of CPNs in the management of non-psychotic patients in the primary care setting include: number of patients treated; number of consultations per patient; length of consultations per patient; and compliance rates with therapy.

However, whilst these factors are important in determining the success of CPNs working in this setting, they do not show the ultimate effect of the intervention on the health of the target population of patients.

Utility-based measures of outcome

Utility-based measures of outcome are used to measure the effectiveness of health care programmes in cost-utility analyses.

In the context of health care, utility is usually referred to as the subjective level of well-being that people experience in different states of health. Measures of utility usually attempt to incorporate some component of quality of life as well as quantity (or length) of life, since it is generally assumed that quality of life is an important feature of the utility that an individual experiences in a specific health state.

Furthermore, to be of practical use in economic evaluations, the measure of utility must be *reducible to a single index*, even though it may be made up of components which reflect the multidimensional nature of health. The most widely used utility-based measure of outcome is the *quality-adjusted life year* (or *QALY*), which provides a method for combining information on the quality and quantity of life arising from a particular health care programme.

Quality-adjusted life years

QALYs combine a measure of the quality of life experienced in a particular health state with a quantitative measure of life years experienced in that state in order to obtain a single measure of lifetime utility. QALYs therefore represent years of life adjusted for the quality of those years of life.

To calculate the number of QALYs resulting from a particular intervention, the number of additional years of life obtained must therefore be combined with a measure of the quality of life. Some method is therefore needed to measure the quality of life experienced by an individual in a particular health state arising from a specific health care intervention.

Measuring quality of life

Measuring quality of life is difficult. Nonetheless, it is important to measure this component of health outcome because many health care programmes are concerned primarily with improving the quality of a patient's life rather than extending its length. In order to be able to calculate the QALYs resulting from a particular health care programme, the valuation of health states is required to generate quality of life scores on a scale in which 'death' equals zero and 'ideal health' equals one. Negative values are possible if any health states are regarded as being worse than death.

There are a number of steps to be taken when measuring quality of life, as follows:

1. identifying the relevant health states to be valued;
2. choosing individuals to obtain utility values from;
3. choosing the technique to be used in eliciting the value of health states;
4. measuring utility values.

Identifying the relevant health states to be valued

In order to establish the extent to which a particular health care programme affects the quality of life of a patient, data need to be collected for a number of health states relevant to a particular health care programme. The frequency and timing of assessments will depend upon the objectives of the economic evaluation, but valuation of some or all of the following health states may be relevant:

1. health state prior to the start of treatment, in order to provide a baseline measure;
2. health state during the period of treatment;
3. health state at the end of treatment;
4. health state after treatment has ended.

EXAMPLE _____

In general, treatment for the illnesses which are the subject of this economic evaluation is assumed to last for anything up to one year. Utility values were obtained from patients before they received treatment (that is, at zero years), at the very end of their treatment (that is, after one year) and after treatment was completed (that is, after two years). It is assumed that the health states of the individuals receiving treatment do not change until the very end of treatment (that is, after one year). It is also assumed that individuals remain in the health state after treatment was completed from the very end of treatment for the rest of their lives (assumed to be a further five years).

Choosing individuals to obtain utility values from

There are three basic approaches to measuring the utility of health states and to choosing individuals to obtain utility values from. The first approach involves finding individuals experiencing the health state of interest (for example, patients with the particular condition) and measuring their utility in that state. The second approach is to describe the condition to individuals who do not have the condition (for example, the general public), usually in the form of an abbreviated written scenario, and to measure their utility for that state. The third approach is a variant of the second, except that subjects already knowledgeable about the health states concerned are used (for example, doctors and nurses) in order to minimise the need for elaborate descriptive scenarios.

Therefore, there are three sets of individuals from whom utility values may be obtained:

1. individuals experiencing the health state of interest;
2. individuals not experiencing the health state of interest, from a general cross-section of the population;
3. individuals not experiencing the health state of interest but who are knowledgeable about that health state.

There are advantages and disadvantages associated with each approach. Using the first approach, patients with the health state of interest are asked to place a utility value on that health state. A number of problems may arise with this. First, in some cases patients may not be able to value their health state owing to its nature, either because they are unconscious, or because the health state precludes coherent thought, as might be the case with certain mental illnesses. Secondly, patients assessed in this way are in a situation of potential conflict of interest because collectively, patients with a particular illness have an incentive to exaggerate the disutility of their condition in order to enhance the cost-effectiveness of prevention and treatment of that illness. Thirdly, if the aim of the economic evaluation being conducted is to compare different treatments for different illnesses which are competing for the same resources, then it may be important to have utility values determined by one set of individuals rather than separate groups of patients.

Using both the second and the third approaches, individuals not experiencing the health state are asked to value it. This leads to obvious problems since the individuals concerned may not truly understand what the health state that they are asked to value is like. This is less likely to be a problem in the third situation, where health professionals knowledgeable about the health state may be asked to place a utility value on that health state. This minimises the problem of describing the relevant health states, though it may lead to conflicts of interest similar to those of the patients.

Ultimately, the correct choice of individual to ask depends upon the viewpoint of the economic evaluation that is being undertaken. If the perspective taken is that of society and the results are pertinent to public policy decisions which will affect all members of society, then utility values would ideally be obtained from informed members of the general public, thus implying the second approach outlined above.

The question of choosing which individuals to obtain utility values from is only an issue if the different groups are known to give different results. Fortunately, as explained by Drummond *et al.* (1987), this has generally not been the case. Most studies have found no differences between the different groups, a few have found only small differences and none have found large differences.

EXAMPLE

Information on utility values was obtained from the patients actually experiencing the problems and receiving either of the two interventions. This method was used because it is more likely that patients actually experiencing these problems are able to give a correct account of their utility values in the relevant health states. Also, whilst these problems do relate to a patient's mental health, it is assumed that because patients are non-psychotic their problems do not preclude coherent thought.

Choosing the technique to be used in eliciting the value of health states

The next stage in calculating the quality of life associated with a particular health state is to choose the technique to be used in eliciting the valuation of that state.

In order to be able to calculate the QALYs resulting from a particular health care programme, the valuation of health states is required to generate quality of life scores on a scale in which 'death' equals zero and 'ideal health' equals one. Negative values are possible if any states are regarded as being worse than death.

Various techniques are available for generating quality of life information. These methods include:

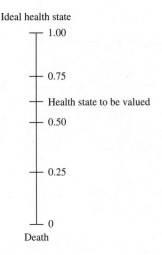

Figure 10.1 Rating scale for health state versus death.

1. Rating scale

A typical rating scale consists of a line on a page with clearly defined endpoints (see Figure 10.1). The line is measured between zero at one end and one at the other, with the 'ideal health state' placed at the 'one' end and the 'death' placed at the 'zero' end. The individual is then asked to value the health state relevant to the outcome of the health care programme which is being evaluated. This is done by placing this health state somewhere on the line in a position which corresponds to the difference in the preferences of the individual between the health state and the other states of 'ideal health state' and 'death'.

2. Time trade-off

The 'ideal health state' is given a utility score of one and 'death' is given a utility score of 'zero'. The individual is then asked to value the health state relevant to the outcome of the health care programme which is being evaluated. This is done by asking the individual how many years in an 'ideal health state' they regard as equivalent to a stated number of years in the specified health state of interest. The bigger the sacrifice of life expectancy they are willing to make, the worse the health state is assumed to be valued (see Figure 10.2).

The individual is offered two alternatives: they may be in the health state of interest for time period P, followed by death; or, they may be in the 'ideal health state' for time Q (which is less than P), followed by death. The time period P is varied until the individual is indifferent between the two alternatives. At this point of indifference, the utility score for the health state of interest is given by the formula Q/P.

3. Standard gamble

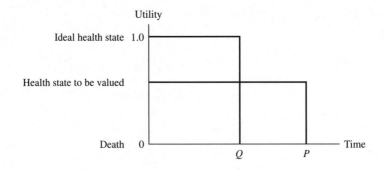

Figure 10.2 Time trade-off for health state versus death.

By this method, individuals are asked what risk of immediate death they would be willing to accept to escape from a specified state of health and to achieve good health. The bigger the acceptable risk, then the worse the poor health state is valued (see Figure 10.3).

The individual is offered two alternatives. With Alternative (1), the individual is offered a treatment with two possible outcomes: either the patient is returned to the 'ideal health state' and lives for an additional T years (which has a probability of occurring of P, where P is between zero and one) or the patient dies immediately (which has a probability of occurring of $1 - P$). With Alternative (2), the individual has the certainty of being in the health state relevant to the outcome of the health care programme which is being evaluated for a time period of T years. The probability P is varied until the individual is indifferent between Alternative (1) and Alternative (2). At this point of indifference, the utility score for the health state of interest is given simply by P.

There are many possible deviations to these three basic methods, each of which has its own advantages and disadvantages. Williams and Kind (1990) give the

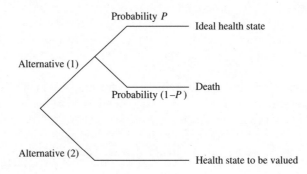

Figure 10.3 Standard gamble for health state versus death.

following criteria for establishing the relative merits of each of these elicitation methods:

1. *face validity*, representing the intuitive appeal of the nature of the choice confronting participants;
2. *comprehensibility*, involving the extent to which individuals understand the valuation task;
3. *internal consistency*, which measures the extent to which the valuations conform to the logically indicated order;
4. *reliability*, which involves the extent to which initial responses given by individuals are replicated when asked to repeat each valuation task;
5. *experimental burden*, which measures the ease with which individuals and interviewers complete the task, and the time taken to collect the data.

A valuation method can be chosen depending on the weight given to each of the above criteria.

EXAMPLE _____

It was decided to use the rating scale method for this economic evaluation since this was thought to be the elicitation method which patients will find easiest to understand. Comprehensibility was therefore deemed to be the most important feature of the elicitation method.

Measuring utility values

Two methods may be used to measure the utility values corresponding to the health states arising from the health care intervention: interviews and self-report questionnaires. Each of these methods has advantages and disadvantages.

Interviews may be conducted by trained interviewers to obtain quality of life data using one of the elicitation methods outlined above. The main advantage of this method is that the interviewer is able to explain clearly how utility values may be elicited, so there is likely to be little chance of misunderstanding or error by the respondent. Correspondingly, data collection is likely to be comprehensive, with minimal missing information. There are, however, a number of disadvantages with this method: first, it is likely to be expensive, since there is a need for trained interviewers, and secondly, it may be impractical if data is required on multiple occasions.

An alternative method to obtaining quality of life information is to collect the required data via *self-report questionnaires*. The main advantage of this method is that they are easy to administer and that they may be constructed so that they take only a little time to complete. The format of such questionnaires is generally designed to be easy to understand and interpret. However, whilst such questionnaires may be designed to be relatively 'user friendly', they still require a trained member of staff to be responsible for administration of the questionnaires and to explain to respondents how to complete the questionnaires. A further disadvantage of this method is that use of self-report questionnaires increases the likelihood of missing data.

EXAMPLE

Interviews were selected as the method for measuring utility values. Each patient was interviewed by a trained interviewer in order to obtain data on their utility in the three health states of interest (namely, before they received treatment at zero years, at the very end of their treatment after one year, and after treatment was completed after two years). Patients were presented with a 'thermometer' (see Figure 10.1) and asked to value their current health state at the times corresponding to each of the health states indicated. In this way, utility values were obtained for each of three health states of interest on a scale from zero to one.

None of the three health states of interest was deemed to be a state worse than death (that is, had a utility value of less than zero), or to be better than the ideal health state (that is, had a utility value of greater than one). Let us suppose that the following mean results were achieved by those receiving treatment by GPs and those receiving treatment by CPNs:

	Utility scores by treatment groups	
Health state	*GPs*	*CPNs*
Before treatment (at zero years)	0.1	0.1
End of treatment (after one year)	0.1	0.1
After completion of treatment (after two years)	0.6	0.7
Ideal health state	1.0	1.0
Death	0.0	0.0

Calculating QALYs

QALYs combine a measure of the quality of life experienced in a particular health state with a quantitative measure of life years in order to obtain a single measure of lifetime utility. QALYs therefore represent years of life adjusted for the quality of those years of life.

With a measure both of life years gained from a particular intervention and of the quality of life in each of these years it is therefore possible to calculate the number of QALYs arising from a particular health care programme.

In order to explain more clearly how QALYs are calculated, four simple statements may be presented:

Statement 1

First, an intervention which results in a patient living for *one* year with a quality of life equal to *one* implies that the intervention results in *one* QALY (that is, 1 year × 1.0 quality of life score = 1 QALY).

Statement 2

Secondly, an intervention which results in a patient living for *two* years with a quality of life equal to *one* implies that the intervention results in *two* QALYs (that is, 2 years × 1.0 quality of life score = 2 QALYs).

Statement 3

Thirdly, an intervention which results in a patient living for *one* year with a quality of life equal to *one half* implies that the intervention results in *one half* of a QALY (that is, 1 year × 0.5 quality of life score = 0.5 QALY).

Statement 4

Fourthly, an intervention which results in a patient living for *two* years with a quality of life equal to *one half* implies that the intervention results in *one* QALY (that is, 2 years × 0.5 quality of life score = 1 QALY).

With these four simple pieces of information it is possible to calculate the QALYs resulting from any health care programme provided information is available on both quantity and quality of life pertaining to that programme.

EXAMPLE

For those individuals receiving traditional GP-based treatment, this will result in patients obtaining 0.1 QALYs for the first year after the start of treatment (that is, 1 year × 0.1 quality of life), and 3 QALYs for the remaining five year of life after the end of treatment (that is 5 years × 0.6 quality of life). Therefore, the total number of QALYs which these individuals will obtain is 3.1.

For those individuals receiving CPN-based treatment, this will result in patients obtaining 0.1 QALYs for the first year after the start of treatment (that is, 1 year × 0.1 quality of life), and 3.5 QALYs for the remaining five year of life after the end of treatment (that is 5 years × 0.7 quality of life). Therefore, the total number of QALYs which these individuals will obtain is 3.6.

(Remember that it is assumed that the health states of the individuals receiving treatment do not change until the very end of treatment [that is,

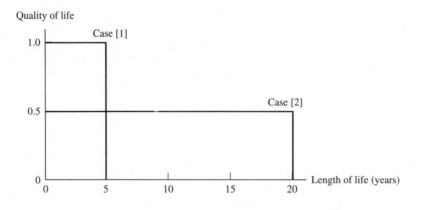

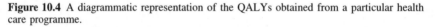

Figure 10.4 A diagrammatic representation of the QALYs obtained from a particular health care programme.

until after one year], and that individuals remain in the health state after treatment was completed from the very end of treatment for the rest of their lives [assumed to be a further five years].)

Diagrammatic representation of QALYs

Estimation of the QALYs obtained from a particular health care intervention may also be presented diagrammatically (see Figure 10.4). For example, after receipt of a particular health care programme an individual will live for another five years with an ideal quality of life score of 1.0, before dying (this is Case [1] in Figure 10.4). After receipt of another different health care programme an alternative individual will live for another twenty years, experiencing a quality of life score of only 0.5 (this is Case [2] in Figure 10.4). Therefore, Case [1] will yield 5 QALYs (that is 5 years × 1.0 quality of life score), and Case (2) will yield 10 QALYs (that is 20 years × 0.5 quality of life score).

EXAMPLE

See Figure 10.5 for a diagrammatic representation of the QALYs obtained from CPNs in the management of non-psychotic patients in the primary care setting.

Valuation of outcome measured in monetary terms

Valuations of outcome measured in monetary terms are used in cost-benefit analyses.

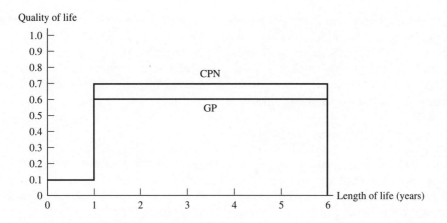

Figure 10.5 A diagrammatic representation of the QALYs obtained from GPs and CPNs for the management of non-psychotic patients in the primary care setting.

There are a number of methods which may be used to place monetary values on the benefits which arise from health care programmes. These may be divided into three main categories: the human capital approach; the observed preferences approach; and the stated preferences approach.

The human capital approach

The concept of 'human capital' conveys the fact that human beings are similar to capital equipment in the sense that they can be expected to yield a flow of productive activity over their years of life. If the value of this productive activity is assumed to be equal to an individual's rate of pay, then the benefits of health care necessary to treat a particular illness can be measured in terms of the flow of income that would have been lost because of that illness if the individual had not been treated. Therefore, the human capital approach basically involves calculating the income forgone because of illness. Should an individual be treated for that illness, then the effectiveness of the treatment measured in monetary terms is that income which would have been lost.

EXAMPLE _____

Suppose an individual is suffering from depressive symptoms which are treated by a CPN but which, if left untreated, would force him to take two weeks off work. If we assume that the value of the productive activity by the individual is equal to his rate of pay, and that the individual earns an income of £10,000 per annum, then the monetary value of CPN-based treatment is estimated to be £385 using the human capital approach (that is, 2/52 per annum potentially off work × £10,000 per annum income).

This provides a relatively simple method of valuing health outcomes in monetary terms. However, there are a number of problems with this approach. For example, valuing health benefits in terms of rates of pay neglects the benefits that accrue to individuals who are not employed, such as housewives and retired people. Also, the human capital approach ignores non-financial costs of pain, anxiety and suffering which are often associated with ill health.

Observed preferences approach

The *observed preferences approach* involves observing individuals' behaviour and using this as a basis for valuing health benefits. One method of doing this is to observe behaviour and attitudes towards risk and then to estimate the personal valuations implict in this behaviour. For example, some people accept large amounts of money to undertake dangerous jobs such as working as steeplejacks or as deep sea divers. Others spend money on providing their cars with additional safety features in order to reduce the risk of injury or death. When the extra income received or the expenditure undertaken is compared with the change in the degree of risk associated with a particular activity then it becomes possible to establish the personal valuations implicit in observed behaviour. Various techniques have been developed associated with scaling risks so that it is possible to convert valuations associated with small changes in risk into full life valuation. In this way, health care interventions which alter an individual's risk of death may be assessed in monetary terms.

Unfortunately, on a practical level, one of the main problems with this approach is the limited number of situations in which attitudes to risk can be observed and measured. This has led to the development of the more explicit stated preferences approach.

Stated preferences approach

The method which is used to measure the outcome of health care programmes in monetary terms via stated preferences is called the *willingness-to-pay* (or *WTP*) approach. This is based on the premise that the maximum amount of money that an individual is willing to pay for a health care programme is an indicator of the value of that programme to that individual.

As we have seen in Chapter 9, through the use of economic evaluation, health care programmes are valued according to their opportunity cost. In simple terms, the concept of opportunity cost means that something is not of value unless an individual is willing to sacrifice something else in order to obtain it. However, it is difficult to ask individuals what health care programmes they would give up in order to have more of another. One way to derive a value for a health care programme is to first ask individuals to *assume* they have to pay for that programme and then ask what is the maximum amount of money they would be willing to give up for it. This is the basic idea behind the WTP approach. The WTP approach therefore measures the strength of preferences of individuals, or how strongly they feel about particular health care programmes. It also uses a unit of measurement with which people are familiar, namely, money.

Questions regarding WTP may be asked in a number of ways. One way is to ask respondents an *open-ended question*. By this method, individuals are directly asked what is the maximum amount of money they would be prepared to pay for a health care programme, without being prompted.

EXAMPLE _____

This question concerns how you personally value treatment by a Community Psychiatric Nurse. Because treatment by Community Psychiatric Nurses uses a lot of health care resources, it may well be the case in future that patients will have to pay a larger proportion of the treatment cost. Assume that this will be the case and that fees will be charged for services provided by a Community Psychiatric Nurse. What is the largest amount of money that you would be prepared to pay per year for the treatment you are currently receiving from the Community Psychiatric Nurse?

I would be prepared to pay a maximum of £......... per year.

A variation on the open-ended question is called the *payment card technique*. In this approach, individuals are presented with a range of values and asked to circle the amount that represents the most they would be willing to pay.

EXAMPLE _____

This question concerns how you personally value treatment by a Community Psychiatric Nurse. Because treatment by Community Psychiatric Nurses uses a lot of health care resources, it may well be the case in future that patients will have to pay a larger proportion of the treatment cost. Assume that this will be the case and that fees will be charged for services provided by a Community Psychiatric Nurse. What is the largest amount of money that you would be prepared to pay per year for the treatment you are currently receiving from the Community Psychiatric Nurse?

	£
Make a tick by each amount you are sure you would pay.	0
	25
Make a cross by each amount you are sure you would not pay.	50
	75
Make a circle around the amount which is the maximum	100
amount you would be willing to pay each year.	125
	150
	200
	250
	300
	400
	500

An alternative to this is a *closed-ended question*, where individuals are asked whether they would pay a specified amount for the health care programme, with possible responses being 'yes' or 'no'. The amount which individuals are asked to accept or reject is varied across respondents and information is obtained from respondents on whether the maximum WTP is greater or less than the value offered to them.

EXAMPLE _____

This question concerns how you personally value treatment by a Community Psychiatric Nurse. Because treatment by Community Psychiatric Nurses uses a lot of health care resources, it may well be the case in future that patients will have to pay a larger proportion of the treatment cost. Assume that this will be the case and that fees will be charged for services provided by a Community Psychiatric Nurse. Would you choose to continue with the treatment you are currently receiving from the Community Psychiatric Nurse if you were charged a fee for doing so of £100* per year?

.... Yes

.... No

* The amount is varied as follows: £0; £25; £50; £75; £100; £125; £150; £200; £250; £300; £400; £500+.

EXAMPLE _____

Let us suppose that after using the payment card technique, it was found that the mean WTP for treatment by CPNs in the primary care setting was £300 per year. The mean WTP for treatment by GPs in the primary care setting was £270.

Obtaining effectiveness data

The second stage to measuring the effectiveness of health care programmes is to obtain effectiveness data on the outcome measure chosen. Data on effectiveness may be obtained in a number of ways, as follows:

1. via clinical trials;
2. via existing research;
3. via expert professional opinion.

Each of these methods may be used to obtain information on the three basic types of outcome measure (that is, common units of outcome relating to measures of physiology, morbidity and mortality; utility-based measures of outcome; and valuation of outcome measured in monetary terms).

Obtaining effectiveness data via clinical trials

In this section, we focus on the general principles and methods of designing, conducting and analysing clinical trials for the purpose of obtaining effectiveness data which may be used in economic evaluations.

The basic approach to measuring effectiveness via clinical trials (which are often also called *intervention studies*) is by means of a comparison between the rates of the outcome of interest in the treatment group and the corresponding rates of outcome in a comparison group or groups.

The ethics, feasibility and cost of clinical trials

With clinical trials, there is an active, deliberate assignment of patients to a particular treatment or health care programme, and there is an active assignment of patients not to that programme, but to some other for the purposes of comparison. Under ideal conditions, the differences in the health outcomes between the two groups may be attributed to the effectiveness of the treatment being assessed. Consequently, for reasons of both ethics and feasibility, there must be sufficient doubt about the particular intervention to be tested to allow withholding it from half the subjects involved in the trial. At the same time, there must be sufficient belief in the potential of the intervention to justify exposing the remaining half of willing and eligible participants involved in the trial.

Ethical considerations therefore preclude the evaluation of many treatments and procedures in clinical trials. Clearly, practices known to be harmful to patients should not be tested via clinical trials, which may put those involved in the trial at risk. Similarly, interventions known to be beneficial to patients should not be withheld from affected individuals who would form the comparison group(s). Problems of *feasibility* may also arise when conducting clinical trials if it is difficult to find a sufficiently large population of individuals willing and eligible to participate in the trial. In addition to the ethical and feasibility considerations of conducting clinical trials there is also the issue of the *cost* of conducting clinical trials. Generally, clinical trials are expensive to conduct, because they are often time-consuming and involve a large number of patients.

Conducting clinical trials

Once issues of ethics, feasibility and cost have been addressed there are a number of issues to consider when designing and conducting clinical trials to ensure that high-quality results are obtained. These include the following:

1. selecting a study population;
2. allocating individuals to study groups;
3. maintaining compliance;

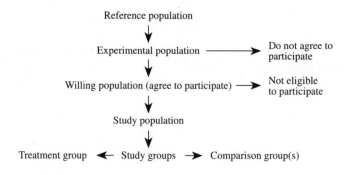

Figure 10.6 Population stages for a clinical trial.

4. ensuring complete follow-up;
5. blinding and use of placebos;
6. choosing the correct sample size.

We shall now address each of these issues in turn.

Selecting a study population

Figure 10.6 presents a flow diagram showing the population hierarchy for a clinical trial. The groups of individuals among whom a clinical trial is conducted are derived from a number of interrelated populations.

Reference population

The *reference population* is the general group of individuals from whom the investigators expect the results of the clinical trial to be applicable. This may be restricted by geography, age, sex or any other characteristic that is thought to modify the existence or magnitude of the effects seen in the trial.

Experimental population

The *experimental population* is the actual group of individuals among whom the trial is conducted. This group should not differ from the the reference population. Three factors are important when determining the experimental population for a clinical trial:

1. to determine whether the proposed experimental population is sufficiently large to achieve the necessary sample size for the trial;
2. to choose an experimental population that will experience a sufficient number of the outcomes or endpoints of interest to permit meaningful comparison between various treatments or procedures within a reasonable period of time;

3. to ensure that it will be possible to obtain complete and accurate follow-up information from the experimental population for the duration of the trial.

Willing population

Once the experimental population has been defined, individuals in that population may then be invited to participate in the trial. Potential participants should be fully informed as to the purposes of the trial, the study procedure and the possible risks and benefits. If appropriate, this briefing should include information that they may be allocated to a group receiving no active treatment and that they may not know the treatment they received until the end of the trial. Those who agree to participate in the trial are called the *willing population.*

After allowing for individuals in the experimental population who are unwilling to participate, the willing population in a clinical trial is often a relatively small and select subgroup of the experimental population. Problems may arise, because those who agree to participate in a clinical trial may be different from those who do not wish to participate in a number of ways that may affect the generalisability of the clinical trial results.

It has been found that those individuals who are willing to participate in clinical trials tend to experience lower morbidity and mortality rates than those who do not (see, for example, Wilhelmsen *et al.*, 1976). This is because so-called *volunteerism* is associated with age, sex, socio-economic status, education and other factors which are likely to influence morbidity and mortality. Therefore, in simple terms, individuals who are willing to participate in a clinical trial are likely to be generally less ill than those who do not agree to participate. Therefore, the subgroup comprising the willing population may not be representative of the population under consideration, and this will affect the ability to generalise the results of the clinical trial to the entire reference population.

If it is possible to obtain effectiveness data for individuals who do not agree to participate in a clinical trial, such information is useful in order to assess the presence and extent of differences between willing and unwilling participants. This will aid in the judgement as to whether the study results are generalisable.

Study population

Those willing to participate are then screened to assess their eligibility for inclusion in the trial. This will be decided according to a set of predetermined eligibility criteria. Reasons for exclusion from the trial may include factors such as a previous history of any of the endpoints relevant to the trial, or contraindications of the study treatment. Those individuals who agree to participate and who are eligible for inclusion in the trial comprise the final *study population.*

Study groups

After the study population has been determined, individuals may be assigned to *study groups*. At this stage, allocation of individuals to study regimens should take place only after individuals in the experimental population have been determined to be eligible for study inclusion and have expressed a willingness to participate.

The aim of a clinical trial is to compare the health care programme to be evaluated to a comparison group or groups. Thus, the effects of the health care programme can be compared with one or more of a variety of groups, such as the following:

1. an alternative health care programme for management of the same condition;
2. another dosage of the same intervention;
3. continuation of the standard health care practice;
4. a placebo.

Individuals who comprise the study population are thus allocated to study groups. Individuals assigned to receive the health care programme being evaluated comprise the *treatment group*. Those who are used as a basis of comparison to this group comprise the *comparison group*.

EXAMPLE

The reference population relevant to this economic evaluation consists of patients who obtain help from their GP for one of the following non-psychotic problems: relationship/family problems; depressive symptoms; anxiety symptoms; phobic anxiety; bereavement; obsessive/compulsive disorder; post-traumatic stress disorder; and morbid jealousy.

The economic evaluation was carried out across five general practices in London, which have a total of 36 GPs. The total number of patients registered at these practices was 62,000. The patients with the problems stated above who seek help from these five general practices form the experimental population. The number of individuals comprising the experimental population was 1,800.

On presentation to their GP with the problems of interest, patients were asked if they would be willing to participate in a clinical trial atttempting to assess the usefulness of CPNs in the primary care setting. Patients were told the aims of the trial, how it was to be conducted, the possible study groups to which they might be allocated and the possible risks and benefits associated with these allocations. After receiving this information, a number of individuals were willing to participate and these individuals comprised the willing population. Five hundred individuals were unwilling to participate in the trial, and therefore the willing population consisted of 1,300 individuals.

Patients who were willing to participate were then screened to assess their eligibility for inclusion in the trial Predetermined eligibility criteria and their rationale were devised to determine eligibility. Criteria for exclusion included factors such as: psychotic patients with the problems of interest (because the evaluation is aimed at the treatment of non-psychotic problems); patients who regularly obtained health care for treatment of unrelated problems (because patients may obtain help in these consultations which would not be recorded); and patients who lived more than ten miles from the GP practices (to enable ease of follow-up). Those individuals who agreed to participate and who were deemed eligible for inclusion comprised the study population. On hundred individuals who had agreed to participate were not eligible to participate according to the exclusion criteria. Therefore, the study population consisted of 1,200 individuals.

Individuals who agreed to participate in the trial and who were eligible to participate were then assigned to study groups. Two study groups were used in this clinical trial:

1. Treatment of non-psychotic patients by CPNs. Patients are allowed to attend their GP if they wish, but they may see a CPN instead should they wish to do so. GPs initially suggest to patients (if appropriate) that they should see the CPN, but treat patients as normal if they decline to do so. CPNs follow their normal procedures and treat patients as they see fit. Individuals assigned to this group comprise the treatment group.
2. Treatment of non-psychotic patients by GPs. Patients continue to see their GP as normal. GPs manage their patients as if treatment by CPNs is not available. This is the current best-practice option. Individuals assigned to this group comprise the comparison group.

Six hundred individuals were assigned to each study group

Allocating individuals to study groups

To maximise the possibility that the groups receiving the different interventions in the clinical trial will be comparable, the assignment of an individual to either the treatment or a comparison group should ideally be made on a *randomised* basis. Random assignment implies that each individual in the study population has exactly the same chance of receiving each of the possible interventions in the clinical trial (that is, each individual has exactly the same chance of entering the treatment group as of entering the comparison group).

When the health outcome being studied is expected to differ among subgroups of the study population with different characteristics (for example, across sexes or across individuals at different stages of illness), then the results of the study might be improved by ensuring that the study groups are approximately equal or balanced with respect to this characteristic. This may be accomplished using a more complex form of randomisation known as *blocking*, where every individual in the study population is classified with respect to each variable considered important before allocation and then randomised within that subgroup.

Randomisation is commonly regarded as the best method of allocating individuals to study groups within clinical trials. This is for a number of reasons. First, investigators involved in the clinical trial are unable to affect the allocation of an individual to a particular study group. Therefore, a potential bias is removed since investigators may be confident that observed differences in study groups are not due to the selection of particular individuals to a particular group.

Secondly, the study groups will, on average, tend to be comparable with respect to all variables except for the interventions being evaluated. This feature of randomisation is extremely important because all baseline characteristics suspected or unsuspected by the investigator that differ between the treatment group and comparison group(s) could potentially confound the relationship between the intervention and the health outcome.

Note that 'on average' in this sense implies that the larger the sample size (that is, the larger the study groups), the more successful the randomisation process will be in distributing characteristics among the study groups: when the sample size is sufficiently large, both known and unknown confounding factors are likely to be distributed equally among study groups. Therefore, randomisation can provide assurance regarding the comparability of the study groups.

EXAMPLE

In order to make the study groups as comparable as possible, individuals were randomly allocated to the study groups so that each individual in the study population had exactly the same chance of receiving each of the possible interventions in the clinical trial. Prior to the commencement of the trial, investigators placed information packs inside sealed envelopes. Also inside these envelopes was information detailing the study group to which the individual who opened that envelope would be assigned. Half the envelopes indicated a CPN allocation, and the other half indicated a GP allocation. The envelopes were identical so that it was not possible to tell one from another. On agreeing to participate in the trial and being found to be eligible, individuals were asked to select, at random from a pile, an envelope which contained their study group.

Maintaining compliance

A clinical trial requires the active participation and co-operation of individuals in the study population. Unfortunately, after agreeing to participate, individuals in a clinical trial may decide to deviate from the trial protocol for a variety of reasons including the development of side-effects, forgetfulness or withdrawing consent to participate.

Non-compliance, as this is called, is also likely to be related to the length of time that individuals allocated to study groups are expected to follow their particular study regimen. Therefore, for any number of reasons, individuals who originally agree to participate in clinical trials may choose not to, or may be forced not to, *comply*.

The higher the degree of *compliance* to study regimens, the greater the extent to which observed differences between those allocated to the treatment and comparison groups reflect real differences in the effects of the health care programme being evaluated. Non-compliance will decrease the ability of the clinical trial to detect any true effect of the health care programme being evaluated. For example, if individuals in the treatment group do not comply, then they become more similar in terms of study regimen to the comparison groups. Consequently, any true magnitude of the effect of the health care programme being evaluated will be obscured.

There are a number of ways in which compliance may be increased among trial participants. These include selecting individuals who are likely to be interested in the outcome of the trial and who will therefore have a much stronger motivation to comply. Other methods of enhancing compliance are frequent contact with participants (by home visit, clinic visit, telephone or post), the use of calendar packs of study medication (in which interventions are labelled for each day they are to be taken), and the use of other incentives such as detailed information not normally available to the general population.

In order to assess the impact of non-compliance, some method of compliance measurement is needed. The simplest way to measure compliance is to rely on self-reporting by study participants. Unfortunately, whether deliberate or not, this may be unsuccessful in eliminating any inaccuracies. An alternative method, which is feasible in some cases, is to use biochemical markers to validate self-reports, in which laboratory tests may be used to detect adherence to the intervention. Unfortunately, some participants in any clinical trial are likely to become non-compliant despite all reasonable efforts to the contrary.

EXAMPLE

Compliance was easily measured in this clinical trial, since it was possible to verify the contacts which any individual patients made with either their GP or the CPN. Compliance was enhanced by frequent contact by trial investigators, mainly by telephone. Because the trial protocol ensured that individuals assigned to the CPN groups were also able to see their GP if they wished, compliance was not a problem.

Ensuring complete follow-up

A crucial issue in the design and conduct of a clinical trial is the ascertainment of the health outcome of interest. The primary objective is to ensure that trial results are not biased by collecting more complete or accurate information from one study group than from another.

To ensure this, there is a need for complete follow-up of study participants for the duration of the trial. For some research questions being addressed, ascertainment of outcomes for the study groups may require only a short follow-up period, in which case it may be relatively easy to maintain contact with study participants during the entire study period. However, if many years of follow-up are needed for a clinical trial, maintaining follow-up and complete ascertainment of health outcomes becomes more difficult.

Complete follow-up is important because otherwise outcomes for part of the study population are not identified and the proportion of outcomes obtained becomes different across study groups. The results obtained may therefore be an over-estimation or underestimation of the true effect of the health care programme being evaluated. To avoid this bias, it is crucial to keep the number of individuals lost over the follow-up period to an absolute minimum.

Blinding and the use of placebos

Another potential problem may occur in the ascertainment of health outcomes in a clinical trial if the knowedge of an individual's study group influences the identification or reporting of relevant clinical events by that individual. This problem is related to the level of subjectivity of the outcomes under study. In clinical trials in which the endpoints of interest include subjective outcomes such as severity of illness, frequency of side effects, increased mobility or decreased pain, this is more likely to be a problem. In these circumstances, it is important to use methods to minimise the likelihood of any systematic difference in the ascertainment of outcomes between study groups.

One approach to this problem is to ensure that participants and investigators are *blind* as far as possible as to the identity of the interventions being assessed until data collection has been completed. In a *double-blind* trial design, neither the participants nor the investigators responsible for data collection know to which study group an individual has been allocated. The ability to conduct double-blind trials relies on having study groups which are as similar as possible.

In some cases, it is not possible to blind both the participants and the investigators. For example, it would be difficult to design a double-blind trial for the evaluation of health care programmes involving substantial changes in lifestyle, or drugs with characteristic side effects. In these circumstances, a *single-blind* or *unblinded* trial may be necessary.

In a single-blind trial design, the investigator is aware of which intervention the participants are receiving, though the participants are not. With an unblinded or *open* trial, both the patients and the investigator know to which study group each patient is assigned.

In many trials examining the effectiveness of drug therapies, the comparison group is often assigned to receive a *placebo*, which is an inert agent indistinguishable from active treatment. By making it difficult to differentiate between the treatment and comparison groups, the use of a placebo will minimise bias in the ascertainment of both subjective disease outcomes and side effects.

One problem with the evaluation of subjective endpoints is the well-documented tendency for individuals to report a favourable response to any treatment received regardless of their study groups and of the actual effectiveness of the intervention they receive. This phenomenon is known as the *placebo effect*. If a study does not use a placebo for a comparison group, then it is impossible to tell whether a subjective outcome is due to actual trial treatments, to the extra attention that participants are receiving or to the belief that the treatment will help. The use of a placebo ensures that all aspects of the interventions offered to study participants are identical except for the actual treatment. Consequently, by comparing the proportion of individuals in the treatment group and placebo groups who report a particular outcome under investigation, the true incidence of treatment-related effects may be determined.

EXAMPLE

In this trial, blinding was not possible, because it was not possible to mask the study groups to which an individual was assigned. The trial was therefore unblinded, or open. The use of a placebo was also not possible.

Choosing the correct sample size

An important issue in any clinical trial is the *sample size* of each study group (that is, the number of individuals allocated to each study group). A clinical trial must have a sufficiently large sample size to be able adequately and reliably to detect small but important differences in outcomes between study groups that may occur.

EXAMPLE

One of the major problems in using clinical trials which use a sample of individuals (the study population) to draw inferences about a larger population (the experimental population) is that *chance* may affect the results observed simply because of random variation across the sample of individuals and the study groups. One of the major determinants of the degree to which chance affects the findings in any particular clinical trial is sample size. If we examined the effectiveness of using CPNs in the management of non-psychotic patients in the primary health care setting compared to GPs by allocating only five individuals to each study group, then the results of the trial may differ substantially from the true results for all individuals in the experimental population simply as a result of chance. Had we obtained results from 2,000 individuals there would be less variability in our estimates of effectiveness and consequently we would be much more likely to draw a valid inference about the experience of the experimental population.

The effects of sample size and the ability to detect a difference in outcome between study groups depend specifically on a number of factors, as follows: selection of a high risk population; length of follow-up period; and compliance.

The ability of a clinical trial to detect differences in outcomes across study groups depends upon the accumulation of adequate endpoints. A primary strategy to ensure the accumulation of an adequate number of endpoints is *selection of a high-risk population*, and to select individuals at an increased risk of developing the outcomes of interest.

A further factor that is likely to affect the accumulation of adequate endpoints is the *length of follow-up period*. The length of time for which participants are followed from the commencement of the trial to assess whether they obtain the health outcomes of interest will have an important effect on detecting differences in health outcomes between treatment and comparison groups.

A third major factor which is likely to affect the ability of a clinical trial to detect differences in outcomes between study groups is *compliance*. This is because the effect of non-compliance is to make the treatment and comparison groups more alike, which has the result of decreasing the ability of the clinical trial to detect any true differences between study groups.

Obtaining effectiveness data via existing research

When it is not possible to conduct a clinical trial in order to obtain information on the effectiveness of a particular health care intervention (for reasons of, for example, ethics, feasibility or cost), then it may be appropriate to look to the existing research for the information required. Obtaining effectiveness data via existing research in this way involves *reviewing the literature* in order to obtain evidence on the effectiveness of a particular health care programme.

EXAMPLE

Suppose no information is available on the effectiveness of CPNs in the treatment of non-psychotic patients in the primary care setting. In this case, it is hoped that a comprehensive literature review will provide estimates of effectiveness and remove any ambiguities or controversy surrounding the effectiveness of the use of CPNs.

There are a number of steps to carrying out a review of the literature:

1. statement of objectives;
2. literature search;
3. comparison of studies found with inclusion and exclusion criteria;
4. data collection;
5. assessment of study quality;
6. pooling of results;
7. sensitivity analysis.

We shall now examine each of these in turn.

Statement of objectives

The main objective of a literature review is to arrive at a general conclusion regarding the effectiveness of the health care programme being evaluated. It is important that the objectives of a review are clearly formulated before the analysis, and that a clear definition of the question to be addressed is given. This should include specific, explicit definitions of the condition of interest, the population concerned, the outcomes of interest and the options considered. Also, a list of the inclusion and exclusion criteria should be given (see below).

EXAMPLE

The objective of this literature review is to assess the effectiveness of CPNs in the management of non-psychotic patients in the primary health care setting. The target group for inclusion into this economic evaluation consists of patients who obtain help from their GP for non-psychotic problems such as: relationship/family problems; depressive symptoms; anxiety symptoms; phobic anxiety; bereavement; obsessive/compulsive disorder; post-traumatic stress disorder; and morbid jealousy. Alternatives considered were: (1) treatment of non-psychotic patients by CPNs; and (2) treatment of non-psychotic patients by GPs.

Literature search

The next step in conducting a literature review consists of identifying all the relevant existing studies. This can be done by computer search of electronic databases such as the MEDLINE database. A hierarchy of key words can be plugged into a computer from a list compiled from the objectives, including factors such as target condition, target population and target measure of outcome.

EXAMPLE

The hierarchy of key words could run as follows: (1) Community Psychiatric Nurses; (2) psychiatric nursing; (3) GPs; (4) primary care; (5) depression; (6) relationship problems; and (7) anxiety symptoms.

This method of searching will narrow down the number of studies available until only those relevant are left. However, one problem is that a computerised search conducted in this way may miss some published titles. To correct for this, the reference lists of retrieved articles can be cross-checked manually to obtain further studies. Also, experts in the particular clinical area may be consulted for information on additional research. By these methods, all relevant published material may be obtained.

A further problem arises from the fact that unpublished studies may not be found by computerised literature searches. This may introduce bias into the review if unpublished studies are systematically different from published studies. Efforts to minimise this potential bias include working from the references of published studies, searching computerised databases of unpublished material and polling investigators in the field.

Comparison of studies found with inclusion and exclusion criteria

Studies found in the literature search may then be retrieved and selected for review on the basis of the *inclusion criteria* and *exclusion criteria*. These criteria will ideally be given at the stage of the statement of objectives and should depend on these specific objectives.

There are no standardised criteria for inclusion of studies in a review, and this would be inappropriate because a review of published studies can be applied to a broad range of topics. Investigators may disagree on the inclusion and exclusion criteria for a particular review. Therefore, inclusion and exclusion criteria and their rationale should be presented and all studies that are found should be provided in the reference list, even those that are excluded.

Some of the variables on which inclusion and exclusion criteria may be based include: study design; sample size; whether the study is published; the type of treatment and comparison therapies; and the outcome of interest. Studies found by the literature search may then be compared to these criteria.

In order to avoid bias in the selection process, the reviewer should be blinded to the study results, and the title, authors and abstracts should be removed from each paper. The use of two or more reviewers blinded in this way allows for the assessment of inter-reviewer agreement.

EXAMPLE

The literature review was restricted to randomised trials of the use of CPNs or psychiatric nurses. Trials of the treatment of psychotic individuals were not included, neither were trials with sample sizes of less than fifty patients per study group. Trials comparing different nursing or GP treatment regimens in which the aim was to produce similar health outcomes in each treatment arm were also not included.

Data collection

Once studies are collected and chosen on the basis of the inclusion and exclusion criteria they may then be reviewed so that the relevant information on effectiveness is abstracted. It is necessary to bring the result of each study selected into a standardised form to allow for comparison between the studies. To this end, *data forms* may be developed to record relevant information such as number of patients per group, outcome in each group and other key descriptive characteristics.

The outcome of interest may be measured by a continuous variable (for example, blood pressure), a quality of life score (for example, that used to calculate QALYs), a categorical variable (for example, mortality), an ordinal variable (for example, tumour stage) or a time-related variable (for example, disease-free survival), which should be delineated at the statement of objectives.

EXAMPLE _____

A data form was developed which recorded: the interventions included in each study; the composition of the treatment and comparison groups; sample sizes; the study setting; the outcome measures used; and study results.

Assessment of study quality

The studies included in the review will undoubtedly be of varying quality, and it is necessary to assess the quality of each study included so that a greater weighting may be given to those studies which are of high quality.

Before assessing study quality, a *quality protocol* may be formulated and studies can then be compared to this. To avoid potential bias, the assessment of study quality requires that the reviewers read only the methods and results of the reports, and all identifying information (such as authors and institutions) should be removed.

One method of assessing the quality of studies would be to assign a quality score ranging from zero to one hundred to each study. These scores may then be used in a number of ways: a previously defined cut-off point can be used to include or exclude studies from the review. Alternatively, these quality scores can be used to weight the individual study in the pooling process.

Although an objective quality scoring system can be used, quality assessment is still a subjective process, and there is therefore a potential for error. To help alleviate this problem, numerous researchers could perform quality assessment for each study, followed by a 'consensus meeting' to discuss agreements.

Various aspects of a study need to be analysed when assessing the quality. These generally refer to the *internal validity*. The internal validity of a study refers to whether the results are likely to reflect a real effect on health outcome or are artefacts due to design. The greater the internal validity, the greater the quality score. The quality score may thus be affected by factors such as the existence of randomisation between study groups, sample size and the use of blinding.

Another important feature to look for in the design of a study is whether the results can be generalised to the wider population. This is known as the *external validity* of a study, and will be affected by the way in which people were selected for the study.

EXAMPLE

All identifying features on each study were removed, before two researchers separately reviewed each study in turn. No contact was allowed between the two reviewers during the review process. The quality protocol asked each reviewer to award each study a mark from zero to one hundred, depending on their opinion of the quality of the study. Reviewers were asked to take into account factors such as the sample size, the composition of the population, the use of blinding, the effects of compliance and the length of follow-up when determining study quality, and the effect that these factors might have on the internal validity of the study. On completion of the assessment of study quality, the reviewers met to establish a consensus of study quality. Greater weighting in the review was given to those studies with a higher quality score.

Pooling of results

Once the quality of each study has been assessed the study results may be synthesised. Traditionally, *narrative reviews* of the literature have been conducted where investigators would consult relevant articles and then make some educated conclusions concerning the results compared. This method has been criticised, however. For example, Jenicek (1989) argues that 'narrative reviews express the personal opinions of their authors and depend heavily on the perspicacity and personal experience of the reviewer'.

In this context, there has been a growth in the use of a quantitative, structured, formal technique known as *meta-analysis* which has been defined by Chalmers and Altman (1995) as the statistical analysis of a large collection of analysis results for the purpose of integrating the findings.

As a first step in conducting a meta-analysis, a graphic display of the results of each individual study is helpful. Depending on the nature of the outcome measured in each meta-analysis, each component study can be displayed graphically showing the differences in outcomes between treatment and comparison groups.

Statistical methods used in meta-analysis compute a weighted average of the results in which the higher-quality trials have more influence than the lower-quality ones. There are a variety of techniques available for this purpose, which can be broadly classified into two models which treat the variability of the results between studies differently.

The *fixed effects model* considers this variability as exclusively due to random variation, on the assumption that there is a single underlying effect of therapy. So, an underlying assumption in using this model to combine individual study results to arrive at a summary measure is that their differences are due to chance alone and therefore all study results are the same (that is, they reflect the same effect).

However, if variations do not seem to be due to chance alone, pooling results will be more complicated, hence the *random effects model*. This model assumes a different underlying effect for each study, therefore taking between-study variation as well as random variation into consideration. So, more formal statistical approaches to investigating variation in study outcomes are available, comparing observed variations to what would be expected simply due to sampling.

Sensitivity analysis

The final stage in conducting a literature review and obtaining effectiveness data via existing research is to conduct a *sensitivity analysis* of the results. Sensitivity analysis is a useful means of exploring how sensitive the results of a literature review are to varying the assumptions made in conducting the review. This may include changing the inclusion and exclusion criteria and changing the methods by which study quality is assessed.

In this way, sensitivity analysis permits the robustness of the results to be tested in light of variations in the key assumptions. By using sensitivity analysis it is possible to show whether the results of a particular study are robust over a range of assumptions or whether the results hinge on the accuracy of particular assumptions.

EXAMPLE _____

To study how the pooled results change when both randomised and non-randomised studies instead of just randomised ones are included in the analysis, a sensitivity analysis was conducted. This was also used to assess the way in which results change when the sample size restriction is removed. This simply involves reanalysis, this time also including data from the now included studies. Comparison of the two sets of results in fact shows that the type of study and the sample size have little effect on the results, in which case disagreement about the inclusion criteria is unimportant.

Obtaining effectiveness data via expert professional opinion

The use of expert professional opinion in economic evaluations is widespread. This is an appropriate method to use for measuring effectiveness in situations where clinical trials are unethical, unfeasible or too costly and where there has been little or no research conducted. Professional opinion may be used to derive effectiveness data on: probability estimates; values for resource utilisation; information on costs; information on utilities and quality of life; practice guidelines; and disease management strategies.

There are several different methods of obtaining expert opinion for the purposes of economic evaluations:

1. Delphi panels;
2. modified Delphi panels;

3. nominal group processes;
4. expert panels.

We shall now examine each of these in turn.

Delphi panels

Conventional *Delphi panels* operate in rounds or stages in an effort to obtain a convergence of opinion in a particular area. There are a number of stages to conducting Delphi panel assessments, as follows:

1. Developing a questionnaire

As the first step, a questionnaire is developed by the investigator, usually with the assistance of an outside expert. This questionnaire asks the questions pertinent to the measures of effectiveness on which data are required. Occasionally, the questionnaire is pilot-tested on one or two experts in order to ensure that the questionnaire is understandable and comprehensive.

2. Selecting the experts

Once the questionnaire has been approved, experts are selected for participation in the study. The main criterion for selection of experts is that they be appropriate for the study under consideration. The criteria for selection of experts and their relevant qualifications and experience should be published along with any results.

There is no minimum or maximum number of members who should be included in the panel, though this is subject to common sense and practical limits.

3. Eliciting answers from the experts

Experts selected for inclusion in the Delphi panel are then provided with the questionnaire, which asks questions necessary to obtain the effectiveness data required. Experts may also be provided with a review of the relevant literature in order to frame their responses.

One distinct feature of the conventional Delphi panel is that there is no face-to-face contact between the expert respondents, although there may be face-to-face contact between the investigator and the respondents. By this method, all responses provided by expert panellists are anonymous to other expert panellists. This ensures that no one respondent is intimidated or dominated by another.

4. Collecting and disseminating results

Results are then collected from each expert and summarised. Usually the responses are tabulated and simple summary statistical measures are reported back to the experts. Included in the summary provided to a particular respondent are their responses as well as some measure of the average for all other panellists.

After all the members of the Delphi panel have had a chance to review their answers against the responses of other members they are given the opportunity to alter their responses. Frequently, severe outliers are asked to provide justification for their positions to the Delphi investigator. This process may be repeated until a consensus is reached among the Delphi panel members, where one is sought.

Modified Delphi panels and nominal group processes

There is no clear definition as to what exactly constitutes a *'modified' Delphi panel*. One possibility is that evaluations may retain many of the conventional Delphi principles with one exception, such as that one of the anonymous rounds is replaced with a face-to-face group discussion between the expert panellists. This may occur as an initial open meeting followed by a second anonymous round, or as an anonymous first round followed by a group meeting in the second round.

Modified Delphi panels conducted in this way have much in common with *nominal group processes*, in which group members discuss a particular topic during the course of a meeting and each member contributes ideas to the discussion. These ideas are then subjected to evaluation by all panel members privately. The results of each panel member's evaluation are tabulated and presented to the larger group. These results may then be re-evaluated until a consensus is reached.

Expert panels

Expert panels are frequently used as an alternative to Delphi panels and nominal group processes. They refer to a group of experts who are selected to answer either in a face-to-face interview or by post, in one round, questions relevant to a particular study. Responses may be queried for additional information once the initial data are collected. However, in contrast to other techniques, this procedure does not occur over several rounds and not all participants need be questioned again. Typically, results provided by panel members are not shared with others in the group. Results may then be averaged and used in the economic evaluation.

Measuring effectiveness

From the discussion in this chapter, there are two components to measuring the effectiveness of health care programmes assessed via economic evaluation: choosing an outcome measure and obtaining effectiveness data.

Corresponding to the different forms of economic evaluation, the three main categories of outcome measures in economic evaluations are: common units of outcome relating to measures of physiology, morbidity or mortality; utility-based units of outcome with qualitative and quantitative components; and valuation of outcome measured in monetary terms. The chosen measure will ultimately depend upon the health care programme being evaluated, and upon the objectives of the evaluation.

The availability of data on the effectiveness of the programmes being assessed is crucial to the accuracy of any economic evaluation. Data on effectiveness may be obtained in a number of ways: via clinical trials; via existing research; and via expert professional opinion. There are numerous advantages and disadvantages associated with each.

In this chapter we have therefore seen various methods by which the effectiveness of health care programmes may be assessed. However, the economic evaluation of health care programmes also requires further information so that meaningful data on cost-effectiveness may be obtained. Specifically, information is required on measuring costs, and this is the subject of the next chapter.

References

Chalmers I. and Altman D.G. (eds.) (1995) *Systematic reviews*. London: BMJ Publishing Group.

Drummond M.F., Stoddart G.L. and Torrance G.W. (1987) *Methods for the economic evaluation of health care programmes*. New York: Oxford Medical Publications.

Jenicek M. (1989) Meta-analysis in medicine: where are we and where do we want to go? *Journal of Clinical Epidemiology* 42: 35–44.

Wilhelmsen L., Ljungberg S. and Wedel H. (1976) A comparison between participants and non-participants in a primary preventive trial. *Journal Chronic Disease* 29: 331–5.

Williams A. and Kind P. (1990) The present state of play about QALYs. In: Hopkins A. (ed.) *Measures of quality of life*. London: Royal College of Physicians.

Suggested further reading

For a discussion of issues involved when choosing an outcome measure for use in an economic evaluation see one of the following:

Drummond M.F., Stoddart G.L. and Torrance G.W. (1987) *Methods for the economic evaluation of health care programmes*. New York: Oxford Medical Publications.

Robinson R. (1993) Economic evaluation and health care. *British Medical Journal* 307: 670–3, 726–8, 793–5, 859–62, 924–6, 994–6.

For issues involved when obtaining effectiveness data via clinical trials see, for example:

Hennekens C.H. and Buring J.E. (1987) *Epidemiology in medicine*. Boston: Little, Brown.

For methods for conducting systematic reviews of the literature and obtaining effectiveness data via existing research see:

Chalmers I. and Altman D.G. (eds.) (1995) *Systematic reviews*. London: BMJ Publishing Group.

For a generic discussion, not necessarily linked to economic evaluation, of obtaining effectiveness data via expert professional opinion, see:

Sackman H. (1975) *Delphi critique: expert opinion, forecasting and group processes.* Lexington MA: Lexington Books.

11   Measuring costs

In this chapter we examine the various ways in which the costs incurred by health care programmes may be measured. Various issues in the measurement of costs are discussed, including identifying the range of resource inputs to include, valuing the unit cost of the resource inputs, measuring the volume of resource use and multiplying the unit cost by the volume of resource use. Where appropriate and useful, examples are provided.

Summary

1. Limited resources have alternative uses. In choosing to use resources one way we are forgoing the opportunity to use them in another and a sacrifice is therefore involved. This sacrifice is called the opportunity cost. The cost of using resources in one way can therefore be measured in terms of the benefits forgone from other competing options.

2. There are four interrelated steps to measuring costs in an economic evaluation: identifying the range of resource inputs to include; valuing the unit cost of the resource inputs; measuring the volume of resource use; and multiplying the unit cost by the volume of resource use.

3. There are four issues that should be taken into consideration when identifying the range of resource inputs to include in an economic evaluation: the viewpoint of the analysis; the extent to which the comparison is restricted to the health care programmes immediately under study; the extent to which some costs are merely likely to confirm results that would be obtained by consideration of a narrower range of costs; and the relative order of magnitude of costs.

4. If an economic evaluation is to consider all the relevant costs from a particular treatment programme, then three main categories of cost should be considered: health service costs; costs borne by patients and their families; and costs borne by the rest of society.

5. Health service costs include: labour costs; non-labour costs; capital costs; and overheads. In an economic evaluation, all health service costs are referred to as direct costs.

6. Costs borne by patients and their families include out-of-pocket expenses such as travel, and any costs resulting from care activities provided by the family or other informal carers. These are both direct cost items. Patients and their families occasionally lose time from work whilst seeking or obtaining health care. Similarly, other socially productive activities, such as voluntary work, housework and informal care, may be sacrificed with the receipt of health care. These are classified as indirect costs. In addition to direct costs and indirect costs, a third category of costs which may be incurred by patients and their families are intangible costs. Intangible costs constitute the pain, anxiety and general unpleasantness associated with the provision and receipt of health care.

7. Costs borne by the rest of society may be incurred when individuals not directly involved in a health care programme experience increased costs because of it.

8. Unit labour costs may be estimated from the gross salary earned by the individual concerned.

9. Unit non-labour costs incurred by the health service may generally be obtained from market prices.

10. Capital costs differ from non-labour costs because they apply to assets which are reusable and which often have a useful life of more than one year. An adjustment to the total cost of the capital asset is therefore required to estimate the cost per year. This is known as the production of an equivalent annual cost. In its simplest form, the calculation of equivalent annual cost involves estimating the lifespan (in years) of the capital asset and dividing the market price of the capital asset by this estimate. There are two additional factors which should be considered in the calculation of capital costs: interest costs and depreciation costs.

11. The term overheads refers to those resources that serve, and may be attributable to, a number of health care programmes. The main problem arising from the valuation of unit overhead costs is that these are generally shared costs and need to be apportioned to individual health care programmes. Estimation of the overhead costs therefore requires an assessment of the proportion of the total overheads used by each individual health care programme. This is achieved using a measure called an allocation basis.

12. Unit costs for out-of-pocket expenses for caring activities may be obtained from market prices.

13. In order to measure the volume of resource use for each cost component it is necessary to measure the physical quantity of the resource input used providing

treatment in the health care programme under consideration. This information may be obtained from a number of sources: via clinical trials; via existing research; via expert professional opinion; and via strictly defined options.

14. When measuring the volume of resource use via clinical trials, there are a number of methods which may be used to collect resource data: time-use diaries; monitoring forms; and questionnaires.

15. The final stage in measuring the costs of a health care programme is to multiply the unit costs of each cost component by the volume of resource use.

16. Once the magnitude of each cost component has been calculated in this way, total costs may then be estimated by adding together all costs incurred from each cost component.

Measuring costs in an economic evaluation

In this chapter we concentrate specifically on methods for measuring costs in economic evaluations. To do this, we first need to describe the concept that economists use as the central criterion for appraisal in economic evaluation, which is called *opportunity cost*.

Opportunity cost

Limited resources have alternative uses. In choosing to use resources one way we are forgoing the opportunity to use them in another and a sacrifice is therefore involved. This sacrifice is called the opportunity cost of a decision. The cost of using resources in one way can therefore be measured in terms of the *benefits forgone* from other competing alternatives.

EXAMPLE

The opportunity cost of providing a particular nursing service (for example, a Community Psychiatric Nurse) is measured in terms of the benefits forgone from the alternative use of those resources (such as, say, providing hysteroscopies). Alternatively, the opportunity cost of providing a Community Psychiatric Nurse is the benefits forgone which would have arisen from other methods of providing the same care (such as via a general practitioner [GP]).

Therefore, the decision to provide a particular nursing service may well have a financial cost. In addition, it will also have an opportunity cost arising from the potential benefits forgone.

EXAMPLE _____

Suppose a Community Psychiatric Nurse is hired to work in a particular primary health care setting at a cost of £20,000. The *financial* cost of the Community Psychiatric Nurse is therefore £20,000. However, suppose that if that money were not spent on providing this nursing service, it would instead be spent providing 50 outpatient hysteroscopies at a cost of £400 each. The opportunity cost of the community psychiatric nurse is the lost potential benefit to the 50 patients who would have received the hysteroscopies had the money been diverted instead to fund those services.

Economic evaluation is the comparative analysis of alternative courses of action, in terms of both their (opportunity) costs and their outcomes, in order to achieve efficiency in the allocation of scarce resources. These methods may be distinguished by the way in which the outcomes or benefits of an intervention are measured. However, what the different forms of economic evaluation have in common is that they all seek to include some measure of the cost of the alternatives examined.

Measuring costs

There are four interrelated steps to measuring costs in an economic evaluation:

1. identifying the range of resource inputs to include;
2. valuing the unit cost of the resource inputs;
3. measuring the volume of resource use;
4. multiplying the unit cost by the volume of resource use.

Once the relevant costs to be included in the analysis have been identified, the measurement of costs may then proceed by estimating the unit cost of a particular resource and then estimating the total volume of that resource used. The unit cost may then be multiplied by the volume of resources used to give the total cost incurred from a particular resource input.

We shall now proceed by examining each of these issues in more detail.

Identifying the range of resource inputs to include

Drummond et al. (1987) delineate four issues that should be taken into consideration when identifying the range of resource inputs to include in an economic evaluation:

1. the viewpoint of the analysis;
2. the extent to which the comparison is restricted to the health care programmes immediately under study;
3. the extent to which some costs are merely likely to confirm results that would be obtained by consideration of a narrower range of costs;
4. the relative order of magnitude of costs.

The viewpoint for the analysis

It is important to specify the viewpoint of an economic evaluation when considering the costs to include because an item may be considered a cost from one point of view, but not from another. As discussed in Chapter 9, there are a number of potential viewpoints that may be taken:

- the patient;
- the third-party payer of services;
- the health care provider (local, regional or national);
- society.

In its simplest form, an economic evaluation might consider the costs and benefits only to patients or only to the local health care provider. However, if this viewpoint alone is considered, this may result in a number of important costs being omitted from the analysis. The viewpoint adopted will generally depend on the decision-making context of the economic evaluation. An economic evaluation designed by, say, the Department of Health to analyse the cost-effectiveness of Community Psychiatric Nurses in the primary care setting is unlikely to be interested in an evaluation which concentrates solely on the costs to patients. More likely, a much wider viewpoint will be preferred which considers wider cost and health outcome implications for the NHS and society.

The societal perspective is the most general and therefore the most preferred viewpoint for an economic evaluation because it ensures that all costs are considered.

The extent to which the comparison is restricted to the health care programmes immediately under study

If the comparison is restricted only to the health care programmes immediately under study, costs common to both need not be considered because they will not affect the choice between the given programmes. Elimination of such costs may save the investigator a considerable amount of time and effort. However, if it is the case that at some later stage a broader comparison may be considered, including other options not yet specified, it might be prudent to consider all costs incurred by each health care programme.

The extent to which some costs are merely likely to confirm results that would be obtained by consideration of a narrower range of costs

Sometimes the consideration of, for example, costs incurred by patients merely confirms a result that might be obtained from, for example, consideration of costs only within the health sector. Therefore, if inclusion of patient costs requires considerable extra effort and the choice of programme would not be changed, it may not be worth while including the costs which complicate the economic evaluation unnecessarily. However, some justification should be provided for the exclusion of these cost components.

The relative order of magnitude of costs

Often it may not be worth investing a substantial amount of time and effort considering costs that are small and therefore unlikely to make any difference to the results of the economic evaluation. However, some justification should be given for the elimination of such costs. It is good practice to identify cost components even if they are not to be formally included in the economic evaluation.

If an economic evaluation is to consider all the relevant costs from a particular health care programme, then three main categories of cost should be considered:

1. health service costs;
2. costs borne by patients and their families;
3. costs borne by the rest of society.

We shall now discuss each of these in turn. A list of the costs pertaining to each of these three categories which may be included in an economic evaluation is provided in Table 11.1.

Identifying health service costs

Health service costs include: labour costs (that is, staff time); non-labour costs (including medical supplies such as drugs); capital costs (incurred from both

Table 11.1 Cost components to be considered in the economic evaluation of health care programmes.

Cost	Cost type
Health service costs	Direct
Labour costs	Direct
Non-labour costs	Direct
Capital costs	Direct
Overheads	Direct
Costs borne by patients and their families	Direct/indirect/intangible
Travel costs	Direct
Out-of-pocket expenses for caring activities	Direct
Production losses	Indirect
Pain	Intangible
Anxiety	Intangible
General unpleasantness	Intangible
Costs borne by the rest of society	Indirect

equipment and buildings); and overheads (such as heating and lighting). These items may be divided into *variable costs*, which may vary according to the level of activity (such as staff costs) and *fixed costs*, which are incurred whatever the level of activity (such as heating and lighting). In an economic evaluation, all health service costs, both fixed and variable, are referred to as *direct costs*.

EXAMPLE

In the economic evaluation of Community Psychiatric Nurses (CPNs) in the primary health care setting, the main health service costs identified for consideration were: CPN time; GP time; medications; telephone; postage; CPN travel; non-psychiatric hospital treatment; other psychiatric treatment; heating and lighting in the GP surgery; and administration costs.

Identifying costs borne by patients and their families

Costs borne by patients and their families include out-of-pocket expenses, such as travel, and any costs resulting from care activities provided by the family or other informal carers. These are both direct cost items. Patients and their families occasionally lose time from work whilst seeking or obtaining health care. Similarly, other socially productive activities, such as voluntary work, housework and informal care, may be sacrificed with the receipt of health care. *Production losses* are therefore incurred by society. These production losses may also be included as costs attributed to a health care programme, though these are classified as *indirect costs*.

Because the estimation and inclusion of indirect costs is not fully accepted by health economists as being relevant in economic evaluations, these costs shall not be examined in detail here. For a comprehensive discussion on the inclusion and calculation of indirect costs see Drummond *et al.* (1987), pp. 78–9.

In addition to direct costs and indirect costs, a third category of costs which may be incurred by patients and their families is *intangible costs*. Intangible costs constitute the pain, anxiety and general unpleasantness associated with the provision and receipt of health care. Unfortunately, by their very definition, intangible costs do not relate to material objects and are thus extremely difficult to quantify. The majority of economic evaluations do not therefore include intangible costs. However, although intangible costs are difficult to quantify, even if they are omitted from the analysis, it is still good practice to identify them in an economic evaluation.

EXAMPLE

Direct costs borne by patients and their families in the receipt of care by CPNs and GPs were identified as follows: travel costs incurred by patients and their families and out-of-pocket expenses for caring activities.

Possible intangible costs which may be relevant in this economic evaluation include the anxiety experienced by patients in the receipt of care. Intangible costs were, however, not included in this analysis.

Identifying costs borne by the rest of society

Costs borne by the rest of society may be incurred when individuals not directly involved in a health care programme experience increased costs because of it. In most cases these effects are very small and do not merit inclusion in the analysis, but there may be some occasions when they are large enough to require attention. These may be classified as a form of indirect cost.

EXAMPLE

No costs borne by the rest of society were identified. Therefore, this cost component was ignored.

EXAMPLE

Therefore, the twelve cost components identified for inclusion in this economic evaluation of CPNs in the primary care setting are as follows:

1. CPN time;
2. GP time;
3. medications;
4. telephone;
5. postage;
6. CPN travel;
7. non-psychiatric hospital treatment;
8. other psychiatric treatment;
9. heating and lighting in GP surgery;
10. administration costs;
11. travel costs incurred by patients and their families;
12. out-of-pocket expenses for caring activities.

Valuing the unit cost of the resource inputs

The valuation of opportunity cost requires a unit cost to be attached to each resource input identified. We shall now discuss methods for the valuation of unit costs, examining each cost component in turn.

Valuing unit health service costs

Labour costs

Labour costs arise from the time inputs of health care professionals and other staff involved directly or indirectly in the provision of the health care programme under consideration. Analysis of labour costs might involve inclusion of the following:

- nurses;
- midwives;
- doctors;
- professions allied to medicine (PAMs);
- health visitors;
- care assistants;
- clerical staff;
- receptionists;
- managerial staff;
- administration staff.

Unit labour costs may be estimated from the gross salary earned by the individual concerned (gross salary is payment before tax, superannuation and National Insurance contributions have been deducted). Gross salaries earned may be obtained from national publications, such as the annual *Report on nursing staff, midwives and health visitors*, or from individual health care providers. The unit cost per hour for each relevant member of staff can be calculated by dividing the gross annual salary by the number of hours worked over this period.

EXAMPLE

From local health care providers, it was ascertained that the average gross salary for CPNs in the Health Authority where the economic evaluation was conducted was £15,648 per annum.

The CPNs were found to work, on average, 48 weeks per annum, 5 days per week and 8 hours per day. Therefore, CPNs work an average of 1,920 hours per annum (that is, 48 weeks $\times$ 5 days $\times$ 8 hours).

On the basis of this information, CPNs are estimated to earn £8.15 per hour (that is, £15,648/1,920 hours).

It was also ascertained from local health care providers that the average gross salary for GPs in the Health Authority where the economic evaluation was conducted was £50,054 per annum.

The GPs were found to work, on average, 49 weeks per annum, 5 days per week and 9 hours per day. Therefore, GPs work an average of 2,205 hours per annum (that is, 49 weeks $\times$ 5 days $\times$ 9 hours).

On the basis of this information, GPs are estimated to earn £22.70 per hour (that is, £50,054/2,205 hours).

Non-labour costs

Non-labour costs incurred by the health service for the provision of health care programmes might include the following:

- medical supplies;
- telephone;
- postage;
- travel.

Unit non-labour costs incurred by the health service may generally be obtained from market prices, which may be taken from a variety of sources.

Standard market prices for pharmaceuticals and other medical supplies may often be derived from publications such as the *British National Formulary* or the *Monthly Index of Medical Specialities*. Market prices for medical supplies not included in these publications may be obtained directly from the manufacturer or from health care providers who are in receipt of the supplies.

Telephone costs and postage costs may be valued using readily available market prices.

Travel costs incurred by health care professionals or other staff may be estimated from various sources. First, the price of petrol for private transport or the fare paid for public transport or private taxis can be used. Secondly, the cost can be estimated using Automobile Association or Royal Automobile Club mileage cost estimates. Thirdly, NHS mileage allowances may be used which are available for calculating the travel reimbursement of NHS staff using private cars for NHS business.

EXAMPLE _____

Medication costs were incurred by patients receiving prescriptions for psychotropic drugs for the treatment of their condition. Unit costs were obtained from the most recent edition of the *Monthly Index of Medical Specialities*, and were estimated to be £5.45 per day.

Telephone costs were incurred for arranging and confirming appointments with patients and for subsequent reminders. Telephone calls were estimated to cost an average of £6 per hour for local daytime calls, obtained from market prices available from the telephone company. The average duration of each telephone call was estimated to be 6 minutes; therefore, the average cost per telephone call was calculated to be £0.60.

Postage costs were also incurred for arranging and confirming appointments with patients and for subsequent reminders. Postage costs were estimated at £0.26 per item, obtained from the Post Office as the price of a first-class stamp.

CPN travel costs were estimated using local NHS mileage allowances available for calculating the travel reimbursement of NHS staff using private cars for NHS business. These unit costs were obtained from local health care providers and estimated to be £0.85 per mile travelled.

Unit costs of non-psychiatric hospital treatment and unit costs of other psychiatric treatment provided to patients were obtained using NHS internal market prices. Inpatient costs, outpatient costs and day case costs were estimated separately. Specifically, these unit costs were obtained from average GP Fundholding extra-contractual referral tariffs, and from average procedure costs for services for all Health Authorities in England and for all Health Boards and NHS Trusts in Scotland. Separate figures for each institution were obtained from the local Health Authority and then aggregated by the investigators. On this basis, non-psychiatric hospital treatment services were estimated to cost £350, £95 and £225 per episode for inpatient, outpatient and day case procedures, respectively. Other psychiatric treatments provided to patients were estimated to cost £425, £115 and £260 per episode for inpatient, outpatient and day case procedures, respectively.

Capital costs

Capital costs are the costs required to purchase major *capital assets* required by a health care programme. They generally include:

- equipment;
- buildings.

Capital costs are a form of non-labour cost. However, they differ from the costs discussed above because they apply to capital assets, which are reusable, and which often have a useful life of more than one year.

EXAMPLE

A GP may wish to buy new premises in order to treat the growing number of patients on her list. This will involve a significant cost to the GP, and the building will have an expected lifetime of greater than one year.

If a capital asset does have a useful life of greater than one year then an adjustment to the total cost of the capital asset is required to estimate the cost per year (and to derive from this a cost per hour which may be used as a unit cost value). This is known as the production of an *equivalent annual cost*. In its simplest form, the calculation of equivalent annual cost involves estimating the lifespan (in years) of the capital asset and dividing the market price of the capital asset by this value.

EXAMPLE

The building which the GP would like to buy costs £75,000. It is also expected to have a useful lifespan of 15 years. Therefore, the cost of the building is calculated to be £5,000 per annum (that is, £75,000/15 years). This calculation does not include interest costs or depreciation costs.

There are two additional factors which should be considered in the calculation of capital costs: *interest costs* and *depreciation costs*. Interest costs should be included even if the capital asset was not acquired with borrowed money because tying up money in a capital asset such as a piece of equipment or a building involves an opportunity cost. Therefore, there is an opportunity cost arising from the funds being tied up in the capital asset. This cost is the lost opportunity to invest the sum of money in some other venture which would yield positive benefits. This opportunity cost is valued by applying an interest rate to the amount of capital invested.

The second component of a capital cost is depreciation cost and this represents the depreciation over time of the capital asset. Depreciation costs arise because of the wear and tear that a capital asset undergoes through use and the consequent reduction in the length of its useful life.

For an in-depth discussion of the calculation of capital costs, including both interest costs and depreciation costs, see Drummond *et al.* (1987), pp. 67–70.

If expenditure on capital assets involves incurring costs that are related to more than one health care programme, then they may require allocation in a similar fashion to overheads, as discussed below.

Overheads

Costs which are unambiguously attributable to a particular health care programme are known as *directly allocatable costs*. These may be directly and immediately apportioned to the health care programme under consideration. The term *overheads* or *overhead costs* refers to those resources that serve, and may be attributable to, a number of health care programmes. Overheads include:

- heating;
- lighting;
- general administration;
- medical records;
- cleaning;
- central laundry services;
- portering services.

The main problem arising from the valuation of unit overhead costs is that these are generally *shared costs* and need to be apportioned to individual health care programmes. Unfortunately, it may be difficult to identify the value of overhead resources used in a health care programme that shares those resources with other health care programmes. Estimation of the overhead costs therefore requires an assessment of the proportion of the total overheads used by each individual health care programme.

Overheads may generally be allocated to health care programmes using a measure called an *allocation basis*. The allocation basis is related to usage of the shared resource, and involves finding a common unit for measuring the proportion of usage of the overhead across health care programmes. Common units of measurement might include: square metres of floor space for the allocation of heating, lighting and cleaning; number of patients treated for general administration and medical records; and the number of patient-hours of health care provided for central laundry services and portering services.

EXAMPLE

Unit costs of heating and lighting are required for those patients treated in the GP setting. Total heating and lighting costs are available for the entire GP practice, but these must be allocated down to heating and lighting costs for a single GP consultation. Unit costs are estimated by calculating the square metres of floor space in the entire building and then calculating the square metres of floor space in the consultation room. The length of time over which the total heating and lighting costs and the average length of one consultation are also required for the allocation procedure.

Total heating and lighting costs are found to be £576 over a twelve-week period. Over this time period, the GP practice is open 5 days a week for 8 hours a day. Therefore, the GP practice is open for 480 hours (that is, 12 weeks × 5 days × 8 hours). Heating and lighting costs are therefore calculated to be £1.20 per hour (that is, £576/480 hours). The GP practice has a total size of 125 square metres, and the GP consultation room has a size of 25 square metres. Therefore, the consultation room is a proportion of 0.2 of the total size of the entire practice (that is, 25/125). Therefore, the consultation room has an average heating and lighting cost per hour of £0.24 (that is, £1.20 per hour/0.2 proportion). If each consultation lasts an average of 15 minutes, then the heating and lighting costs for one GP consultation are calculated as £0.06 (that is, £0.24 per hour × one quarter of an hour).

Administration costs are estimated using a similar procedure, though these overheads may be allocated on the basis of the number of patients treated and on the number of times they are treated.

Administration costs are incurred because the health care provider is required to employ an administration secretary in order to arrange appointments and for the upkeep of medical records. This administration secretary earns a gross salary of £10,236 per annum, and is responsible for the administration of 7,874 patients. On average, each patient contacts the health care provider twice per annum, and so there are therefore 15,748 contacts per annum. On this basis, the administration cost is calculated to be £0.65 per patient per GP or CPN contact (that is, £10,236/15,748 contacts).

When calculating overhead costs, two issues may apply. First, if there is evidence that the health care programme under consideration uses shared resources that would have been incurred without that health care programme and would not have been diverted from any other use, then an opportunity cost of zero can be assumed.

EXAMPLE _____

If a spare office in the GP surgery is used in order to provide a base for CPNs, and this room would not have been used otherwise, then an opportunity cost of zero can be assumed.

Similarly, no overhead cost for heating and lighting is incurred if the GP practice would have been heated and lit anyway.

Secondly, if it is not practical to estimate the amount of overhead resources used by a particular health care programme, then a subjective judgement may be used to estimate the 'add-on' cost for shared resources. This add-on cost could be considered to be from, for example, 5 to 40 per cent on top of all other costs, depending on the range and type of overheads identified.

Valuing unit costs borne by patients and their families

Travel costs

Travel costs incurred by patients and their families may be estimated from various sources, in much the same way as estimating travel costs for health care professionals and other staff: the price of petrol for private transport or the fare paid for public transport or private taxis can be used; alternatively, costs may be estimated using Automobile Association or Royal Automobile Club mileage cost estimates.

EXAMPLE _____

Unit costs of travel incurred by patients and their families were estimated using public transport prices, since this was the most popular mode of transport used by patients. The unit cost of bus travel was obtained from local bus service providers and was found to be £1.10 per mile travelled.

Out-of-pocket expenses for caring activities

In addition to travel costs there may be other out-of-pocket expenses incurred by the patients and their families, such as payment for over-the-counter medicines, charges payable for the receipt of prescription medicines, or payments for any other goods or services which may be purchased by patients and their families for the treatment of a particular illness.

Unit costs for out-of-pocket expenses for caring activities may generally be obtained from market prices, available from either the retailer or the manufacturer of the good or service in question.

EXAMPLE _____

Out-of-pocket expenses incurred by patients and their families arose from the purchase of over-the-counter medications from pharmacists. These medications were mainly weak painkilling medicines. Unit costs were obtained from a retailer of these medications and were estimated to be £1.25 per day.

Using price as a proxy for cost

Empirically, price is often important as a means of estimating the costs of different options. Unfortunately, the price of a good and the cost of producing that good may not necessarily be the same. In the National Health Service the price of health care in the internal market is based, in theory, on average procedure cost. The fundamental principles set out by the National Health Service Management Executive (NHSME, 1990) for the establishment of costs and prices are as follows:

1. prices should be based on average costs;
2. costs should generally be arrived at on a full cost basis;
3. there should be no planned cross-subsidisation between contracts.

Unfortunately, in practice, owing to the lack of available cost data, and differences in definitions and terminology, prices may often not reflect true costs (MacKerrell, 1993). Therefore, caution should be exercised when using price as a proxy for cost.

EXAMPLE

Data on the unit costs for each of the twelve cost components identified for inclusion in the economic evaluation of CPNs in the primary care setting are summarised in Table 11.2.

Table 11.2 Unit costs of each cost component.

	Cost component	Unit cost
(1)	CPN time	£8.15 per hour
(2)	GP time	£22.70 per hour
(3)	medications	£5.45 per day
(4)	telephone	£0.60 per telephone call
(5)	postage	£0.26 per item
(6)	CPN travel	£0.85 per mile
(7)	non-psychiatric hospital treatment	£350.00 per episode (inpatient)
		£95.00 per episode (outpatient)
		£225.00 per episode (day case)
(8)	other psychiatric treatment	£425.00 per episode (inpatient)
		£115.00 per episode (outpatient)
		£260.00 per episode (day case)
(9)	heating and lighting in GP surgery	£0.06 per GP consultation
(10)	administration costs	£0.65 per GP or CPN contact
(11)	travel costs incurred by patients and their families	£1.10 per mile
(12)	out-of-pocket expenses for caring activities	£1.25 per day

Measuring the volume of resource use

In order to measure the volume of resource use for each cost component it is necessary to measure the physical quantity of the resource input used in the health care programme under consideration. Possible units of measurement for the volume of resource use for each cost component are presented in Table 11.3.

In a similar fashion to collecting data on effectiveness, this information may be obtained from a number of sources:

1. via clinical trials;
2. via existing research;
3. via expert professional opinion.

Additionally, a fourth method for measuring the volume of resource use is discussed by Tolley and Rowland (1995), namely:

4. via strictly defined options.

Each of these methods may be used to measure the volume of resource use pertaining to each of the cost components classified above (that is, labour costs, non-labour costs, capital costs, overheads, travel costs and out-of-pocket expenses for caring activities).

Table 11.3 Units of measurement of resource use, by cost component.

Cost component	Unit of measurement of resource use
Health service costs:	
Labour costs	
Nurses, midwives, doctors, professions allied to medicine, health visitors, care assistants, clerical staff, receptionists, managerial staff, administration staff	Number of hours worked
Non-labour costs	
Medical supplies	Quantity of items used
Telephone	Number of telephone calls made
Postage	Number of items posted
Travel costs	Number of miles travelled
Capital costs	
Equipment	Number of times/minutes used
Buildings	Length of time occupied
Overheads	
Heating	Proportion of total floor space occupied
Lighting	Proportion of total floor space occupied
General administration	Proportion of total patients treated
Medical records	Proportion of total patients treated
Cleaning	Proportion of total floor space occupied
Central laundry services	Proportion of total patients treated
Portering services	Proportion of total patients treated
Costs borne by patients and their families:	
Travel costs	Number of miles travelled
Out-of-pocket expenses for caring activities	Quantity of items used

Measuring the volume of resource use via clinical trials

The basic approach to measuring the volume of resource use via clinical trials is by means of a comparison between the treatment group and a comparison group or groups.

With clinical trials, there is an active, deliberate assignment of patients to a particular treatment or health care programme, and there is an active assignment of patients not to that programme, but to some other for the purposes of comparison. Under ideal conditions, the differences in the resource use between the two groups may be attributed to the effectiveness of the treatment being assessed.

There are a number of issues to consider when designing and conducting clinical trials to ensure that high-quality results are obtained. These include the following:

1. selecting a study population;
2. allocating individuals to study groups;
3. maintaining compliance;
4. ensuring complete follow-up;
5. blinding and use of placebos;
6. choosing the correct sample size.

For a more detailed exposition of the issues involved in conducting clinical trials, see Chapter 10.

When measuring the volume of resource use via clinical trials, there are a number of methods which may be used to collect resource data, specifically:

1. time-use diaries;
2. monitoring forms;
3. questionnaires.

We shall now discuss the use of each of these in turn, though to do so it is necessary first to distinguish between *prospective* data collection techniques and *retrospective* data collection techniques. Prospective data collection involves measuring resource use identified at the time that treatment is provided, whereas retrospective data collection involves measuring resource use after treatment has been provided.

Time-use diaries

Time-use diaries may be used to collect data on the volume of resource use necessary for calculation of labour costs by recording information on the number of hours that a health care professional or other member of staff devotes to a particular activity.

Time-use diaries therefore involve individuals regularly recording their time input into an activity. This may then be used to identify time spent on key activities, such as time spent interacting with patients or time spent in planning meetings and administration.

Clearly, the accuracy of the data recorded will depend upon the frequency with which the individual completes entries in the diary. Accuracy may be increased if data are recorded at frequent intervals (for example, hourly), though this involves a high level of commitment on the part of the individual concerned. It may be more feasible to encourage entry completion on a daily, two-daily or even weekly basis, though this is likely to entail some loss in precision.

The duration over which a time-use diary is completed can also affect the reliability of this method. A period of at least one year may be required in order to reduce the impact of weekly variations in time use. However, clinical trials may not be conducted over this length of time, and if they are, the use of such an instrument is likely to be difficult to administer, to be costly to implement and to require goodwill from participants. Long time periods pose problems of 'participant fatigue' resulting in errors in the recording of time use and low completion compliance, especially for more detailed diaries.

Shorter time periods have lower administrative costs and place fewer demands on participants, resulting in more incentives to complete a time-use diary satisfactorily. The minimum acceptable period is likely to vary across health care programmes, though a time period of less than two weeks is unlikely to produce meaningful data. A major problem with choosing only a limited time period is the potential for choosing a period in which the time spent by health care professionals and other staff on key activities is not typical of the normal workload distribution, thus resulting in a form of bias. For this reason, if only short time periods for the completion of time-use diaries are to be considered, it is advisable that the individual concerned completes the diary in two or three different time periods spread over the course of the trial in order to reduce the probability of bias.

EXAMPLE

An example of a time-use diary is presented in Table 11.4. For instance, on 16 October, Jane Robinson spent 90 minutes performing administrative tasks, 15 minutes in indirect contact with patients (primarily telephone contacts), 165 minutes in direct contact with patients, 80 minutes travelling and 125 minutes on a training course.

Monitoring forms

Monitoring forms can be used for the collection of prospective data via clinical trials and are particularly useful for obtaining data on the volume of resource use for non-labour costs.

Monitoring forms can therefore be used to record the volume of resource use of medical supplies, telephone, postage, travel costs, capital costs and overheads associated with the health care programme being evaluated, and travel costs and out-of-pocket expenses for caring activities incurred by patients and their families. This method can be used in much the same way as a time-use diary above, and issues concerning the frequency of completion and the duration of the completion period equally apply.

Table 11.4 An example of a time-use diary.

Name: Jane Robinson							
Job title: Community Psychiatric Nurse							
Key: D = direct patient contact; I = indirect patient contact; C = training course; P = planning; A = administration; T = travelling.							
DATE	1	2	3	4	5	6	7	8
15 Oct.	P, 60	D, 245	I, 45	T, 95				
16 Oct.	A, 90	I, 15	D, 165	T, 80	C, 125			
17 Oct.	C, 170	T, 65	D, 325	I, 25				

Table 11.5 An example of a monitoring form.

Patient	Location of contact	Length of contact	Distance travelled	Treatment inputs	Other inputs
Roger Brown	Patient's home	25 minutes	3 miles	Leaflet	Postage
Nancy Clark	Patient's home	45 minutes	1 mile	–	–
Helen Smith	Telephone	10 minutes	–	–	Telephone

EXAMPLE _____

An example of a monitoring form is presented in Table 11.5.

Questionnaires

Questionnaires can be used for the collection of retrospective data on the volume of resource use. They may be used to collect data for all cost components in much the same way that time-use diaries and monitoring forms may be used.

Two methods may be used to collect data on the volume of resource use via questionnaires: interviews and self-reporting. Each of these methods has advantages and disadvantages.

Face-to-face interviews may be conducted by interviewers with health care professionals and other staff in order to elicit data on the volume of resource use. The main advantage of this method is that the interviewer is able to explain clearly exactly what is being asked, so that data collection is likely to be comprehensive, with minimal missing information. There are, however, a number of disadvantages with this method, since it is likely to be expensive, and it may be impractical if data are required on multiple occasions.

An alternative method to obtaining these data is to use self-report questionnaires. The main advantage of this method is that they are easy to administer and that they may be constructed so that they take only a little time to complete. The format of such questionnaires is generally designed to be easy to understand and interpret. However, use of self-report questionnaires increases the likelihood of missing data.

The timing of the questionnaire is also important. It is advisable to collect information as soon after the particular health care programme has been administered as possible. Otherwise, there are likely to be errors in recall.

Measuring the volume of resource use via existing research

When it is not possible to conduct a clinical trial in order to obtain information on the volume of resource use arising from a particular health care intervention, then it may be appropriate to look to the existing research for the information required. Obtaining data via existing research in this way involves reviewing the literature in order to obtain evidence on the volume of resource use of a particular health care programme.

There are a number of steps to carrying out a review of the literature:

1. statement of objectives;
2. literature search;
3. comparison of studies found with inclusion and exclusion criteria;
4. data collection;
5. assessment of study quality;
6. pooling of results;
7. sensitivity analysis.

For a detailed discussion of methods for measuring the volume of resource use via existing research, see Chapter 10.

Apart from reviews of the published literature, routine records and documentation often collected by health care purchasers and providers provide an invaluable source of information on the volume of resource use. Hospital activity systems may be in place to record the labour and non-labour inputs used in the provision of a particular health care programme. Additionally, health care purchasers and providers may keep and regularly update computer databases with details of all patient consultations, drugs prescribed, treatments provided and final health outcomes. If records such as these are kept, they can prove a useful source of information on the volume of resources used by a particular health care programme.

Measuring the volume of resource use via expert professional opinion

The use of expert professional opinion in economic evaluations is widespread. This is an appropriate method to use for measuring the volume of resource use in situations where clinical trials are unethical, unfeasible or too costly and where there has been little or no previous research conducted.

There are several different methods of obtaining expert opinion for the purposes of economic evaluations, listed as follows:

1. Delphi panels;
2. modified Delphi panels;
3. nominal group processes;
4. expert panels.

The most formal method for measuring the volume of resource use via expert opinion is through the use of Delphi panels. There are a number of stages to conducting Delphi panel assessments, as follows:

1. developing a questionnaire;
2. selecting the experts;
3. eliciting answers from the experts;
4. collecting and disseminating results.

For a more detailed discussion of methods for measuring the volume of resource use via expert professional opinion, see Chapter 10.

Measuring the volume of resource use via strictly defined options

A requirement of certain health care programmes is that the treatment options provided to patients have strictly defined boundaries. In this case, it becomes possible to estimate the volume of resource use for each cost component without the need for explicit data collection. A monitoring exercise could be undertaken to check that treatment is being provided as specified in the protocol.

EXAMPLE _____

Treatment by CPNs might be defined as follows: each patient receives an initial session with the CPN of 30 minutes' duration in their own home, where an information leaflet will be provided. Two weeks later, a 15-minute

Table 11.6 Volume of resource use for each cost component.

	Cost component	Volume of resource use CPN	GP
(1)	CPN time	5.5 hours	0 hours
(2)	GP time	1.0 hour	4.5 hours
(3)	medications	3 days	9 days
(4)	telephone	12 calls	1 call
(5)	postage	24 items	2 items
(6)	CPN travel	36 miles	0 miles
(7)	non-psychiatric hospital treatment		
	(a) inpatient	0 episodes	0 episodes
	(b) outpatient	0 episodes	0 episodes
	(c) day care	0 episodes	0 episodes
(8)	other psychiatric treatment		
	(a) inpatient	0 episodes	0 episodes
	(b) outpatient	3 episodes	2 episodes
	(c) day care	1 episode	1 episode
(9)	heating and lighting in GP surgery	4 consultations	18 consultations
(10)	administration costs	15 contacts	18 contacts
(11)	travel costs incurred by patients and their families	12 miles	36 miles
(12)	out-of-pocket expenses for caring activities	15 days	10 days

follow-up session will be provided, again in the patient's own home. Every two weeks subsequent to that, the CPN will contact the patient by telephone, and once a month, an information letter and reminder will be posted to the patient.

EXAMPLE

Using time-use diaries, monitoring forms and self-report questionnaires, a clinical trial of the use of CPNs in the primary health care setting for the treatment of non-psychotic patients obtained various data on the volume of resource use for each of the twelve cost components in this economic evaluation. The time period over which the volume of resource use was considered was one year. Average results per patient were collected for patients receiving treatment from CPNs and for patients receiving treatment from GPs. Results are presented in Table 11.6.

Multiplying the unit cost by the volume of resource use

The final stage in measuring the costs of a health care programme is to multiply the unit costs of each cost component by the volume of resource use. This calculation gives an estimate of the magnitude of each cost component.

Table 11.7 Multiplying the unit cost by the volume of resource use for each cost component.

[1]	Cost component [2]	Unit cost [3]	Volume of resource use [4] CPN	[5] GP	Unit cost × volume of resource use [6] CPN	[7] GP
(1)	CPN time	£8.15	5.5	0	£44.83	£0.00
(2)	GP time	£22.70	1.0	4.5	£22.70	£102.15
(3)	medications	£5.45	3	9	£16.35	£49.05
(4)	telephone	£0.60	12	1	£7.20	£0.60
(5)	postage:	£0.26	24	2	£6.24	£0.52
(6)	CPN travel	£0.85	36	0	£30.60	£0.00
(7)	non-psychiatric hospital treatment					
	(a) inpatient	£350.00	0	0	£0.00	£0.00
	(b) outpatient	£95.00	0	0	£0.00	£0.00
	(c) day care	£225.00	0	0	£0.00	£0.00
(8)	other psychiatric treatment					
	(a) inpatient	£425.00	0	0	£0.00	£0.00
	(b) outpatient	£115.00	3	2	£345.00	£230.00
	(c) day care	£260.00	1	1	£260.00	£260.00
(9)	heating and lighting in GP surgery	£0.06	4	18	£0.24	£1.08
(10)	administration costs	£0.65	15	18	£9.75	£11.70
(11)	travel costs incurred by patients and their families	£1.10	12	36	£13.20	£39.60
(12)	out-of-pocket expenses for caring activities	£1.25	15	10	£18.75	£12.50
	Total cost				£775.10	£707.22

EXAMPLE

Unit costs multiplied by the volume of resource use for each cost component are presented in Table 11.7, Columns [6] and [7].

Finally, once the magnitude of costs for each cost component has been calculated in this way, total costs may then be estimated by adding together all the costs incurred from each cost component.

EXAMPLE

By adding all the costs in Column [6], the total cost per patient for treatment by a CPN over a one-year period is £775.10. From Column [7], the total cost per patient for treatment by a GP over a one-year period is £707.22.

Measuring costs

From the discussion in this chapter, we can see that there are four components to measuring the costs of health care programmes assessed via economic evaluation:

identifying the range of resource inputs to include; valuing the unit cost of the resource inputs; measuring the volume of resource use; and multiplying the unit cost by the volume of resource use.

Once the relevant costs to be included in the analysis have been identified, cost measurement then proceeds by estimating the unit cost of a particular resource and then estimating the total volume of that resource used. The unit cost may then be multiplied by the volume of resources used to give the total cost incurred from a particular resource input.

In this chapter we have thus seen various methods by which the costs of health care programmes may be assessed. However, the economic evaluation of health care programmes requires that scarce health care resources are not allocated solely on the basis of costs, but on the basis of cost-effectiveness. Therefore, it now becomes relevant to combine data on costs and effectiveness, discussed in this and the previous chapter, in order to measure cost-effectiveness. This will be the subject of Chapter 12.

References

Drummond M.F., Stoddart G.L. and Torrance G.W. (1987) *Methods for the economic evaluation of health care programs*. New York: Oxford Medical Publications.

MacKerrell D.K. (1993) Contract pricing: a management opportunity. In: Tilley I. (ed.) *Managing the internal market*. London: Paul Chapman.

NHSME (1990) *Costing and pricing contracts*. London: HMSO.

Tolley K. and Rowland N. (1995) *Evaluating the cost-effectiveness of counselling in health care*. London: Routledge.

Suggested further reading

For a discussion of issues involved in measuring costs in an economic evaluation see one of the following:

Drummond M.F., Stoddart G.L. and Torrance G.W. (1987) *Methods for the economic evaluation of health care programs*. New York: Oxford Medical Publications.

Robinson R. (1993) Economic evaluation and health care. *British Medical Journal* 307: 726–8.

12   Measuring cost-effectiveness

In this chapter we bring together the analysis and discussion of preceding chapters to consider methods for measuring the cost-effectiveness of health care programmes. Most importantly, this chapter concentrates on the construction of cost-effectiveness ratios and on ways of interpreting the results of economic evaluations. Where appropriate, examples are provided.

Summary

1. There are a number of steps to measuring cost-effectiveness in an economic evaluation: adjusting costs and outcomes for differential timing; constructing cost-effectiveness ratios; allowing for uncertainty; and constructing cost-effectiveness league tables.

2. We are not indifferent to the timing of costs and benefits, and we generally prefer to postpone costs and bring benefits forward in time. Therefore, it is argued that costs and outcomes which occur in the future should have a lower value compared to those which occur in the present. This assumption is based on the notion of time preference. The most widely accepted means of incorporating time preference into an economic evaluation is to use discounting, and to discount costs and consequences occurring in the future to present values. There are a number of reasons for discounting: psychological time preference; uncertainty and risk; diminishing marginal utility of income; and the opportunity cost of investment.

3. The methodology used to discount the costs involves four stages: select a discount rate; estimate the expected time profile for future costs; multiply the costs by the appropriate discount factor obtained using a discount table; and add together the discounted costs incurred in each year.

4. Whilst it is generally accepted that future costs should be discounted in an economic evaluation, there is considerable debate surrounding the issue of whether to discount health benefits such as quality-adjusted life years. Since there is controversy surrounding whether health benefits should be discounted, in practice it is usual to

discount health benefits initially at a prespecified value and then to conduct a sensitivity analysis and vary the discount rate.

5. In order to assess the cost-effectiveness of health care programmes it is necessary to estimate the marginal or incremental costs and the marginal or incremental benefits of the health care programme which is the subject of the economic evaluation (the experimental programme) against some alternative for comparison (the comparison programme).

6. If costs increase and benefits decrease with the introduction of the experimental programme, then, on cost-effectiveness grounds, the decision-maker would reject the experimental programme since it cannot be a cost-effective use of resources. In this situation, the comparison programme is said to dominate the experimental programme. If costs decrease and benefits increase with the introduction of the experimental programme, then, on cost-effectiveness grounds, the decision-maker would accept the experimental programme since it must be a cost-effective use of resources. In this situation, the experimental programme is said to dominate the comparison programme. However, if costs increase and benefits increase with the introduction of the experimental programme, or, if costs decrease and benefits decrease with the introduction of the experimental programme, then, in order to facilitate the comparison of alternatives, it is necessary to construct a cost-effectiveness ratio.

7. In order to construct a cost-effectiveness ratio, it is necessary to divide the marginal or incremental costs of the experimental programme relative to the comparison programme by the marginal or incremental benefits of the experimental programme relative to the comparison programme. Once the cost-effectiveness ratio has been constructed, it is then up to the health care decision-maker to decide whether the additional costs incurred by the experimental programme are worth the additional benefits: the cost-effectiveness ratio may be compared with a critical cost-effectiveness ratio, which is the prespecified cost per unit of outcome that the experimental programme must not exceed in order to be considered cost-effective.

8. There are three areas in any economic evaluation in which uncertainty is likely to arise: in measuring effectiveness; in measuring costs; and in the choice of discount rate. Specifically, uncertainty may arise for the following reasons: because the data sources are inadequate; because the estimates are specific to a particular locality or site and the investigators wish to generalise the results across a number of different sites; because the estimates are specific to a particular time; or because the analytical techniques employed are open to debate.

9. The traditional manner to control for uncertainty is through the use of sensitivity analysis. There are three stages to conducting a sensitivity analysis: consider which of the estimates in the economic evaluation are open to debate; select upper and lower boundaries for the estimates in the economic evaluation which are

subject to debate; and recalculate the results of the economic evaluation using different values for the variables concerned.

10. There are three basic types of sensitivity analysis: simple sensitivity analysis; extreme scenarios sensitivity analysis; and threshold sensitivity analysis.

11. When information is available on the costs and effectiveness of different health care programmes, and where effectiveness is measured in commensurate units, then it becomes possible to rank health care programmes in terms of the magnitude of their cost-effectiveness ratio, thus resulting in the formation of a cost-effectiveness league table. This is possible with, for example, cost-utility analysis where outcomes are measured in terms of QALYs. Alternatives may then be expressed in terms of their incremental costs per QALY gained, and the health care programme with the lowest incremental cost per QALY gained is the most cost-effective use of resources.

12. The ultimate use of a cost-effectiveness league table is to guide resource allocation decisions: that is, to seek to shift scarce health care resources away from the provision of health care programmes that are costly in terms of the additional health benefits that they produce, towards health care programmes that incur a relatively low additional cost for each additional unit of health benefit that they produce.

13. One of the most ambitious applications of cost-effectiveness league tables has been the so-called Oregon Experiment, which sought to produce an explicit cost-effectiveness league table for the prioritisation of approximately 1,600 health care programmes provided by the Medicaid scheme in the state of Oregon, US.

14. The comparison necessary for the use of cost-effectiveness league tables requires homogeneity in the study methods employed so that the ranking of health care programmes is solely a function of their relative cost-effectiveness and is independent of the methods used in the original economic evaluations on which the league table is based. Methodological features which are particularly important in the construction of league tables are: year of analysis; range of costs included; choice of health care programme for comparison; study setting; and discount rate.

15. Economic evaluation provides a clear framework for the allocation of scarce health care resources. However, there are a number of limitations with economic evaluation techniques: the use of economic evaluation as a decision-making tool; the precision of results in an economic evaluation; the consistency of results in an economic evaluation; the economic evaluation of economic evaluations; and the use of resources saved in an economic evaluation.

Measuring cost-effectiveness in an economic evaluation

In this chapter we concentrate specifically on methods for measuring cost-effectiveness in economic evaluations. There are four components to measuring the cost-effectiveness of health care programmes, as follows:

1. adjusting costs and outcomes for differential timing;
2. constructing cost-effectiveness ratios;
3. allowing for uncertainty;
4. constructing cost-effectiveness league tables.

Adjusting costs and outcomes for differential timing

Discounting

An important issue in any economic evaluation relates to the fact that the costs and consequences arising from a particular health care programme may have different time profiles. For example, a screening programme for the prevention of a disease may incur substantial present-day costs, with the consequences only materialising some time in the future.

Similarly, the costs and consequences of different health care programmes which form the basis for comparison in an economic evaluation may also have different time profiles. For example, a screening programme for the prevention of a disease may incur substantial present-day costs with the consequences materialising some time in the future, whereas direct treatment for a chronic illness may incur both immediate costs and immediate benefits.

On a conceptual level, it is argued that, as individuals, we are not indifferent to the timing of costs and benefits, and that we prefer to postpone costs and bring benefits forward in time. Thus, a general principle of economic evaluation is that people prefer to delay costs and desire immediate benefits. Hence, it is argued that costs and outcomes which occur in the future should have a lower value compared to those which occur in the present.

This assumption is based on the notion of *time preference*. The most widely accepted means of incorporating time preference into an economic evaluation is to use *discounting*, and to discount costs and consequences occurring in the future to *present values*.

Reasons for discounting

There are a number of reasons for incorporating discounting into an economic evaluation, including: psychological time preference; uncertainty and risk; diminishing marginal utility of income; and the opportunity cost of investment.

1. Psychological time preference. One justification for discounting arises from the fact that individuals tend to attach less importance to the future, even when there is no rational reason for doing so.
2. Uncertainty and risk. A second justification for discounting is couched in terms of risk and uncertainty. Often, uncertainty and risk are both functions of temporal distance: the more distant in time a particular event, the less certain we may be that it will occur and of its magnitude. We therefore place a higher value on the present, of which we are more certain.
3. Diminishing marginal utility of income. It is generally the case that over time the economy will grow and individuals will become better off as their income rises. In a growing economy, where individuals will be better off in the future, the concept of diminishing marginal utility of income implies that we will derive more satisfaction from an event now (when we have less income) than in the future (when we will have more income).
4. The opportunity cost of investment. The most orthodox justification for discounting is presented in terms of opportunity cost. This is because the amount of money invested in a particular health care programme may instead be invested in an alternative project, which will itself involve a return on the amount of money invested. There is therefore an opportunity cost involved in providing a particular health care programme arising from this potential rate of return on the alternative investment uses of the resources that would be utilised on the programme.

Now we have seen the rationale behind discounting, we shall proceed to discuss how to incorporate discounting into an economic evaluation. For the purposes of this discussion, it is useful to examine issues concerning discounting costs and discounting health benefits separately. We shall first examine methods for discounting costs, which involve the use of a *discounting formula*.

The discounting formula

The use of discounting has the effect of giving less weight to future events. Economic evaluation weights costs with a *discount rate*, denoted by the letter r, according to the year in which they accrue, before adding them up and expressing total costs in *present value* terms (that is, values are expressed in terms of the current year). The discounting formula which may be used for this process is presented in Appendix 12.1.

Fortunately, the application of discounting to economic evaluation does not require close familiarity with the discounting formula since most economics, financial and accounting textbooks include *discount tables*. These tables indicate *discount factors* for calculating the present value of future costs at different discount rates. A discount table is presented in Table 12.1, and this shows the discount factors for various discount rates and years in which costs are incurred. To calculate discounted costs, simply multiply the undiscounted costs by the relevant discount factor.

Table 12.1 Discount factors for calculating the present value of future costs

Year	1%	2%	3%	4%	5%	6%	7%	8%	Discount rate 9%	10%	11%	12%	13%	14%	15%
0	1.0000	1.0000	1.0000	1.0000	1.0000	1.0000	1.0000	1.0000	1.0000	1.0000	1.0000	1.0000	1.0000	1.0000	1.0000
1	0.9901	0.9804	0.9709	0.9615	0.9524	0.9434	0.9346	0.9259	0.9174	0.9091	0.9009	0.8929	0.8850	0.8772	0.8696
2	0.9803	0.9612	0.9426	0.9246	0.9070	0.8900	0.8734	0.8573	0.8417	0.8264	0.8116	0.7972	0.7831	0.7695	0.7561
3	0.9706	0.9423	0.9151	0.8890	0.8638	0.8396	0.8163	0.7938	0.7722	0.7513	0.7312	0.7118	0.6931	0.6750	0.6575
4	0.9610	0.9238	0.8885	0.8548	0.8227	0.7921	0.7629	0.7350	0.7084	0.6830	0.6587	0.6355	0.6133	0.5921	0.5718
5	0.9515	0.9057	0.8626	0.8219	0.7835	0.7473	0.7130	0.6806	0.6499	0.6209	0.5935	0.5674	0.5428	0.5194	0.4972
6	0.9420	0.8880	0.8375	0.7903	0.7462	0.7050	0.6663	0.6302	0.5963	0.5645	0.5346	0.5066	0.4803	0.4556	0.4323
7	0.9327	0.8706	0.8131	0.7599	0.7107	0.6651	0.6227	0.5835	0.5470	0.5132	0.4817	0.4523	0.4251	0.3996	0.3759
8	0.9235	0.8535	0.7894	0.7307	0.6768	0.6274	0.5820	0.5403	0.5019	0.4665	0.4339	0.4039	0.3762	0.3506	0.3269
9	0.9143	0.8368	0.7664	0.7026	0.6446	0.5919	0.5439	0.5002	0.4604	0.4241	0.3909	0.3606	0.3329	0.3075	0.2843
10	0.9053	0.8203	0.7441	0.6756	0.6139	0.5584	0.5083	0.4632	0.4224	0.3855	0.3522	0.3220	0.2946	0.2697	0.2472
11	0.8963	0.8043	0.7224	0.6496	0.5847	0.5268	0.4751	0.4289	0.3875	0.3505	0.3173	0.2875	0.2607	0.2366	0.2149
12	0.8874	0.7885	0.7014	0.6246	0.5568	0.4970	0.4440	0.3971	0.3555	0.3186	0.2858	0.2567	0.2307	0.2076	0.1869
13	0.8787	0.7730	0.6810	0.6006	0.5303	0.4688	0.4150	0.3677	0.3262	0.2897	0.2575	0.2292	0.2042	0.1821	0.1625
14	0.8700	0.7579	0.6611	0.5775	0.5051	0.4423	0.3878	0.3405	0.2992	0.2633	0.2320	0.2046	0.1807	0.1597	0.1413
15	0.8613	0.7430	0.6419	0.5553	0.4810	0.4173	0.3624	0.3152	0.2745	0.2394	0.2090	0.1827	0.1599	0.1401	0.1229
16	0.8528	0.7284	0.6232	0.5339	0.4581	0.3936	0.3387	0.2919	0.2519	0.2176	0.1883	0.1631	0.1415	0.1229	0.1069
17	0.8444	0.7142	0.6050	0.5134	0.4363	0.3714	0.3166	0.2703	0.2311	0.1978	0.1696	0.1456	0.1252	0.1078	0.0929
18	0.8360	0.7002	0.5874	0.4936	0.4155	0.3503	0.2959	0.2502	0.2120	0.1799	0.1528	0.1300	0.1108	0.0946	0.0808
19	0.8277	0.6864	0.5703	0.4746	0.3957	0.3305	0.2765	0.2317	0.1945	0.1635	0.1377	0.1161	0.0981	0.0829	0.0703
20	0.8195	0.6730	0.5537	0.4564	0.3769	0.3118	0.2584	0.2145	0.1784	0.1486	0.1240	0.1037	0.0868	0.0728	0.0611
21	0.8114	0.6598	0.5375	0.4388	0.3589	0.2942	0.2415	0.1987	0.1637	0.1351	0.1117	0.0926	0.0768	0.0638	0.0531
22	0.8034	0.6468	0.5219	0.4220	0.3418	0.2775	0.2257	0.1839	0.1502	0.1228	0.1007	0.0826	0.0680	0.0560	0.0462
23	0.7954	0.6342	0.5067	0.4057	0.3256	0.2618	0.2109	0.1703	0.1378	0.1117	0.0907	0.0738	0.0601	0.0491	0.0402
24	0.7876	0.6217	0.4919	0.3901	0.3101	0.2470	0.1971	0.1577	0.1264	0.1015	0.0817	0.0659	0.0532	0.0431	0.0349
25	0.7798	0.6095	0.4776	0.3751	0.2953	0.2330	0.1842	0.1460	0.1160	0.0923	0.0736	0.0588	0.0471	0.0378	0.0304
26	0.7720	0.5976	0.4637	0.3607	0.2812	0.2198	0.1722	0.1352	0.1064	0.0839	0.0663	0.0525	0.0417	0.0331	0.0264
27	0.7644	0.5859	0.4502	0.3468	0.2678	0.2074	0.1609	0.1252	0.0976	0.0763	0.0597	0.0469	0.0369	0.0291	0.0230
28	0.7568	0.5744	0.4371	0.3335	0.2551	0.1956	0.1504	0.1159	0.0895	0.0693	0.0538	0.0419	0.0326	0.0255	0.0200
29	0.7493	0.5631	0.4243	0.3207	0.2429	0.1846	0.1406	0.1073	0.0822	0.0630	0.0485	0.0374	0.0289	0.0224	0.0174
30	0.7419	0.5521	0.4120	0.3083	0.2314	0.1741	0.1314	0.0994	0.0754	0.0573	0.0437	0.0334	0.0256	0.0196	0.0151
35	0.7059	0.5000	0.3554	0.2534	0.1813	0.1301	0.0937	0.0676	0.0490	0.0356	0.0259	0.0189	0.0139	0.0102	0.0075
40	0.6717	0.4529	0.3066	0.2083	0.1420	0.0972	0.0668	0.0460	0.0318	0.0221	0.0154	0.0107	0.0075	0.0053	0.0037
45	0.6391	0.4102	0.2644	0.1712	0.1113	0.0727	0.0476	0.0313	0.0207	0.0137	0.0091	0.0061	0.0041	0.0027	0.0019
50	0.6080	0.3715	0.2281	0.1407	0.0872	0.0543	0.0339	0.0213	0.0134	0.0085	0.0054	0.0035	0.0022	0.0014	0.0009

It is usual for discounting to operate on an annual basis. This means that any costs which are incurred within one year from the introduction of a health care programme are classified as being in the present time period and are therefore not subjected to discounting. With regard to the discount formula, such costs are said to occur in year zero and therefore have a discount factor of one. Therefore, costs arising from health care programmes which have a duration and effect of less than one year need not be discounted.

Choice of discount rate

The degree of time preference is represented by a discount rate, r. Clearly the choice of discount rate is important, because this will affect the magnitude of costs in an economic evaluation. The larger the value of r, then the less weight is given to future events, and so the present value of costs incurred in the future is smaller. Conversely, the smaller the value of r, then the more weight is given to future events, and so the present value of costs incurred in the future is greater. We can see this from the discounting table presented in Table 12.1. For any given year in which a cost might be incurred, we can see that as the discount rate is increased from 1 per cent to 15 per cent, so the discount factor decreases.

There is controversy surrounding the choice of discount rate to be used in economic evaluations. In practice, it is usually admissible to select a central best estimate and then to vary this systematically in a sensitivity analysis to determine the impact of the choice on the study conclusions. The criteria to use in selecting a central value for the discount rate and the range of values for the sensitivity analysis should:

1. be consistent with economic theory;
2. include any government recommended rates;
3. include rates that have been used in other published studies to which the results may be compared; or
4. be consistent with current practice.

In general, the baseline discount rate adopted by most economic evaluations of health care programmes within the National Health Service in the UK is that used by HM Treasury for appraising investment in public sector projects. At the present time, this discount rate is 6 per cent. However, given the sensitivity of the results of an economic evaluation to the choice of discount rate, and the fact that the rate chosen will affect the cost ranking of different projects with different time profiles, it is good practice to calculate costs using a range of discount rates. There is no agreement regarding the best range of discount rates to use for this, though it would be normal to vary the discount rate between 0 per cent (that is, no discounting) and 15 per cent.

Table 12.2 Undiscounted and discounted costs of CPN treatment and GP treatment for non-psychotic patients in the primary care setting, by the year in which they occur (costs discounted at an annual rate of 6 per cent).

(1) Year	Undiscounted costs		(4) Discount factor	Discounted costs	
	(2) Cost of CPN treatment	(3) Cost of GP treatment		(5) Cost of CPN treatment	(6) Cost of GP treatment
0	5,000	30,000	1.0000	5,000	30,000
1	11,000	25,000	0.9434	10,377	23,585
2	17,000	20,000	0.8900	15,130	17,800
3	22,000	15,000	0.8396	18,471	12,594
4	26,000	10,000	0.7921	20,595	7,921
5	31,000	5,000	0.7473	23,166	3,737
Total	112,000	105,000		92,739	95,637

Column (5) = Column (2) × Discount factor
Column (6) = Column (3) × Discount factor

EXAMPLE _____

We can analyse the effects of discounting on the costs of managing non-psychotic patients in the primary health care setting either by a Community Psychiatric Nurse (CPN)-based programme or by a general practitioner (GP)-based programme. Let us suppose that both of these health care programmes run for a time period of six years. The total costs of each programme (that is, the total costs across all patients treated) may be identified by the year in which they occur, and are presented in Table 12.2. Column (1) shows the time period, and Columns (2) and (3) show the costs incurred by the CPN-based programme and the GP-based programme, respectively, in each of these time periods. For example, the CPN-based programme incurs a cost of £5,000 in year 0 (the present time period), and costs of £11,000, £17,000, £22,000, £26,000 and £31,000 in years 1, 2, 3, 4 and 5, respectively. These are annual undiscounted costs, and by adding these together we can see that the total undiscounted cost of the CPN-based programme across all patients treated is £112,000 over the six-year period. A direct comparison of the total costs of each programme in this way would show the CPN-based programme to be more expensive than the GP-based programme, with total undiscounted costs of £112,000 versus £105,000.

However, the costs of the CPN-based programme and the GP-based programme have different time profiles. Because we are not indifferent to this differential timing, a more relevant comparison of the two health care programmes would involve adjusting for the differential timing of resource outlays by discounting future costs to present values.

Suppose we select a discount rate of 6 per cent to adjust future costs to present values. We can now use Table 12.1 to obtain discount factors for the costs of each programme, by the year in which they are incurred. From

Table 12.1, we can see that, at a discount rate of 6 per cent, discount factors for years 0, 1, 2, 3, 4 and 5 are 1.0000, 0.9434, 0.8900, 0.8396, 0.7921 and 0.7473, respectively (also presented in Table 12.2, Column (4)). To calculate annual discounted costs, we must multiply the cost incurred in each year by the relevant discount factor for that year. On this basis, the discounted costs of the CPN-based programme are presented in Table 12.2, Column (5): year 0, £5,000 (that is, £5,000 × 1.0000); year 1, £10,377 (that is, £11,000 × 0.9434); year 2, £15,130 (that is, £17,000 × 0.8900); year 3, £18,471 (that is, £22,000 × 0.8396); year 4, £20,595 (that is, £26,000 × 0.7921); and year 5, £23,166 (that is, £31,000 × 0.7473). We can now add together these discounted annual costs to give a total discounted cost of the CPN-based programme of £92,739.

Therefore, the present value of the cost of the CPN-based programme is £92,739. Calculated in the same way, the present value of the cost of the GP-based programme is £95,637 (Table 12.2, Column (6)). Therefore, when time preference is taken into account, the CPN-based programme becomes cheaper than the GP-based programme.

In summary, the methodology used to discount the costs incurred by a health care programme involves four stages:

1. select a discount rate;
2. estimate the expected time profile for future costs (that is, estimate the magnitude of costs likely to be incurred by a health care programme, by the year in which they will be incurred);
3. multiply the costs by the appropriate discount factor obtained using a discount table;
4. add together the discounted costs incurred in each year.

Discounting benefits

Whilst it is generally accepted that future costs should be discounted in an economic evaluation, there is considerable debate surrounding the issue of whether to discount health benefits such as quality-adjusted life years.

This debate has arisen for various reasons. A key feature, however, is that health outcomes are not usually expressed in monetary terms: it is generally accepted that a sum of money received in the present is worth more than that same sum of money received in the future, and this is why we discount costs expressed in monetary terms. However, it may be argued that health benefits are not quantifiable in monetary terms and are therefore 'non-tradable'.

The debate therefore concentrates on the issue of whether individuals have a time preference for receiving health benefits now rather than in the future in the same way that they might have a time preference for gaining monetary benefits now rather than later in life. Arguments both for and against this view are plausible, and the issue is currently unresolved.

Since it is usual for discounting to operate on an annual basis, health benefits which have a duration and effect of less than one year would not normally be discounted anyway. Therefore, the issue of whether to discount health benefits only becomes important if the health care programme under consideration produces benefits which last for a time period of more than one year.

In order to explain more clearly the effects of discounting health benefits, four simple statements may be presented. First, the effect of not discounting health benefits is to improve the cost-effectiveness of health care programmes. Therefore:

1. If health benefits are *discounted*, then health care programmes will become *less* cost-effective, because discounting has the effect of *decreasing* the magnitude of the health benefits.
2. If health benefits are *not discounted*, then health care programmes will become *more* cost-effective, because not discounting has the effect of *increasing* the magnitude of the health benefits.

However, whilst the decision regarding whether to discount health benefits will change the cost-effectiveness of health care programmes, it may also change the cost-effectiveness of different health care programmes *relative to each other* (that is, it may affect the *relative* cost-effectiveness of health care programmes). Discounting health benefits tends to make those health care programmes with benefits realised in the future *less* cost-effective relative to those with benefits realised in the present (which are unlikely to be affected by discounting). Therefore:

3. *Not discounting* health benefits will *improve* the cost-effectiveness of health care programmes with benefits realised in the future *relative* to those with benefits realised in the present.
4. *Discounting* health benefits will *diminish* the cost-effectiveness of health care programmes with benefits realised in the future *relative* to those with benefits realised in the present.

Since there is controversy surrounding whether health benefits should be discounted, in practice it is usual initially to discount health benefits at the discount rate recommended by HM Treasury (currently 6 per cent) and then to conduct a sensitivity analysis and vary the discount rate between 0 per cent (that is, no discounting) and 15 per cent.

Constructing cost-effectiveness ratios

Marginal analysis and incremental analysis

Whilst they are similar in meaning, there is a growing distinction between the terms *marginal* and *incremental* in the context of economic evaluation, as follows:

1. a *marginal analysis* considers the costs and the benefits arising from the *contraction* or *extension* of a particular health care programme;
2. an *incremental analysis* considers the costs and benefits arising from changes *across* health care programmes.

EXAMPLE

The decision to extend CPN-based treatment for the management of non-psychotic patients in the primary care setting to a larger geographical area will involve a marginal analysis because the treatment itself does not change. A change from GP-based treatment to CPN-based treatment in a given geographical area will involve an incremental analysis, because the treatment programme itself changes.

Economic evaluation is concerned with identifying the point at which the costs arising from a particular allocation of resources exceed the benefits. A means of identifying the precise allocation at which costs exceed benefits is to consider the marginal or incremental changes in costs and benefits as the provision of health care changes. By considering these marginal or incremental changes, economic evaluation can identify the point at which the additional costs of an intervention become greater than the additional benefits received. We are therefore interested in the *marginal cost* or *incremental cost* and the *marginal benefit* or *incremental benefit* of different alternatives, defined as follows:

1. marginal or incremental costs are defined as the change in total costs resulting from a change in the provision of a particular health care programme;
2. marginal or incremental benefits are defined as the change in total benefits resulting from a change in the provision of a particular health care programme.

Resources should be allocated so that the additional cost of producing a level of provision of the health care programme (that is, the marginal or incremental cost) equals the additional benefit gained (that is, the marginal or incremental benefit). If the additional costs are greater than the additional benefit then this implies that resources are being wasted and provision of that health care programme should be curtailed. Conversely, if the additional benefits are greater than the additional costs then this implies that even greater benefits may be made, and provision of that health care programme should be increased.

Domination

In order to assess the cost-effectiveness of health care programmes it is therefore necessary to estimate the marginal or incremental costs and the marginal or incremental benefits of the health care programme which is the subject of the economic evaluation (hereafter called the *experimental programme*) against some alternative for comparison (hereafter called the *comparison programme*).

When the relative costs and benefits of these alternatives are compared, four possible scenarios may arise, as follows:

Scenario 1

The costs of the experimental programme are *greater* than the costs of the comparison programme, and the benefits of the experimental programme are *greater* than the benefits of the comparison programme. In this situation, *costs increase* and *benefits increase* with the introduction of the experimental programme, and incremental or marginal costs are *positive* and incremental or marginal benefits are *positive*.

Scenario 2

The costs of the experimental programme are *less* than the costs of the comparison programme, and the benefits of the experimental programme are *less* than the benefits of the comparison programme. In this situation, *costs decrease* and *benefits decrease* with the introduction of the experimental programme, and incremental or marginal costs are *negative* and incremental or marginal benefits are *negative*.

Scenario 3

The costs of the experimental programme are *greater* than the costs of the comparison programme, and the benefits of the experimental programme are *less* than the benefits of the comparison programme. In this situation, *costs increase* and *benefits decrease* with the introduction of the experimental programme, and incremental or marginal costs are *positive* and incremental or marginal benefits are *negative*.

Scenario 4

The costs of the experimental programme are *less* than the costs of the comparison programme, and the benefits of the experimental programme are *greater* than the benefits of the comparison programme. In this situation, *costs decrease* and *benefits increase* with the introduction of the experimental programme, and incremental or marginal costs are *negative* and incremental or marginal benefits are *positive*.

Each of these scenarios is portrayed diagrammatically in Figure 12.1. Suppose a comparison programme with costs and benefits C_c and B_c, respectively, described by the point x. Costs and benefits of the experimental programme are likely to differ from those of the comparison programme so that the combination of costs and benefits may be described by a position in one of the four quadrants, A, B, C or D, which corresponds to each of the scenarios described above, as follows:

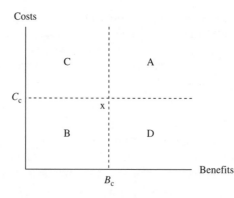

Figure 12.1 Costs and benefits of experimental versus comparison health care programmes.

1. An increase in costs and an increase in benefits with the introduction of the experimental programme describes Scenario 1, and is shown by a shift to quadrant A.
2. A decrease in costs and a decrease in benefits with the introduction of the experimental programme describes Scenario 2, and is shown by a shift to quadrant B.
3. An increase in costs and a decrease in benefits with the introduction of the experimental programme describes Scenario 3, and is shown by a shift to quadrant C.
4. A decrease in costs and an increase in benefits with the introduction of the experimental programme describes Scenario 4, and is shown by a shift to quadrant D.

If costs increase and benefits decrease with the introduction of the experimental programme (Scenario 3), then, on cost-effectiveness grounds, the decision regarding whether to implement the experimental programme is clear-cut: *reject* the experimental programme and *do not implement* it since it cannot be a cost-effective use of resources if it is more costly and less effective than the alternative. In this situation, the comparison programme is said to *dominate* the experimental programme.

If costs decrease and benefits increase with the introduction of the experimental programme (Scenario 4), then, on cost-effectiveness grounds, the decision regarding whether to implement the experimental programme is also clear-cut: *accept* the experimental programme and *implement* it since it must be a cost-effective use of resources if it is less costly and more effective than the alternative. In this situation, the experimental programme is said to *dominate* the comparison programme.

In both these situations, the decision regarding whether to implement the experimental programme is relatively easy. However, if costs increase and benefits increase with the introduction of the experimental programme (Scenario 1), or if costs decrease and benefits decrease with the introduction of the experimental programme (Scenario 2), then the decision is not so straightforward.

In both these situations, in order to facilitate the comparison of alternatives, it is necessary to construct a *cost-effectiveness ratio*.

Cost-effectiveness ratios

If costs increase and benefits increase with the introduction of the experimental programme (Scenario 1) or if costs decrease and benefits decrease with the introduction of the experimental programme (Scenario 2), then it is necessary to construct a cost-effectiveness ratio in order to examine whether the experimental programme compares favourably with other health care programmes which are competing for the same limited health care resources. If the cost-effectiveness ratio of the experimental programme *does* compare favourably then, on cost-effectiveness grounds, the experimental programme should be implemented.

The cost-effectiveness ratios which may be constructed are similar for each form of economic evaluation. However, so that the construction methods are made clear, it is worth examining each form of economic evaluation separately.

Cost-minimisation analysis

If the form of economic evaluation used is *cost-minimisation analysis* then the construction of cost-effectiveness ratios is not possible because the health programmes under consideration have the same outcomes and only the costs are measured. In this case, costs are measured in monetary terms, and the health care programme which incurs the least cost is the most cost-effective. Therefore, on cost-effectiveness grounds, this is the health care programme that should be implemented.

Cost-effectiveness analysis

If the form of economic evaluation used is *cost-effectiveness analysis*, then costs are measured in monetary units and outcomes are measured in commensurate units of physiology, morbidity or mortality. In this case, the cost-effectiveness ratio, R_e, is calculated using the following formula:

$$R_e = (C_e - C_c)/(E_e - E_c) \tag{12.1}$$

where C_e is the cost of the experimental programme (measured in monetary units), C_c is the cost of the comparison programme (measured in monetary units), E_e is the effect of the experimental programme (measured in commensurate units of physiology, morbidity or mortality) and E_c is the effect of the comparison programme (also measured in commensurate units of physiology, morbidity or mortality). $C_e - C_c$ is the marginal or incremental cost of the experimental programme, and $E_e - E_c$ is the marginal or incremental benefit of the experimental programme.

Once the cost-effectiveness ratio has been constructed, it is then up to the health care decision-maker involved to decide whether the additional costs incurred by the experimental programme are worth the additional benefits. More formally, the cost-effectiveness ratio may be compared with a *critical cost-effectiveness ratio*, denoted by $1/g$, which is the prespecified cost per unit of outcome that the experimental programme *must not exceed* in order to be considered cost-effective, and therefore to be implemented.

Therefore, on cost-effectiveness grounds, the experimental programme should be implemented provided that:

$$R_e \leq 1/g \qquad (12.2)$$

Cost-utility analysis

If the form of economic evaluation used is *cost-utility analysis*, then costs are measured in monetary units and outcomes are measured in units of utility. In this case, the cost-effectiveness ratio, R_u, is calculated using the following formula:

$$R_u = (C_e - C_c)/(U_e - U_c) \qquad (12.3)$$

where C_e is the cost of the experimental programme (measured in monetary units), C_c is the cost of the comparison programme (measured in monetary units), U_e is the effect of the experimental programme (measured in units of utility) and U_c is the effect of the comparison programme (also measured in units of utility). $C_e - C_c$ is the marginal or incremental cost of the experimental programme, and $U_e - U_c$ is the marginal or incremental benefit of the experimental programme.

Once the cost-effectiveness ratio has been constructed, it is once again up to the health care decision-maker involved to decide whether the additional costs incurred by the experimental programme are worth the additional benefits. More formally, on cost-effectiveness grounds, the experimental programme should be implemented provided that:

$$R_u \leq 1/g \qquad (12.4)$$

where $1/g$ is the critical cost-effectiveness ratio.

Cost–benefit analysis

If the form of economic evaluation used is *cost–benefit analysis*, then both costs and benefits are measured in monetary units. In this case, the cost-effectiveness ratio, R_b, is calculated using the following formula:

$$R_b = (C_e - C_c)/(B_e - B_c) \qquad (12.5)$$

where C_e is the cost of the experimental programme (measured in monetary units), C_c is the cost of the comparison programme (measured in monetary units), B_e is the effect of the experimental programme (measured in monetary units), and B_c is the effect of the comparison programme (also measured in monetary units). $C_e - C_c$ is the marginal or incremental cost of the experimental programme, and $B_e - B_c$ is the marginal or incremental benefit of the experimental programme.

Once the cost-effectiveness ratio has been constructed, it is then up to the health care decision-maker involved to decide whether the additional costs incurred by the experimental programme are worth the additional benefits. This occurs when:

$$R_b \leq 1/g \qquad (12.6)$$

where $1/g$ is the critical cost-effectiveness ratio.

The use of cost–benefit analysis has an additional advantage in that, unlike the other forms of economic evaluation, it enables the *net benefit* of a treatment (that is, the extent to which the marginal or incremental benefits exceed the marginal or incremental costs) to be estimated. Net benefits are calculated using a formula derived from Equations 12.5 and 12.6. This formula and its derivation are presented in Appendix 12.2.

EXAMPLE

Using the hypothetical example in Chapters 10 and 11, we calculated the effectiveness and costs of CPN-based treatment and GP-based treatment for the management of non-psychotic patients in the primary care setting. Suppose that we now wish to bring together these pieces of information in order to assess the cost-effectiveness of these two strategies. Let us assume that we wish to conduct a cost-utility analysis, where outcomes are measured in terms of quality adjusted life years (QALYs).

From Chapter 10, the total number of QALYs which patients receiving traditional GP-based treatment obtain is 3.1. The total number of QALYs which patients receiving CPN-based treatment obtain is 3.6.

From Chapter 11, the total cost per patient for treatment by a GP was estimated to be £707.22. The total cost per patient for treatment by a CPN was estimated to be £775.10.

We can now substitute these values into Equation 12.3 above, which is the appropriate formula for constructing cost-effectiveness ratios in a cost-utility analysis. Let CPN-based treatment be the experimental programme and GP-based treatment be the comparison programme. On this basis we know the following information:

$C_e = £775.10$
$C_c = £707.22$
$U_e = 3.6$ QALYs
$U_c = 3.1$ QALYs

Therefore, the cost-effectiveness ratio, R_u, is calculated as follows:

$$R_u = (775.10 - 707.22)/(3.6 - 3.1)$$
$$= 67.88/0.5$$
$$= 135.76$$

Therefore, the incremental cost per QALY gained by CPN-based treatment relative to GP-based treatment is £135.76. In other words, it costs an additional £135.76 to gain one additional QALY from the shift from GP-based treatment to CPN-based treatment in the management of non-psychotic patients in the primary care setting.

The critical cost-effectiveness ratio

Clearly, the value of the critical cost-effectiveness ratio, denoted by $1/g$, is a key feature in the decision regarding whether to implement a particular health care programme.

The value $1/g$ is the cut-off ratio for cost-effectiveness that is acceptable to a health care decision-maker for the implementation of a particular health care programme. Typically, $1/g$ will represent the cost-effectiveness ratio of the *least desirable health care programme which is currently provided*. That is, $1/g$ represents the cost-effectiveness ratio of the *first health care programme that would be contracted or reduced or would no longer be provided if resources were to decrease*. Therefore, any health care programme which is more cost-effective than this least desirable health care programme will be implemented instead.

In the discussion above, the value of the critical cost-effectiveness is formally stated as an explicit value, $1/g$, which is some figure expressed in monetary units. In reality, however, health care decision-makers may not explicitly state a value for the critical cost-effectiveness ratio in this way. However, a value for $1/g$ may at least be derived implicitly from the decision-making process by which health care programmes are implemented.

EXAMPLE

Once the cost-effectiveness ratio has been constructed, it is then up to the health care decision-maker involved to decide whether the additional costs incurred by the experimental programme are worth the additional benefits. Let us suppose in this case that the decision-maker involved is a GP Fundholder who must decide whether to provide services for non-psychotic patients herself, or to employ a CPN. In this instance, the GP Fundholder has decided to base her decision on the most cost-effective option. A cost-effectiveness ratio is constructed as above, which indicates an incremental cost per QALY gained of CPN-based treatment relative to GP-based treatment of £135.76. This cost-effectiveness ratio may be compared with a critical cost-effectiveness ratio which is the prespecified level of cost-effectiveness that CPN-based treatment must not exceed in order to be considered cost-effective. The GP Fundholder concerned set the critical cost-effectiveness ratio at £220. This value may then be inserted into Equation 12.4 above, as follows:

$$R_u = £135.76$$
$$1/g = £220$$

Therefore, since $R_u < 1/g$ (that is, since £135.76 < £220), the CPN-based programme is considered to be cost-effective, and is therefore implemented.

Constructing cost-effectiveness ratios when the comparison programme has no costs and no benefits

In certain situations, it may be the case that the comparison programme has no costs and no benefits. In this case, the cost-effectiveness ratios presented in Equations 12.1, 12.3 and 12.5 may be adjusted to Equations 12.1a, 12.3a and 12.5a, respectively, depending on the form of economic evaluation used:

$$R_e = C_e/E_e \qquad (12.1a)$$

$$R_u = C_e/U_e \qquad (12.3a)$$

$$R_b = C_e/B_e \qquad (12.5a)$$

This modification is possible because C_c, E_c, U_c and B_c all equal zero if the comparison programme has no costs and no benefits. This has the effect of simplifying the construction of the cost-effectiveness ratio.

The economic evaluation may then proceed in the same way as before, and the cost-effectiveness ratios constructed using Equations 12.1a, 12.3a and 12.5a may be compared with the critical cost-effectiveness ratio as described in Equations 12.2, 12.4 or 12.6, depending upon the form of economic evaluation used. It is therefore possible to see whether, on cost-effectiveness grounds, the experimental programme should be implemented.

This simplification of cost-effectiveness ratios should only be used when there is evidence that the comparison programme has no costs and no benefits. In reality, this is likely to occur only very rarely. Even when the comparison programme is a 'do-nothing' strategy where no intervention is used as the basis for comparison, there are still likely to be costs and benefits arising from the comparison programme.

Comparing more than two health care programmes

So far we have examined the construction of cost-effectiveness ratios in the context of only one experimental programme which is compared to a comparison programme. When conducting an economic evaluation, however, it may be the case that we in fact wish to compare more than two health care programmes: we may wish to assess the cost-effectiveness of more than one experimental programme, which we wish to compare to the comparison programme.

In this case, the cost-effectiveness of each experimental programme is calculated separately relative to the comparison programme using Equations 12.1, 12.3 or 12.5 above, depending on the form of economic evaluation used.

Once the cost-effectiveness ratio for each experimental programme has been constructed relative to the comparison programme, the experimental programme with the *lowest* cost-effectiveness ratio is the *most cost-effective*. In other words, this is the experimental programme which, on cost-effectiveness grounds, should be implemented *before* any of the other experimental programmes.

However, whilst this is the most cost-effective experimental programme and should be implemented before the other experimental programmes, the cost-effectiveness ratio of this experimental programme should still be compared to the critical cost-effectiveness ratio, $1/g$, in order to see if it should be implemented at all. The methodology for doing this is described in Equations 12.2, 12.4 or 12.6, depending upon the form of economic evaluation used. If the most cost-effective experimental programme has a cost-effectiveness ratio that *does not exceed* the critical cost-effectiveness ratio, then, on cost-effectiveness grounds, this experimental programme should be implemented.

Allowing for uncertainty

The existence of uncertainty in economic evaluations

Given the difficulties in measuring costs and effectiveness, most economic evaluations have addressed the issue of uncertainty surrounding estimates calculated within analyses. Tolley and Rowland (1995) delineate three areas in any economic evaluation in which uncertainty is likely to arise: uncertainty in measuring effectiveness; uncertainty in measuring costs; and uncertainty in the choice of discount rate.

1. Uncertainty in measuring effectiveness

Uncertainty in measuring effectiveness may arise as a consequence of imprecision in the measurement process. Specifically, uncertainty in measuring effectiveness may arise with the following:

(a) choosing an outcome measure;
(b) obtaining effectiveness data.

2. Uncertainty in measuring costs

Uncertainty in measuring costs may also arise as a consequence of imprecision in one or more parts of the costing process. Specifically, uncertainty in measuring costs may arise with the following:

(a) identification of the range of resource inputs to include;
(b) valuation of the unit cost of the resource inputs;
(c) measurement of the volume of resource use.

3. Uncertainty in the choice of discount rate

Uncertainty may also arise in the choice of discount rate. As discussed in the previous section, a problem inherent in the discounting process is the choice of discount rate to use. In general, the baseline discount rate adopted by most economic evaluations of health care programmes within the NHS is that used by HM Treasury for appraising investment in public sector projects, which at the present time is 6 per cent. Costs may then be calculated using a range of discount rates between 0 per cent and 15 per cent.

With regard to these three areas in which uncertainty is likely to arise, uncertainty regarding the true value of an estimate may occur for a number of specific reasons, including the following:

1. because the data sources are inadequate;
2. because the estimates are specific to a particular locality or site and the investigators wish to generalise the results across a number of different sites;
3. because the estimates are specific to a particular time; or
4. because the analytical techniques employed are open to debate (for example, whether to discount health benefits).

The traditional manner to control for uncertainty is through the use of *sensitivity analysis*.

Sensitivity analysis

Sensitivity analysis is an often crude but useful means of exploring how sensitive the results of an economic evaluation are to varying cost and effectiveness values. For example, an investigator may feel that particular costing data are not reliable, and may use sensitivity analysis to establish the importance of such data to the result of the study. To do so the investigator may alter the value of the costing parameter by, for example, doubling, trebling or halving the value to assess the importance of this parameter in reaching a final result.

Such an approach may be unhelpful if there is no information on the expected variation in the parameter values. However, if there is information on the variance of these values, then this may be used to set intervals around baseline values which may be used to recalculate cost-effectiveness results.

Therefore sensitivity analysis permits the robustness of results to be tested in light of variations in the values of the key variables. There are three stages which may be taken when conducting a sensitivity analysis:

1. Consider which of the estimates in the economic evaluation are open to debate because:

    (a) the data sources are inadequate;

    (b) the estimates are specific to a particular locality or site and the investigators wish to generalise the results across a number of different sites;

    (c) the estimates are specific to a particular time; or

    (d) the analytical techniques employed are open to controversy.

2. Select upper and lower boundaries for the estimates in the economic evaluation which are subject to debate. These boundaries may be based on a possible range of values which may be obtained by the following:

    (a) via clinical trials;

    (b) via existing research; or

    (c) via expert professional opinion.

3. Recalculate the results of the economic evaluation using different values for the variable concerned.

Types of sensitivity analysis

Using these three stages, there are three basic types of sensitivity analysis: simple sensitivity analysis; extreme scenarios sensitivity analysis; and threshold sensitivity analysis.

1. Simple sensitivity analysis

This entails varying each of the uncertain estimates used in the economic evaluation in turn to see how it affects the overall results.

2. Extreme scenarios sensitivity analysis

This approach entails identification of extreme estimates of costs and effectiveness so that cost-effectiveness may be calculated under the most optimistic (that is, low cost and high effectiveness) and the most pessimistic (that is, high cost and low effectiveness) assumptions. This method involves combining different assumptions considered in a simple sensitivity analysis, so that an overall best-case scenario and worst-case scenario may be calculated.

3. Threshold sensitivity analysis

If two treatments are being compared, and one is more cost-effective than the other, this form of sensitivity analysis entails altering certain key variables assumed in the economic evaluation until the rank ordering of the cost-effectiveness of the two treatments is changed.

By using these three different types of sensitivity analysis, it is possible to show whether the results of a particular economic evaluation are robust over a range of assumptions or whether the cost-effectiveness results hinge on the accuracy of any one particular assumption. A clear identification of the uncertain or controversial estimates and a discussion of the ways in which different assumptions regarding these estimates would impact on the cost-effectiveness results should be incorporated into any economic evaluation.

Constructing cost-effectiveness league tables

Information from economic evaluations can be extremely useful in clarifying choices between different health care programmes: interventions may be selected according to the magnitude of their cost-effectiveness ratio, with those health care programmes with the lowest cost-effectiveness ratio being the most cost-effective and therefore the most desirable health care programmes to implement.

When information is available on the costs and effectiveness of different health care programmes, and where effectiveness is measured in *commensurate* units, then it becomes possible to rank health care programmes in terms of the magnitude of their cost-effectiveness ratio, thus resulting in the formation of a *cost-effectiveness league table*.

Clearly, the construction of cost-effectiveness league tables is possible only if outcomes are measured in commensurate units so that there is scope for comparison across different interventions for different illnesses. This is possible with cost-utility analysis where outcomes are measured in terms of a utility-based measure of outcome such as quality adjusted life years (QALYs). Alternatives may then be expressed in terms of their incremental costs per QALY gained, and the health care programme with the lowest incremental cost per QALY gained is the most cost-effective use of resources.

Health care programmes may therefore be ranked in a cost-effectiveness league table (or often, more specifically, a cost per QALY league table) in order to determine their relative cost-effectiveness of the use of health services resources.

The ultimate use of a cost-effectiveness league table is to guide resource allocation decisions: that is, to seek to shift scarce health care resources away from the provision of health care programmes that are costly in terms of the additional health benefits that they produce towards health care programmes that incur a relatively low additional cost for each additional unit of health benefit that they produce.

An example of a cost-effectiveness league table is presented in Table 12.3, where the cost-effectiveness of various health care programmes is expressed as the incremental cost per QALY gained. This combines cost-effectiveness data obtained from a number of different economic evaluations, and shows considerable variation in cost-effectiveness. In the most extreme cases, cholesterol testing and treatment by diet for adults aged 40–69 costs £220 for one additional QALY gained, whereas erythropoietin for anaemia in patients receiving dialysis costs over 500 times more than this for the same health benefit: £126,290 for one additional QALY gained.

If health care resources were to be allocated solely on the basis of cost-effectiveness, decision-makers would therefore seek to provide health care programmes which feature high up the league table, such as cholesterol testing and

Table 12.3 A cost-effectiveness league table for various health care programmes.

Treatment	Incremental cost per QALY gained (£)
Cholesterol testing and treatment by diet (adults aged 40–69 years)	220
Neurosurgical intervention for head injury	240
Advice to stop smoking from general practitioner	270
Neurosurgical intervention for subarachnoid haemorrhage	490
Antihypertensive treatment to prevent stroke (aged 45–64)	940
Pacemaker implantation	1,100
Valve replacement for aortic stenosis	1,140
Hip replacement	1,180
Cholesterol testing and treatment	1,480
Coronary artery bypass graft (patients with left main vessel disease and severe angina)	2,090
Kidney transplant	4,710
Breast cancer screening	5,780
Heart transplant	7,840
Cholesterol testing and treatment (incrementally) of all adults aged 25–39 years	14,150
Home haemodialysis	17,260
Coronary artery bypass graft (patients with one vessel disease and moderate angina)	18,830
Continuous ambulatory peritoneal dialysis	19,870
Hospital haemodialysis	21,970
Neurosurgical intervention for malignant intracranial tumours	107,780
Erythropoietin for anaemia in patients receiving dialysis (assuming no increase in survival)	126,290

Source: Maynard, 1991.

treatment by diet in adults aged 40–69, and to move health care resources away from the provision of health care programmes which are further down the league table, such as erythropoietin for anaemia in patients receiving dialysis. Thus the implication of data presented in cost-effectiveness league tables is that resources should be invested in health care programmes higher up the table that produce additional health benefits at relatively low additional cost.

Problems with cost-effectiveness league tables

The implication of the use of cost-effectiveness league tables is that decision-makers should choose to invest in health care programmes which produce additional health benefits at relatively low additional cost. However, the comparison necessary for this choice requires *homogeneity* in the study methods employed. That is, the methods used to obtain cost-effectiveness data from the different economic evaluations which provide the basis for the league table need to be the same.

In other words, the ranking of health care programmes in a cost-effectiveness league table is intended to be a function solely of the relative cost-effectiveness of each health care programme, and is therefore supposed to be independent of the methods used in the original economic evaluations on which the league table is based.

Mason *et al.* (1993) list a number of methodological features which are particularly important in the construction of league tables (ideally, each of these features should be the same across all economic evaluations that provide data which are incorporated into a cost-effectiveness league table):

1. year of analysis;
2. range of costs included;
3. choice of health care programme for comparison;
4. study setting;
5. discount rate.

We shall examine briefly the importance of these features on the accurate interpretation and use of cost-effectiveness league tables.

Year of analysis

The year in which an economic evaluation is conducted reflects the state of knowledge regarding the costs and effectiveness of different health care programmes existing at that time. Because knowledge increases over time, so health care improves as medical technology becomes more advanced. Therefore, one might expect that an economic evaluation conducted recently is likely to find a health care programme more cost-effective than an economic evaluation of the same health care programme conducted at an earlier date.

Range of costs included

If one economic evaluation includes a narrower range of costs than another, then it would be unsurprising if that health care programme were found to be more cost-effective than the other, which includes a wider range of costs. If the range of costs differs across the economic evaluations which are used to construct cost-effectiveness league tables, then the rank ordering in the league table is unlikely to be solely a function of the relative cost-effectiveness of each health care programme.

Choice of health care programme for comparison

Economic evaluations are likely to differ with respect to the choice of comparison programme from which the cost-effectiveness ratio is calculated. However, clearly the choice of this comparison programme may have an impact on the rank ordering of individual health care programmes in a cost-effectiveness league table. For instance, some health care programmes may be compared with a 'do-nothing' alternative. Others may be compared with the current best practice option, and some with a minimum intervention. Others may consider the effect of expanding services to larger groups of patients. Where the health care programme used for comparison differs across economic evaluations, then the rank ordering in a cost-effectiveness league table may reflect this rather than relative cost-effectiveness.

Study setting

Further problems are encountered if cost-effectiveness league tables use data from economic evaluations conducted in different countries. This is because methods of health care provision will probably differ across those countries. For instance, differences exist between countries in clinical practice, the availability and cost of health care resources, and the incentives facing health care professionals and health care institutions. Therefore, considerable care should taken when including the results of economic evaluations from different countries in the same cost-effectiveness league table because the rank ordering of health care programmes is unlikely to be a feature solely of relative cost-effectiveness

Discount rate

Clearly the choice of discount rate used to discount both costs and benefits will have an impact on the relative cost-effectiveness of health care programmes used in the construction of cost-effectiveness league tables. An effort should be made to use economic evaluations which use the same discount rate, or this may affect the rank ordering of health care programmes.

Ideally, each of these features should be the same across all economic evaluations that provide data which are incorporated into a cost-effectiveness league table. The methods used in different economic evaluations are then more likely to be the same, so that the ranking of health care programmes in a cost-effectiveness league table is more likely to be a function of the relative cost-effectiveness of each health care programme, rather than the study methods employed.

The Oregon Experiment

One of the most ambitious applications of cost-effectiveness league tables has been the so-called *Oregon Experiment*, which sought to produce an explicit cost-effectiveness league table for the prioritisation of health care programmes provided by the Medicaid scheme in the state of Oregon, US.

In July 1989 the Oregon legislature passed the Oregon Basic Health Services Act, which was a programme designed to ensure that every individual in Oregon would receive at least a basic standard of health care. A central feature of the programme was to set priorities for the provision of health care programmes. The Act created the Oregon Health Services Commission, which had a remit to produce a ranked list of health care programmes that could be used to define the basic health care package for coverage by the Medicaid scheme.

In the initial phase of the priority-setting process, the Commission conducted a huge cost-utility analysis. The first stage of this analysis involved defining the health care programmes to be ranked. The Commission defined a service as a specific treatment or procedure applied to a specific diagnosis or condition, so that each service was defined by a condition and treatment pair. The initial list condensed all possible condition and treatment pairs into approximately 1,600 services.

Once the services were defined, the next stage in the priority-setting process was to calculate a cost-utility ratio for each service. For estimates of the cost of each service the Commission used the charges for the treatment, including all medications and ancillary services, based on local Medicaid and health insurance records.

To estimate the utility derived from each service, the Commission developed a formula based on a set of health and functional states called the *Quality of Well-Being Scale* (or *QWB scale*). This scale defines 24 health or functional states ranging from perfect health to death. Examples are: 'loss of consciousness, such as seizure, fainting, or coma'; 'burn over large areas of face, body, arms, or legs'; 'general tiredness, weakness, or weight loss'; and 'spells of feeling upset, being depressed, or of crying'.

Each QWB state was assigned a weight to reflect the quality of life associated with any symptoms or limitations related to that category. Weights for QWB states were anchored by zero (corresponding to 'death') and one (corresponding to 'no significant decrement in quality of life').

To estimate utility values, the Commission asked panels of physicians to estimate the patient age at which the condition occurred, the duration of the benefit from treatment, and the probabilities of various types of outcomes associated both with and without treatment. The physician panels based their estimates primarily on the existing literature, but they used clinical judgements when necessary.

The weights for various QWB states were obtained from a random telephone survey of 1,001 Oregon citizens, supplemented by surveys of people in special categories, such as people who were economically and educationally disadvantaged, bedridden or chronically depressed.

This produced a ranking of some 1,600 services in a cost-effectiveness league table. The state's legislature then determined the total annual Medicaid budget. This had the effect of drawing a budget line on the cost-effectiveness league table (which was equivalent to the value of the critical cost-effectiveness ratio, $1/g$, discussed above). Specific services were to be covered in order of their appearance on the league table until the budget was exhausted. Those services which fell below the budget line were to be dropped from coverage by the Medicaid scheme.

A provisional cost-effectiveness league table derived by this approach was released in May 1990 and was widely criticised by Commission members, outside reviewers and the general public. The immediate reaction was that many of the rankings were clinically counterintuitive, assigning higher priorities to some services that were clearly less important than other, lower-ranked services.

In response to apparent inconsistencies like these, the Commission identified several technical problems: first, some services were defined too broadly; secondly, the duration of the benefits of treatment was inaccurately estimated; and thirdly, cost data were incomplete or inaccurate.

The problems in obtaining reliable cost and effectiveness data led to the provisional cost-effectiveness league table being set aside. Subsequently, a revised list of 709 services based on quality of life but not cost data was published in April 1992. However, in response to federal government objections to the use of quality of life scores, yet another list was produced in November 1992. This list comprises 688 services, but was based on only three outcome measures: the probability of death; the probability of an asymptomatic health state; and the probability of a symptomatic health state.

As the Oregon Health Services Commission itself determined, the initial method it used to set priorities using economic evaluation techniques and cost-effectiveness league tables was crude. There were many *technical* problems in the construction of the league table that caused it to generate counterintuitive results which were deemed unacceptable. However, in spite of these problems, it was argued that there was nothing inherent in the methods of economic evaluation employed that rendered it incapable of being used in a priority-setting exercise (Eddy, 1991). Rather, the problems encountered were technical, *not conceptual*, and revolved around inadequate data sources.

Given the problems associated with the use of economic evaluation as a means of allocating scarce resources found in the Oregon Experiment, we may now further discuss some possible limitations of economic evaluation.

Limitations of economic evaluation

Economic evaluation provides a clear framework for the allocation of scarce health care resources. However, there are a number of limitations with economic evaluation techniques, and various reasons why the implementation of such techniques should be treated with caution.

Clearly there are many potential problems with the use of economic evaluation, and these might include the following:

1. the limitations of economic evaluation in decision-making;
2. the precision of results in an economic evaluation;
3. the consistency of results in an economic evaluation;
4. the need for economic evaluations of economic evaluations;
5. the inappropriate use of resources saved in an economic evaluation.

We shall now discuss each of these in turn.

The limitations of economic evaluation in decision-making

First, economic evaluation can be used only as a *tool* for allocating scarce health care resources. Information on cost-effectiveness provides only one piece of information which may be used in the health care decision-making process. Ultimately, deciding what treatments are to be provided and the nature of that provision are questions to be answered by health care decision-makers, who may well deem factors other than cost-effectiveness to be more important. Such other factors might include public and media pressure, and ethical and political considerations. These factors may mean that recommendations derived from an economic evaluation are not integrated into practice. For example, Centrewall (1981) states that '[c]ost–benefit analysis offers medical programs many advantages – organisation, cohesion and data – but it will not say what will be done. That is up to us.'

Related to this issue is the fact that economic evaluations do not usually incorporate the importance of the distribution of costs and consequences to particular population groups (such as the elderly or the young) into the analysis. However, in some cases, that distribution may be an important factor in deciding whether to allocate resources in a particular way. It *is* possible to weight the costs and outcomes arising from health care programmes to different population groups, though this is not normally done within the confines of the economic evaluation. Rather, it is left to the health care decision-maker.

The precision of results in an economic evaluation

A second limitation of economic evaluation relates to the precision of results generated. Centrewall (1981) states that 'any medical program that is ambiguous enough to require cost–benefit analysis is too ambiguous to be resolved by cost–benefit analysis'.

Economic evaluations often require investigators to base analyses to a greater or lesser extent on informed judgements and best guesses. Indeed, we have seen that when measuring costs and outcomes, in the absence of any other source of information, it may be necessary to obtain data via expert professional opinion. Whilst formal methods do exist for doing this, it implies that methods used to measure costs and effectiveness are often not as rigorous as investigators would ideally like. As Fein states (1977): '[t]he numbers have the danger of implying a false precision, and the more so since some of them are subjective'.

The consistency of results in an economic evaluation

A third limitation of economic evaluation is that results are unlikely to be consistent across all settings to which they are applied. As Vladeck (1984) states: '[i]t would be truly surprising if one service were found to be more cost-effective than another for all patients under all circumstances in all settings'. This compromises the extent to which the results of an economic evaluation may be translated into other settings, and implies that care must be taken when extrapolating the results of economic evaluations.

The need for economic evaluations of economic evaluations

Fourthly, any economic evaluation is, in itself, a costly activity. It therefore follows that even economic evaluations should be subjected to economic evaluation. As stated by Fuchs (1980): '[s]ometimes the application of systematic analysis would not be worth the costs. After all, CBA/CEA [cost-benefit analysis/cost-effectiveness analysis] itself involves the use of scarce resources, and their costs may outweigh the benefit of additional information.'

The inappropriate use of resources saved in an economic evaluation

Fifthly, the use of economic evaluation assumes that any resources that are freed or saved by switching to the provision of cost-effective health care programmes will not be wasted, but will instead be used in some alternative worthwhile health care programme. However, as stated by Drummond et al. (1987): '[t]his assumption warrants careful scrutiny, for if the freed resources are consumed by other, ineffective or unevaluated, programmes, then not only is there no saving, but overall health system costs will actually increase without any assurance of additional improvements in the health status of the population'.

There are therefore numerous limitations which may arise with the use of economic evaluation. However, so that the number of methodological and technical problems is minimised, a critical appraisal for assessing economic evaluations is presented in Appendix 12.3. This may be used to assess the quality of economic evaluations and for formulating and assessing research proposals.

Conclusion

In this chapter we have seen how economic evaluation may be used to allocate scarce resources among health care programmes competing for the same limited resources. By measuring their costs and by measuring their effectiveness, the cost-effectiveness of health care programmes may be calculated. This provides a method for solving the questions relating to the basic economic problem:

1. What health care interventions or treatments should be made available?

Through the use of economic evaluation, health care decision-makers may decide which interventions or treatments should be provided by implementing the most cost-effective health care programmes: that is, by implementing those health care programmes that dominate others, and by implementing those with the most favourable cost-effectiveness ratios.

2. How should these treatments be provided?

Economic evaluation also tells us how these treatments should be provided: health care programmes should be provided by the most cost-effective means available.

3. Who should receive these treatments?

In its ultimate use, economic evaluation also tells us for whom these treatments should be provided: health care programmes should be provided to those individuals who achieve the most additional benefit per additional unit of cost, that is, those patients who are the most cost-effective to treat.

Therefore, within the framework of economic evaluation, the health care programmes which will be implemented are those that entail the most cost-effective use of resources, that is, those which maximise the additional benefits over the additional costs.

Appendix 12.1

The discounting formula

Suppose a health care programme with undiscounted costs, by the year in which they occur, as follows:

Year 0	Year 1	Year 2	Year 3	...	Year n
C_0	C_1	C_2	C_3	...	C_n

So that total undiscounted costs, TC_u, are estimated as follows:

$$TC_u = C_0 + C_1 + C_2 + C_3 + ... + C_n$$

This may be summarised as

$$TC_u = \Sigma C_i$$

where C_i are the costs which are incurred in year i and 'Σ' means 'sum of'.

Given this information, discounted costs of the health care programme are calculated as follows:

Year 0	Year 1	Year 2	Year 3	...	Year n
C_0	$C_1/(1+r)$	$C_2/(1+r)^2$	$C_3/(1+r)^3$	...	$C_n/(1+r)^n$

So that total discounted costs, TC_d, are estimated as follows:

$$TC_d = C_0 + C_1/(1+r) + C_2/(1+r)^2 + C_3/(1+r)^3 + ... + C_n/(1+r)^n$$

This may be summarised as

$$TC_d = \Sigma C_i/(1+r)^i$$

where C_i are the costs which are incurred in year i, r is the discount rate and 'Σ' means 'sum of'.

The factor $1/(1 + r)^i$ is known as the *discount factor* and can be obtained from any given value of r.

For example, suppose the undiscounted costs incurred by a health care programme in Years 0, 1 and 2 are £125, £150 and £175, respectively. This implies a total undiscounted cost of £450.

That is, $C_0 = £125$, $C_1 = £150$, and $C_2 = £175$. Therefore, $TC_u = £450$ (that is, £125 + £150 + £175).

Now suppose we wish to discount these costs using a discount rate of 6 per cent. The discounted costs incurred by the health care programme in Years 0, 1 and 2 are calculated as follows:

$$C_0 = £125$$
$$C_1 = £150/(1 + 0.06) = £150/(1.06) = £142$$
$$C_2 = £175/(1 + 0.06)^2 = £175/(1.06)^2 = £175/(1.1236) = £156$$

This implies a total discounted cost of £423. Therefore, $TC_d = £423$ (that is, £125 + £142 + £156).

Appendix 12.2

Calculating net benefit

From Equations 12.5 and 12.6 we have the following:

$$R_b = (C_e - C_c)/(B_e - B_c) \tag{12.5}$$

and

$$R_b \leq 1/g \tag{12.6}$$

where R_b is the cost-effectiveness ratio, C_e is the cost of the experimental programme (measured in monetary units), C_c is the cost of the comparison programme (measured in monetary units), B_e is the effect of the experimental programme (measured in monetary units) and B_c is the effect of the comparison programme (also measured in monetary units). $C_e - C_c$ is the marginal or incremental cost of the experimental programme, $B_e - B_c$ is the marginal or incremental benefit of the experimental programme. $1/g$ is the critical cost-effectiveness ratio.

These two pieces of information indicate that the experimental programme should be implemented provided that the ratio of additional costs to additional benefits does not exceed some prespecified level. That is, Equations 12.5 and 12.6 may be combined, and the experimental programme should be implemented provided that:

$$(C_e - C_c)/(B_e - B_c) \leq 1/g \tag{12.7}$$

We may now reformulate Equation 12.7 by multiplying both sides by g:

$$(C_e - C_c) \times g/(B_e - B_c) \leq 1 \tag{12.8}$$

and then by multiplying both sides by $B_e - B_c$:

$$(C_e - C_c) \times g \leq B_e - B_c \qquad (12.9)$$

Equation 12.9 may then be expanded to give:

$$(C_e \times g) - (C_c \times g) \leq B_e - B_c \qquad (12.10)$$

which may then be rearranged to give:

$$B_c - (C_c \times g) \leq B_e - (C_e \times g) \qquad (12.11)$$

or, similarly:

$$B_e - (C_e \times g) \geq B_c - (C_c \times g) \qquad (12.12)$$

Equation 12.12 may be rearranged as follows:

$$[B_e - (C_e \times g)] - [B_c - (C_c \times g)] \geq 0 \qquad (12.13)$$

Equation 12.13 says that the experimental programme should be implemented provided the *net benefits* are greater than zero.

Appendix 12.3

Critical appraisal of an economic evaluation: a suggested checklist

In order to aid in the assessment of the quality of an economic evaluation, a ten-point checklist has been developed by Drummond *et al.* (1987):[1]

1. **Was a well-defined question posed in answerable form?**

    1.1 Did the study examine both the costs and effects of the service(s) or programme(s)?
    1.2 Did the study involve a comparison of alternatives?
    1.3 Was a viewpoint for the analysis stated and was the study placed in any particular decision-making context?

2. **Was a comprehensive description of the competing alternatives given? (i.e. can you tell who? did what? to whom? where? and how often?)**

    2.1 Were any important alternatives omitted?
    2.2 Was (Should) a 'do-nothing' alternative (be) considered?

3. **Was there evidence that the programme's effectiveness had been established?**

    3.1 Has this been done through a randomised, controlled clinical trial? If not, how strong was the evidence of effectiveness?

---

[1] By permission of Oxford University Press.

4. Were all important and relevant costs and consequences for each alternative identified?

4.1 Was the range wide enough for the research question at hand?

4.2 Did the costs cover all relevant viewpoints? (Possible viewpoints include the community or social viewpoint, and those of patients and third party payers. Other viewpoints may also be relevant depending upon the particular analysis.)

4.3 Were capital costs, as well as operating costs, included?

5. Were costs and consequences measured accurately in appropriate physical units? (e.g. hours of nursing time, number of physician visits, lost work-days, gained life-years)

5.1 Were any of the identified items omitted from measurement? If so, does this mean that they carry no weight in the subsequent analysis?

5.2 Were there any special circumstances (e.g. joint use of resources) that made measurement difficult? Were these circumstances handled appropriately?

6. Were costs and consequences valued credibly?

6.1 Were the sources of all values clearly identified? (Possible sources include market values, patient or client preferences and views, policymakers' views and health professionals' judgements.)

6.2 Were market values employed for changes involving resources gained or depleted?

6.3 Where market values were absent (e.g. volunteer labour), or market values did not reflect actual values (such as clinic space donated at a reduced rate), were adjustments made to approximate market values?

7. Were costs and consequences adjusted for differential timing?

7.1 Were costs and consequences which occur in the future 'discounted' to their present values?

7.2 Was any justification given for the discount rate used?

8. Was an incremental analysis of costs and consequences of alternatives performed?

8.1 Were the additional (incremental) costs generated by one alternative over another compared to the additional effects, benefits or utilities generated?

9. Was a sensitivity analysis performed?

9.1 Was a justification provided for the ranges of values (for key study parameters) employed in the sensitivity analysis?

9.2 Were the study results sensitive to changes in the values (within the assumed range)?

10. Did the presentation and discussion of study results include all issues of concern to users?

10.1 Were the conclusions of the analysis based on some overall index or ratio of costs to consequences (e.g. cost-effectiveness ratio)? If so, was the index interpreted intelligently or in a mechanistic fashion?

10.2 Were the results compared with those of others who have investigated the same question?

10.3 Did the study discuss the generalisability of the results to other settings and patient/client groups?

10.4 Did the study allude to, or take account of, other important factors in the choice or decision under consideration (e.g. distribution of costs and consequences, or relevant ethical issues)?

10.5 Did the study discuss issues of implementation, such as the feasibility of adopting the 'preferred' programme given existing financial or other constraints, and whether any freed resources could be redeployed to other worthwhile programmes?

This checklist is not intended to be all-encompassing, and many well conducted economic evaluations may fail at least some of the points on the checklist. However, as a starting point for the assessment of an economic evaluation, such a checklist is useful. It is also a helpful starting point for formulating and assessing research proposals for economic evaluations.

References

Centrewall B.S. (1981) Cost-benefit analysis and heart transplantation. *New England Journal of Medicine* 304: 901–3.

Drummond M.F., Stoddart G.L. and Torrance G.W. (1987) *Methods for the economic evaluation of health care programmes*. New York: Oxford Medical Publications.

Eddy D.M. (1991) Oregon's methods: did cost-effectiveness analysis fail? *Journal of the American Medical Association* 266: 2135–41.

Fein R. (1977) But on the other hand: high blood pressure, economics and equity. *New England Journal of Medicine* 296: 751–3.

Fuchs V.R. (1980) What is CBA/CEA, and why are they doing this to us? *New England Journal of Medicine* 303: 937–8.

Mason J.M., Drummond M.F. and Torrance G.W. (1993) Some guidelines on the use of cost-effectiveness league tables. *British Medical Journal* 306: 570–2.

Maynard A. (1991) Developing the health care market. *The Economic Journal* 101: 1277–86.

Tolley K. and Rowland N. (1995) *Evaluating the cost-effectiveness of counselling in health care*. London: Routledge.

Vladeck B.C. (1984) The limits of cost-effectiveness. *American Journal of Public Health* 74: 652–3.

Suggested further reading

For a discussion of the rationale behind discounting see:

Goodin R.E. (1976) Discounting discounting. *Journal of Public Policy* 2: 53–72.

For the arguments both for and against discounting health benefits see the following:

Cairns J. (1992) Discounting and health benefits: another perspective. *Health Economics* 1: 76–9.
Parsonage M. and Neuberger H. (1992) Discounting and health benefits. *Health Economics* 1: 71–6.

For a discussion of the construction of cost-effectiveness ratios see, for example:

Phelps C.E. and Mushlin A. (1991) On the (near) equivalence of cost-effectiveness and cost-benefit analysis. *International Journal of Technology Assessment and Health Care* 7: 12–21.

For an introduction to cost-effectiveness league tables and priority setting see:

Mason J.M., Drummond M.F. and Torrance G.W. (1993) Some guidelines on the use of cost-effectiveness league tables. *British Medical Journal* 306: 570–2.

For a discussion of the Oregon Experiment see:

Eddy D.M. (1991) Oregon's methods: did cost-effectiveness analysis fail? *Journal of the American Medical Association* 266: 2135–41.

Index